Serono Symposia Publications from Raven Press
Volume 50

THE MOLECULAR AND CELLULAR
ENDOCRINOLOGY OF THE TESTIS

Serono Symposia Publications from Raven Press

Serono Symposia Publications from Raven Press
Volume 50

The Molecular and Cellular Endocrinology of the Testis

Editors

B.A. Cooke
Royal Free Hospital School of Medicine
Dept. of Biochemistry and Chemistry
Rowland Hill Street
London NW3 2PF
England

R.M. Sharpe
MRC Reproductive Biology Unit
Centre for Reproductive Biology
37 Chalmers St.
Edinburgh EH3 9EW
Scotland

Raven Press ■ New York

Raven Press, 1185 Avenue of the Americas, New York, New York 10036

THE MOLECULAR AND CELLULAR ENDOCRINOLOGY OF
THE TESTIS
(Symposia Publications from Raven Press; v. 50)

International Standard Book Number 0-88167-418-4
Library of Congress Catalog Number 87-043293

Printed in Rome, Italy
by Christengraf

Preface

This book contains the Proceedings of the 5th European Workschop on the Molecular and Cellular Endocrinology of the Testis held in Brighton, England between 13th and 16th April 1988. This Workshop continued in the tradition of these biannual meetings. For the first time however, we were fortunate in having the Workshop included as an official Ares Serono Symposium. The subjects covered ranged from molecular mechanisms of hormone action to clinical andrology. The current main areas of research were reflected in the choice of symposium lectures which included inhibin, toxicology, and paracrine and autocrine control mechanisms. In order to draw parallels between different endocrine systems we invited speakers for the symposua who do not necessarily work on the testis.

All participants of the Workshop had the opportunity to contribute to the now traditional "Mini Poster" book; the result was a feast of high quality posters which reflected the very high standards of work on the testis being carried out in Europe. As on previous occasions, each participants received a copy of this book before the meeting so that they could contribute and benefit from well-informed discussions during the Workshop. Some of the authors of the miniposters were asked to present their data as oral communications. These presentations together with the symposium lectures are included in these Proceedings of the Workshop.

We would like to thank the other members of the Local Organizing Committee, Drs P. Foster and F.C. Wu for their contributions in planning the programme and selecting the short papers.

Special thanks are due to the other members of the Permanent Scientific Commitee of the European Study Group for Molecular and Cellular Endocrinology of the Testis (Drs V. Hansson (N), I. Huhtaniemi (SF), E. Nieschlag (FRG), M.E. Ritzen (S), F.F.G. Rommerts (NL), J.M. Saez (F), M. Stefanini (I) and to Dr. I. Fritz (Canada) who heroically summarized the Workshop at the close of the meeting.

We also wish to thank Dr F.F.G. Rommerts for his highly entertaining evening lecture entitled "Testomania" – the text of which is included in this book. We apologise to him for some editorial censorship!

B.A. COOKE
R.M. SHARPE

Contents

IV. Factors controlling blood and lymph flow and hormone secretion

VIII. Control of spermatogenesis

IX. Paracrine and autocrine control mechanisms

Contributors

Dr D.R.E. Abayasekara
Department of Biochemistry
Royal Free Hospital of Medicine
Rowland Hill Street
London NW3 2PF

Dr R.J. Aitken
MRC Reproductive Biology Unit
Centre for Reproductive Biology
37 Chalmers Street
Edinburgh EH3 9EW
UK

Dr O. Avallet
INSERM U 307
Hopital Debrousse
69322 Lyon
France

Dr C.W. Bardin
The Population Council
1230 York Avenue
New York
NY 10021
USA

Dr J.M.S. Bartlett
Max Planck Clinical Research Unit for
Reproductive Medicine and Institutte of
Reproductive Medicine
Westfalish-Wilhelms Universitat
Steinfurter Strasse 107
D4400 Munster
Fed. Republic of Germany

Dr A. Bergh
Department of Anatomy
University of Umea
S-901 87 Umea
Sweden

Dr L. Birnbaumer
Department of Physiology
and Molecular Biophysics
Baylor College of Medicine
Houston
TX 77030
USA

Dr C. Boitani
Institute of Histology and
General Embryology
University La Sapienza of Rome
Via Scarpa 14
00161 Rome
Italy

Dr A.C. Brownie
Department of Biochemistry
State University of New York at Buffalo
Buffalo
N.Y. 14214
USA

Dr D.M. de Kretser
Department of Anatomy
Monash University
Melbourne
Victoria 3168
Australia

Dr P.J. den Boer
Department of Biocheministry II
Medical Faculty
Erasmus University Rotterdam
P.O. Box Box 1738
The Netherlands

Dr G. Edwards
Reproductive Research Group
Physiological Sciences
University of Manchester
Manchester M13 9PT
UK

Dr I.B. Fritz
Banting and Best Department of
Medical Research
University of Toronto
Charles H. Best Institute
112 College St.
Toronto
Ontario
Canada M5G 1L6

Dr A. Frøysa
Institute of Medical Biochemistry
University of Oslo
0317 Oslo 3
Norway

Dr P.M.D. Foster
ICI Central Toxicology Laboratory
Alderley park
Macclesfield
Cheshire
SK10 4TJ

Dr R.B. Heap
A.F.R.C. Institute of Animal
Physiology and Genetics Research
Babraham
Cambridge CB2 4AT

Dr A.J. Holloway
Institute of Zoology
Zoological Society of London
Regents Park
London NW1 4RY

Dr O. Hovatta
Infertility Clinic of the Finnish
Population and Family Welfare
Federation
"Vaestoliitto"
SF-00100 Helsinki

Dr A.J.W. Hsueh
Department of Reproductive
Medicine M-025
School of Medicine
University of California
San Diego
La Jolla
California 92093
USA

Dr A. Jassin
Department of Immunology
London Hospital Medical College
Turner Street
London E1 2AD
UK

Dr B. Jegou
Laboratoire de Biologie de la
Reproduction
UA CNRS 256
Université de Rennes I
Campus de Beaulieu
35042 Rennes Cedex
France

Dr J.B. Kerr
Department of Anatomy
Monash University
Victoria 3168
Melbourne
Australia

Dr Z. Krawczyk
Department of Tumor Biology
Institute of Oncology
44-100 Gliwice
Poland

Dr S. Maddocks
MRC Reproductive Biology
37 Chalmers Street
Edinburgh EH3 9EW
Scotland
UK

Dr J.P. Mather
Genetech Inc.
South San Francisco
USA

Dr E. Nieschlag
Max Planck Clinical Research Unit for
Reproductive Medicine and Institute of
Reproductive Medicine
Westfalische-Wilhelms Universitat
Steinfurter Str. 107
D4400 Munster
Federal Republic of Germany

Dr F. Palombi
Istituto di Istologia ed Embriologia
Generale
Via A. Scarpa 14
00161 Roma, Italy

Miss E.A. Platts
Department of Biochemistry
Royal Free Hospital Medical School
University of London
Rowland Hill St.
London
UK

Dr F.F.G. Rommerts
Department of Biochemistry (Chemical
Endocrinology) Medical Faculty
Erasmus University Rotterdam
P.O. Box 1738
3000 DR Rotterdam
The Netherlands

Dr M. Schumacher
Institute for Hormone and Fertility
Research
Grandweg 64
2000 Hamburg 54
Fed. Rep. Germany

Dr E.R. Simpson
Department of Obstetrics & Gynecology
& Biocheministry
The Cecil H. & Ida Green Center
for Reproductive Biology Sciences
University of Texas
Southwestern Medical Center
Dallas
TX 75235
USA

Dr M.H.F. Sullivan
Department of Biochemistry
Royal Free Hospital Medical School
University of London
Rowland Hill Street
London
UK

Dr O. Soder
Pediatric Endocrilogy Unit
Karolinska Institute
S-104 01
Stockholm
Sweden

Dr A.M.W. Toebosch
Department of Biochemistry
Erasmus University Rotterdam
P.O. Box 1738
3000 DR Rotterdam
The Netherlands

Dr M. van Noort
Department of Biochemistry
Division of Chemical Endocrinology
Faculty of Medicine
Erasmus University Utrecht
P.O. Box 80054
3508 TB Utrecht
The Netherlands

Dr G. Verhoeven
Laboratory for Experimental Medicine
and Endocrinology
Gasthuisberg
Onderwijs en Navorsing
Herestraat 49
B-3000
Leuven
Belgium

Dr F.C.W. Wu
MRC Reproductive Biology Unit
Centre for Reproductive Biology
37 Chalmers Street
Edinburgh EH3 9EW
Scotland
United Kingdom

Testomania

F.F.G. Rommerts*

*Department of Biochemistry (Chemical Endocrinology),
Medical Faculty, Erasmus University Rotterdam,
P.O. Box 1738, 3000 DR Rotterdam, The Netherlands*

INTRODUCTION

Reproduction is a well recognized feature of living creatures and the evolution of many species has greatly benefitted from the process of bisexual reproduction. For mankind, reproduction and sexuality have played an important role in the development and maintenance (and also the fall) of cultures, and it is therefore not surprising that even today gonadal activities have a major influence on our current thinking and behavior.

For many ages males have dominated in civilizations. Since it was also known that male characteristics depend on the testis which is exposed in most mammalian species, the testis has attracted relatively much attention and much more than the ovary.

This overappreciation of the male sex-organ can be conceived as a clear manifestation of testomania. On the occasion of the V European Workshop on the Molecular and Cellular Endocrinology of the Testis, this mondial testicular preoccupation will be scrutinized. The thesis will be developed that testomania has always influenced mankind in the past and will continue to do so in the years to come. Since the manifestations of this frequently denied or suppressed process are not always easily recognizable, the eye of the experienced beholder can be of great help. In this brief chapter attempts will be made to uncover the hidden testomanic influences in our society of today and in the past.

The plates and a subjective view will show that the function of the testis is not limited to the production of spermatozoa and steroids. Hopefully, this new look on testis function will be a stimulus to continue testis research and the organization of testis workshops, since both have contributed so much to our knowledge about the functional aspects of the lowest male endocrine organ, which is so highly esteemed.

HISTORICAL AND CONTEMPORARY ASPECTS

For ages fertility and reproduction have been considered as manifestations of divine powers and sex organs such as the testes

*F.F.G.R. is an established testis investigator

were worshipped as symbols of procreation. A good example is the ancient Greek mother-goddess Artemis, known by the Romans as Diana, who was decorated with fifteen to thirty large bulbous objects, shaped somewhat like eggs and situated just above the waist (1, and see also Figure 1).

Since Christian times these objects have been described as breasts. However, careful scientific examination revealed that there was no sign of nipples and consequently the breast hypothesis had to be rejected. Recent investigations by Austrian researchers revealed that the egg-shaped objects were testicles of bulls (1). From an historical point of view this discovery illustrates the early appreciation of testicular function, and from a technical point of view it shows that it may take many years of careful and elaborate research before testomanic influences can be recognized.

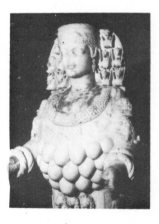

FIG. 1. "Artemis"

In this respect it also seems relevant to question several hypotheses on the egg searching and eating habits around Easter. Hopefully this topic will also be thoroughly re-investigated by the Austrian scientists. More historical information and references on testicular symbols, testis adoration and the consequences of castration can be found in "Ruminations on the testis" (12) and "Historical aspects of the study on the testis" (2).

Old writings such as the Authorized Version of the Bible, show clearly that mankind has always been extremely interested in the testis but references were often evasive, euphemistic or sometimes misleading.

Newly acquired information on the possible correlation between testis size and copulatory frequency in apes has recently given enough courage to investigators to publish results of studies on human behaviour and testicular size and a digest of these studies was recently published in Nature (7).

Since measurements of testis size by orchidometry in living subjects are difficult to standardize, testis weights were determined at autopsy (Fig. 2). Interesting differences were observed between different ethnic groups but the variations in size could not be explained. An explicit test revealed no relation between size and copulatory frequency in Korean men , (10). Further investigations on the possible causal links between testis size and genetic traits, hormone levels or human behavior are required. Moreover the apparent differences in left and right testis weight also warrants serious study (see also figure 7 and context).

The importance of the testis (left or right) can also be recognized in words connected with legal customs. The word "testis" is derived from the Latin word "testis" meaning "witness". The testis is therefore the third party when witnesses had to "testify" and in some civilizations the witness was required to place his hand on his or somebody else's testis while testifying (2). Women could not be witnesses. Testament is another example of the testomanic influence on vocabulary.

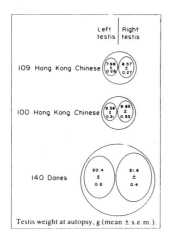

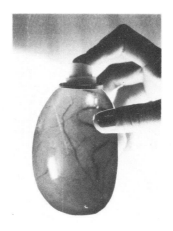

FIG. 2. Testis weights (grams) of various ethnic groups at autopsy

FIG. 3. Testicular spray: a delightful delicatestis

Not only the organ itself in physical appearance, or in words, has received and still receives wide attention, but also dramatic effects of testicular products on intellectual and physical activities have been described.

In 150 A.D. Aretaeus of Cappadocia formulated that "it is the semen, when possessed of vitality which makes us to be men, hot, well braced in limbs, well voiced, spirited, strong to think and act" (13).

In 1889 Brown-Sequard advocated that injections of extracts from animal testis could produce rejuvenation (3).

Today the procedure for administration of powerful extracts has been modernized but the expectations are still old-fashionedly positive (see figure 3).

Investigations on the relation between sex-hormone levels and life style are being continued today with particular emphasis on the aging man (5). This probably also reflects the

age of the investigators who nowadays live longer and can
therefore study the more touchy projects.

The deep concern and preoccupation of men with the testicles as
has already been emphasized, was more or less constant in all
ages, but manifestations of these personal feelings have not
always been accepted in western societies. In some cases
misleading or false suggestions about the influence of the testis
on human behaviour have been made.

In the Victorian period clergymen even denied the existence of
the testis in men (Figure 4) and from a careful inspection of the
famous picture of the Mona Lisa, a Dutch researcher has concluded
that it is almost certain that on the first draft of tne "Mona
Lisa" the person must have carried a big testis. This discovery
explains the secret smile of this most likely sexually abberant,
person.

Although the society and religion in some periods have attempted
to play down the testicular addiction, also called today
(hemi)castration, and in some cases almost eradicated the
existence of the scrotal organ (see Figure 4), the continuous
importance of the testis shape or content can still be recognized
in sculpture (figure 5), in sports (figure 6), music (rumba balls)
and politics (left or right predominance, figure 7) and in many
other activities of human life such as ballooning and gastronomy

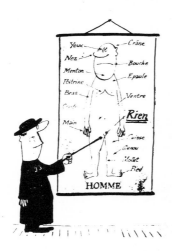

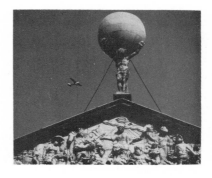

FIG. 4. Atlas of human body   FIG. 5. Royal Palace, Amsterdam
anno 1850.

no figures are shown). The ubiquitous occurrence and importance of the testis is also reflected in the inclusion of the word testis in the appendix (p. 208) of the famous book "What Literate Americans Know".

These examples illustrate the fundamental importance of the testis for the quality of life. The best proof for this statement is the following observation: Men castrated after birth live longer and are less afflicted by (fatal) prostatic diseases. However, there are no reports that large numbers of men voluntarily undergo this beneficial therapy early in life.

An active functioning testis is thus strongly desired. Sometimes, however, a price must be paid for these benefits of testicular origin (Figure 8).

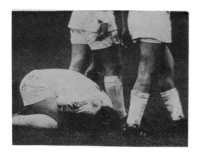

FIG. 6. Testomania in soccer.

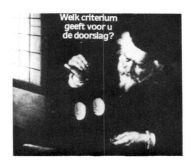

FIG. 7. Testomania in politics. Translated Dutch text: "which criterion is of most importance?"

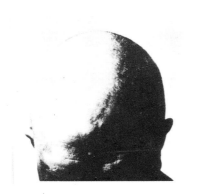

FIG. 8. The skull (superficial view).

Although in general many men and women would like to correct bald-headedness, testomanics would probably prefer this condition (Figure 8).

This strong preference for a testis directed (re)productive life style is not restricted to men, but can also - and much better - be observed in other mammals. The marsupial mouse is a particularly good example. This animal which lives for only 11 months has a very brief though very intense two weeks period of sexual activity. This brief once in-a-lifetime and intense reproductive activity is known as big-bang reproduction (6).

Again a price has to be paid for this (re)productive lifestyle and this time the highest price: within a period of two weeks regression of sexual organs and diseases occur and at the end of the period all animals are dead.

This testis directed behavioral pattern of short duration is probably one of the best expressions of testomania. The central role of the testis in this mouse-life and the submissiveness of the body to the testis perfectly illustrates the importance of the testis for the propagation and life-style of mammalian species. Inside the testis spermatozoa develop and chromosomes are rearranged during the meiotic process. The testis can therefore be considered as the genetic laboratory for optimization of the evolutionary process and in the Darwinian view the male human body is just a carrier for the testis. Darwin can therefore be considered as the most fundamental testomanic that has lived so far.

Since the testis is of such fundamental importance for the production of gametes, optimally functioning systems for communication inside and between testicular cells must be very old and have probably evolved more than 600 million years ago (8). Evolution proven regulatory systems operating in the testis most probably have been utilized in organs originating later in evolution. Consequently many testicular regulatory molecules and systems operate in many organs and especially in the brain which is a relatively young organ. In the universal language of chemistry this statement will create no problems (11). Even at a cell biological level this view can be accepted without too many difficulties. However it is obvious that the biological expressions of these conserved regulatory systems in brain and testis are different and in physiological terms this statement may create some confusion. What remains however is that from an evolutionary testomanic point of view, brain function is derived from testis function and new findings on regulation of brain function made in the last 10 years should be interpreted accordingly: Steroids synthesized de novo from cholesterol in the brain should not be called <u>neuro</u> steroids (9). Similarly, products from the pro-opiomelanocortin precursor in the male brain should not be considered as <u>neuro</u>-peptides. Since both the steroid and the peptide producing capacity are of testicular origin (14,4) the prefix "TESTO"- instead of "NEURO" should be used now and in the future.

Irrespective of what today is considered to be the most important organ for mankind, it must be clear from this essay that testis and brain have many common properties. It is therefore proposed to abandon the idea of two separated organs, the brain and the testis, only connected by a thin brain-testis axis. Instead an integrated organ is proposed: the NEURO-TESTIS which convincingly depicts the derivation of the brain from the testis and the basis for our current thinking (see Fig. 9).

Detailed investigations on hormonally controlled testicular regulatory systems at the (patho) physiological, cellular or biochemical levels are necessary, not only for a better understanding of testis function but of more importance, for a better understanding of mankind.

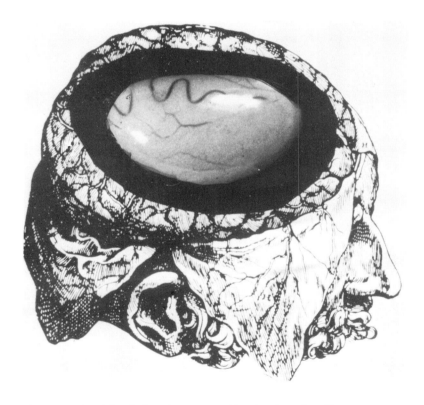

FIG. 9. Neurotestis (also known as the Mastergland)

Integration of the information and theories gathered by many scientists is required and testis workshops will facilitate this enormous task which is clearly beyond the capabilities of individual shoulders. An integrated knowledge of the fundamental laws of testicular cellular sociology (8) is of great value for laymen, scientists in general and sociologists in particular, but it is of paramount importance for testis researchers. These research activities warrant identification as a new sub-branch of science: Testomania.

ACKNOWLEDGEMENT

I am deeply indebted to the many friends and colleagues who have stimulated my interest in the subject of this investigation and have helped me in finding clues to unexpected sources of inspiration and information. Acknowledgements are also made to future sponsors of this research.

REFERENCES

1. Attenborough, D. (1987): In: The First Eden: The Mediterrainean World of Man, pp. 105-11. British Broadcasting Corporation, London.
2. Bremner, W.J. (1981): In: The Testis, edited by H.G. Burger and D.M. de Kretser, Historical aspects on the study of the testis, pp. 1-5. Raven Press, New York.
3. Brown-Sequard, C.E. (1889): Experience demontrant la puissance dynamogenique chez l'homme d'un liquide extrait de testicules d'animaux. Arch. Phys. Norm. Pathol. 21:651-659.
4. Chen, C-L.C., Mather, J.P., Morris, P.L., and Bardin, C.W. (1984): Expression of pro-opiomelanocortin-like gene in the testis and epididymis. Proc. Natl. Acad. Sci., USA 81: 5672-5675.
5. Deslypere, J.P., and. Vermeulen, A. (1984): Leydig cell function in normal men: effect of age, life style, residence, diet and activity. J. Clin. Endocrinol. and Metabolism 59, 955-962.
6. Diamond, J.M. (1982): Big-bang reproduction and ageing in male marsupial mice. Nature 298, 115-116.
7. Diamond, J.M. (1986): Variation in human testis size. Nature 320, 488-489.
8. Fritz, I.B. (1984): In: Recent Progress in cellular Endocrinology of the testis: edited by J.M. Saez, M.G. Forest, A. Dacord and J. Bertrand, Past, present and future of molecular and cellular endocrinology of the testis, pp. 15-54. INSERM, Paris.
9. Hu, Z.Y., Bourreau, E., Jung-Testas, I., Robel, P., and Baulieu, E-E. (1987): Neurosteroids: Oligodendrocyte mitochondria convert cholesterol to pregnenolone. Proc. Natl. Acad. Sci. USA., 84:8215-8219.
10. Kim, D.H., and Lee, H.Y. (1982): No relation between testis size and copulatory frequency in Korean men. J. Korean Med. Ass., 25: 135-138.

11. Kornberg, A. (1987): The Two Cultures: Chemistry and Biology, Biochemistry 26: 6888-6891.
12. Mack, W.S. (1964): Ruminations on the testis. Proc. Royal Soc. Med. 57:47-51.
13. Rolleston, H.D. (1963): In: The Endocrine glands in health and disease, Oxford University Press., London (Quote).
14. Rommerts, F.F.G., Molenaar, R., Themmen, A.P.N., and van der Molen, H.J. (1986): In: Hormones and cell regulation: Hormonal regulation of testicular steroidogenesis via different transducing systems, edited by J. Nunez et al. , pp. 97-109, INSERM, Paris.

Inhibin and Related Peptides

D.M. de Kretser, D.M. Robertson, G.P. Risbridger,
G. Gonzales, A. Drummond and H.G. Burger*

Department of Anatomy, Monash University, Melbourne, Victoria, 3168, Australia;
*Medical Research Centre, Prince Henry's Hospital,
Melbourne, Victoria, 3004, Australia

The long interval of 53 years between the development of the inhibin hypothesis (33) and the isolation of inhibin from bovine follicular fluid (bFF) (44) has been followed by a rapid development of knowledge in this field. The 58 kDa form of inhibin initially isolated from bFF was composed of two dissimilar subunits now termed α and β. Subsequently several investigators isolated a 32 kDa form of inhibin from porcine follicular fluid (28,40,43) which was composed of α and β subunits. Ling et al (28) in fact isolated two types of inhibin termed A and B which were later (31) shown to be composed of identical α subunits linked to differing β subunits termed β_A (Inhibin A) and β_B (Inhibin B). The relationship of the 58 kDa form to the 32 kDa form was clarified by the cloning of the genes which independently control the α and β subunits (18,31). The difference in molecular weights is due to a larger α subunit in the 58 kDa form, the smaller α subunit of the 32 kDa form resulting from a proteolytic cleavage at a Arg-Arg bond. Evidence exists to suggest that this processing occurs when the molecule encounters serum (35). To date the sequences of bovine, porcine, human, ovine, and rat inhibin have been derived by molecular cloning techniques (6,13,18,31,32,51).

The complexity of this field increased with the isolation from porcine follicular fluid of two proteins with the capacity to stimulate FSH secretion (29,54). The two proteins were shown to be dimers of the β subunit of inhibin and are termed Activin A (β_A-β_A) and Activin AB (β_A-β_B). To date no evidence exists to indicate whether activin circulates in blood although it is clear that the predominant action of the ovary on FSH is inhibitory since castration removes a tonic inhibitory control of FSH. The mechanisms by which the granulosa cell synthesizes inhibin or activin remain unknown particularly in view of the fact that the synthesis of the α and β subunits are controlled by separate genes.

The complexity of this field has increased further with the isolation, from bovine and porcine follicular fluid, of a structurally unrelated protein which has the capacity to inhibin FSH secretion by pituitary cells (45,56). This protein, termed FSH suppressing protein (FSP) or follistatin is structurally unrelated to inhibin and its action *in vitro* cannot be neutralized by inhibin specific antisera. Estimations of the relative activity of FSP to inhibin range from 10-30%, though these potencies were determined by two different pituitary bioassays, namely the cell content and basal release systems respectively (45,56).

<u>Bioassays</u> Most investigators have utilized a rat pituitary cell culture system for measuring inhibin based on either changes in basal secretion of FSH into the medium (12) or in the FSH cell content (48). In situations where inhibin, activin or FSP coexist in a medium or tissue fluid, the specificity of the *in vitro* bioassay for measuring inhibin must now be qualified. Though the mechanisms by which inhibin, activin and FSP modify FSH secretion are largely unknown, the coexistence of inhibin and FSP would lead to falsely elevated inhibin potencies and falsely lowered estimations when inhibin and activin are present together. If bioassays are to be employed to determine the presence and potency of inhibin, FSP and activin, then fractionation of the medium using such techniques as reverse phase high pressure liquid chromatography (HPLC) prior to assay will be necessary. Even with such a technique, clear separation is often difficult as these substances have very similar Rfs. These difficulties make it essential that specific and sensitive radioimmunoassays are developed for these three factors.

<u>Radioimmunoassays:</u> Two approaches have been taken in developing radioimmunoassays for inhibin. Our laboratory has used the purified, intact bovine molecule, either in its 58 kDa or 31 kDa forms, for immunization. This has enabled the development of three antisera (Nos. #474, #749, #1989) capable of use in radioimmunoassays. Although raised against bovine inhibin, all were suitable for use in heterologous assays (34, 36, 46). The antiserum 1989, when used with iodinated 31 kDa inhibin as tracer, can be used to measure inhibin in human, rat, ovine and monkey tissue fluids (17,46,47). All these antisera have no significant cross-reactivity to the inhibin-related peptides such as activin, FSP, anti-Mullerian hormone and transforming growth factor β. A similar approach has been used by Hasegawa and colleagues (22) who raised antisera to intact porcine inhibin which were capable of measuring circulating inhibin levels in rats, pigs and cows.

Other laboratories have used the approach of immunization against small peptides synthesized to short sequences of the inhibin subunits (42). In view of the remarkable conservation of the sequence of the β subunit, to date the most successful sequence for raising antisera is 1-26 sequence of the α subunit of porcine inhibin. These antisera have been applied to the measurement of porcine, rat and ovine inhibin (5,42) but have not been suitable for human inhibin radioimmunoassays. Unfortunately many of these assays have not reported their results in terms of standards using the entire native molecule but rather have used the 1-26 α peptide as standard. In addition no data are available to indicate their specificity relative to the subunits of inhibin.

One of the issues that confronts all radioimmunoassays is the cross-reactivity of antisera with the individual subunits (α, β_A, β_B) of the inhibin molecule. Since each subunit is controlled by separate genes, there is a strong possibility that the sites of synthesis, the Sertoli cells and granulosa cells and serum may contain free α or β subunit in addition to inhibin and activin. Consequently, antisera which cross-react significantly with the α or β subunits will lead to an overestimation of inhibin levels. Furthermore, the observation that the adrenal cortex contains only the α subunit (6) suggests that secretion from this source may augment plasma levels of α subunits.

The antisera raised against the native inhibin molecule in our laboratory have been tested against the free α and β_A subunits prepared by reduction and alkylation of the intact molecule, and no significant cross-reactivity has been detected. However, it is possible that this chemical process may have altered the tertiary structure of the molecule such that it differs from native subunits and may therefore not truly reflect their inherent cross-reactivity. A source of pure α or β subunit, isolated from tissue fluids or produced by recombinant techniques, would be a valuable resource for testing the specificity of antisera. Those antisera raised to peptides synthesized from sequences of the α subunit have theoretically a greater potential for cross-reactivity to free α subunit.

Studies of inhibin in the male:
Site of production: There is general agreement using both bioassay and radioimmunoassay measurements, that inhibin is secreted by the Sertoli cell (5,27,49,53). Further support for this view comes from the immunocytochemical localization of inhibin in the Sertoli cells (7,39). Secretion occurs across both basal and apical surfaces of the cell *in vitro* as shown by growing Sertoli cells in bicameral chambers (50). *In vivo* evidence of apical Sertoli cell secretion comes from the rise in intratesticular inhibin levels after short-term (20-24 hrs) efferent duct ligation (1).

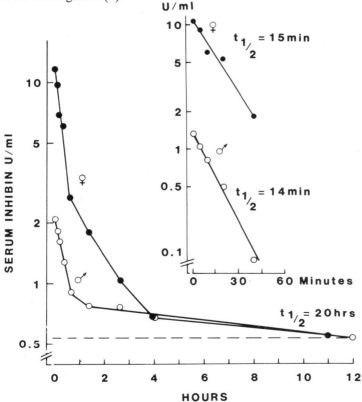

Fig. 1. The disappearance of inhibin from the circulation in male and female rats after castration.   Reproduced with permission from Robertson, 1988 (ref. 47).

Proof that the testis is the major source of circulating inhibin comes from the rapid decline of serum levels after castration (47). Inhibin levels decline with an initial half-time of 13 min (Fig.1)   though the second component of disappearance is more prolonged.

Control of Inhibin Secretion: Inhibin secretion from   immature Sertoli cells in culture is stimulated by FSH through cyclic AMP dependent mechanisms (5,27). Hypophysectomy results in a decline in intratesticular inhibin levels as measured by bioassay (2). The levels decline slowly being 79% of control at 7 days and reaching 30% of controls six weeks post-hypox.   When rats, hypophysectomized four weeks earlier are treated with FSH a significant stimulation of inhibin levels occurs but testosterone had no significant effect. Our recent studies (21) have shown that isolated seminiferous tubules from adult rats also show a dose-dependent stimulation by FSH indicating that the adult testis is capable of responding to FSH.   It is of interest that the secretion of inhibin, both in cultures of immature Sertoli cells and adult seminiferous tubules, continues for prolonged periods in culture in the absence of FSH (21,27,53).

Studies in the human have also added support for the control of inhibin secretion by FSH. Clomiphene citrate, given to normal men stimulated inhibin secretion presumably through the rise in FSH that occurs (52). McLachlan *et al* (37) observed that normal men given 200 mg of testosterone enanthate weekly had a significant fall in serum inhibin levels. When FSH was given together with testosterone, the suppressed inhibin levels increased significantly. Surprisingly, when LH was used instead of FSH, a significant rise of inhibin secretion also occurred. Since no receptors for LH are found on Sertoli cells, the action of LH presumably involved the Leydig cell as an intermediary.

The role of testosterone in the control of inhibin secretion has been a point of controversy. Le Gac & de Kretser (27) found no effect of testosterone on inhibin secretion as measured by bioassay, by immature Sertoli cells in culture. However, Verhoeven and Franchimont (55) using similar systems, noted a stimulation of inhibin secretion.   Recently, several investigators have reinvestigated the action of testosterone on Sertoli cell inhibin secretion and noted no action at physiological levels of testosterone and an inhibition of basal secretion (4,50) and FSH induced inhibin secretion (21) at doses of 10^{-5}M testosterone. These data suggest a minimal suppressive role of testosterone on inhibin secretion, a view supported by our studies using the Leydig cell cytotoxin ethane dimethane sulphonate (EDS). When given a single dose of EDS, known to render the testis devoid of Leydig cells,   to adult rats, we noted a significant rise of inhibin levels *in vivo* 7-14 days later (9). However when testosterone was replaced in varying doses (2-5 cm implants or 22.5 cm implants) serum inhibin levels were still elevated suggesting that testosterone per se may not be the specific inhibitor removed by the destruction of the Leydig cells. Rather, the data suggest that some inhibitory factor made by the Leydig cells other than testosterone had been removed.

The role of testosterone has been complicated further by the observation that inhibin secretion is significantly stimulated after a single injection of a high dose of hCG (100 IU) (10).   That hCG acts through the Leydig cells is supported by the observation that when hCG is given to rats in which the

Leydig cells had been destroyed by EDS, no rise in inhibin occurred. Since all of the data indicate that testosterone either has no action or inhibits inhibin secretion, the nature of the Leydig cell stimulus for inhibin requires further investigation.

Other factors may have a role in controlling inhibin secretion. Epidermal growth factor has been shown to stimulate inhibin secretion by immature Sertoli cells and to synergize with FSH in this action. These investigations also noted an inhibitory effect of β endorphin on FSH-induced inhibin secretion.

The role of inhibin in the feedback control of FSH: The need for a specific feedback regulator of FSH has been contested over the past 50 years. Since McCullagh's (33) postulate that inhibin was a feedback regulator of FSH, a number of studies have supported the view that the principal role in feedback is played by testosterone. There is no doubt that testosterone can suppress FSH as well as LH levels in man (3,26) and other species (8). In all of these studies the delivery of testosterone could not be described as physiological since either injections or implants were utilized. In addition, although testosterone levels were maintained within the normal range, these levels were supraphysiological based on the observation of prostatic hypertrophy.

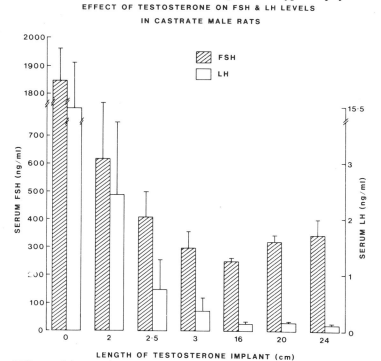

**EFFECT OF TESTOSTERONE ON FSH & LH LEVELS
IN CASTRATE MALE RATS**

Fig. 2. Effect of increasing doses of testosterone on serum FSH and LH in castrate rats is shown. Reproduced with permission from de Kretser *et al* 1987, Serono Symposia. 42: p149.

Furthermore, although FSH levels in castrate rats were suppressed to the normal range, they could not be lowered to the levels found in hypophysectomised rats despite elevation of serum testosterone levels five fold above normal (8) (Fig.2).

Passive immunization with an antiserum to testosterone resulted in elevation of LH levels at low doses and elevation of both FSH and LH at higher doses (30). Supporting evidence that testosterone played a significant role in controlling FSH secretion emerged from the destruction of Leydig cells by EDS which lowered testosterone but resulted in the elevation of FSH to approximately half castrate levels (24,25). Clearly some other factor exerted a restraining influence on FSH levels preventing their rise to the castrate range. The maintenance of inhibin levels in these EDS-treated rats is suggestive that inhibin is the factor controlling FSH (9). Further support for this view can be deduced from the fact that when EDS is given to cryptorchid rats, whose serum and testicular inhibin levels are low and serum FSH levels are elevated to 50% of castrate, the removal of testosterone results in FSH rapidly rising to castrate levels (41). Consequently in rodents, a dual control of FSH by inhibin and testosterone appears to be the physiological control mechanism. A similar mechanism appears likely in primates in view of the recent paper by Dubey *et al* (11). They showed that in arcuate nucleus lesioned monkeys maintained on a constant pulsatile regime of GnRH, testosterone could prevent the castration induced rise of LH but not FSH.

There have been limited studies to date of the action of purified inhibin *in vivo*. Findlay *et al* (16) demonstrated that pure 31 kDa inhibin produced a suppression of FSH when given to ovarectomized sheep providing evidence that the isolated hormone was bioactive *in vivo*. Whether the site of action is at the pituitary alone or at the hypothalamus as well must remain unanswered. Since the inhibin isolation procedures utilized a bioassay based on an action at the pituitary cell, this site of action is well accepted.

The mechanism by which inhibin acts on gonadotrophin secretion has been explored using pure 31 kDa and 58 kDa inhibin both of which show similar patterns of action. Experiments with pure 31 kDa inhibin have demonstrated effects on both basal and GnRH secretion of FSH and to a lesser extent LH (14,20). The effect on basal FSH represents the primary action of inhibin (IC_{50} =7 pM) apparently by selectively blocking tonic FSH synthesis. This may be the result of the slow partial suppression of the mRNA for the β subunit of FSH as shown by Mercer *et al* (38) using ovine follicular fluid as an impure source of inhibin. No change was noted in the levels of mRNA for either the β subunit of LH or the common α subunit of both LH and FSH. An additional action of inhibin was the enhancement of the intracellular degradation of both FSH and LH presumably through the process by which lysosomes breakdown intracellular secretory granules, a mechanism termed crinophagy (14).

The suppressive effect of inhibin on GnRH-induced gonadotrophin secretion represents partly the action of inhibin on the suppression of FSH synthesis. However experiments reveal that inhibin suppresses the release of FSH and LH by a common mechanism (15). The latter is demonstrable by the 2-4 fold greater concentrations of GnRH required to release a standard amount of FSH and LH in the presence of inhibin and secondly by the 35% decrease in the maximum amount of FSH and LH that can be released by excess GnRH. The process by which these changes are mediated is unclear. Inhibin does not compete with GnRH for the GnRH receptor but in unstimulated cultures it causes a 50% decrease in the number of GnRH receptors - with no changes in receptor affinity (57).

Intratesticular actions: The studies by Franchimont *et al* (19) provided data to indicate that impure preparations of inhibin caused a suppression of tritiated thymidine uptake into DNA by spermatogonial cells in culture. However to date no confirmation of this data is available using pure inhibin preparations.

The potential that inhibin may act as an intracompartmental regulator has been explored in our own laboratory and that of Hsueh. We have found that inhibin had no effect on testosterone secretion by Percoll purifed Leydig cells in short term cultures (20 hrs). However Hsueh *et al* (23) noted that inhibin stimulated and activin suppressed, LH induced testosterone production by Leydig cells from neonatal rats or testicular cell prepared from adult hypophysectomized rats. These cells were not Percoll purified and in both experiments the cultures were long term; 48-72 hours for the neonatal interstitial cells and 8-9 days for the cells from the hypophysectomized rats. The reasons for the conflicting results needs exploration. Two factors may have contributed to the differing results (i) the longer term cultures used by Hsueh *et al* (23) and (ii) purified Leydig cells used in our studies.

Conclusions: Considerable progress has occurred since the isolation of inhibin but much of the knowledge gained has resulted from *in vitro* experiments. This is due to the very limited supplies of pure inhibin available from native sources. Further *in vivo* studies will depend on improvements in purification programmes or the production of recombinant inhibin. The isolation of activin and FSP have raised new problems in the measurement of inhibin bioassay potencies and demonstrates the need for specific radioimmunoassays with minimal cross-reactivities to inhibin-related peptides or the inhibin subunits.

References

1. Au, C.L., Robertson, D.M. & de Kretser, D.M. (1984): J. Reprod. Fert., 71: 259-265.
2. Au, C.L., Robertson, D.M. & de Kretser, D.M. (1985): J. Endocr., 105: 1-6.
3. Baker, H.W.G., Bremner, W.J., Burger, H.G., de Kretser, D.M., Dulmanis, A., Eddie, L.W., Hudson, B., Keogh, E.J., Lee, V.W.K. & Rennie, G.C. (1976): Recent Progr. Hormone Res., 32: 429-476
4. Bardin, C.W., Morris, P.L., Chen, C.L., Shaha, C., Voglmayr, J., Rivier, J., Spiess, J. & Vale, W.W. (1987): In: "Inhibin Non-steroidal regulation of Follicle Stimulating Hormone Secretion, edited by H.G. Burger, D.M. de Kretser, J.K. Findlay, M. Igarashi. pp. 179-190. Raven Press, New York.
5. Bicsak, T., Vale, W., Vaughan, J., Tucker, E., Cappel, S. & Hsueh, A.J.W. (1987): Mol. Cell. Endocrinol., 49: 211-217.
6. Crawford, R.J., Hammond, V.E., Evans, B.A., Coghlan, J.P., Haralambidis, J., Hudson, B., Penschow, J.D., Richards, R.I. & Tregear, G.W. (1987): Mol. Endorinol. (in press).
7. Cuevas, P., Ying, S.Y., Ling, N., Ueno, N., Esch, F. & Guillemin, R. (1987):

Biochem. Biophys. Res. Commun. 142: 23-30.
8. Decker, M.H., Loriaux, D.L. & Cutler, G.B. (1981): Endocrinology., 108: 1035-1039.
9. de Kretser, D.M., O'Leary, P.O., Irby, D.C. & Risbridger, G.P. (1988): Int. J. Androl. (submitted).
10. Drummond, A.E., Risbridger, G.P. & de Kretser, D.M. (1988): Endocrinology. (submitted).
11. Dubey, A.K., Zeleznik, A.J. & Plant, T.M. (1987): Endocrinology, 121: 2229-2237.
12. Eddie, L.W., Baker, H.W.G., Dulmanis, A., Higginson, R.E. & Hudson, B. (1979): J. Endocrinol. 81: 49-60.
13. Esch, F.S., Shimasaki, S., Cooksey, K., Mercado, M., Mason, A.J., Ying, S.Y. & Ling, N. (1987): Mol. Endocrinol. 1: 849-855.
14. Farnworth, P.G., Robertson, D.M., de Kretser, D.M. & Burger, H.G. (1988): Endocrinology. (in press).
15. Farnworth, P.G., Robertson, D.M., de Kretser, D.M. & Burger, H.G. (1988): J. Endocrinol. (submitted).
16. Findlay, J.K., Robertson, D.M. & Clarke, I.J. (1987): J. Reprod. Fert. 80: 455-461.
17. Findlay, J.K., Quigg, H., Juholet, P., Katsahambas, S., Clarke, I.J., Doughton, B. & Robertson, D.M. (1988) Proc. 70th Ann. Meet. of US Endocrine Society. (in press).
18. Forage, R.G., Ring, J.M., Brown, R.W., McInerney, B.V., Cobon, G.S., Gregson, R.P., Robertson, D.M., Morgan, F.J., Hearn, M.T.W., Findlay, J.K., Wettenhall, R.E.H., Burger, H.G. & de Kretser, D.M. (1986): Proc. Natl. Acad. Sci. USA 83: 3091-3095.
19. Franchimont, P., Croze, F., Demoulin, A., Bologne, R. & Hustin, J. (1981): Acta Endocrinol. 98: 312-320.
20. Fukuda, M., Miyamoto, K., Hasegawa, Y., Ibuki, Y. & Igarashi, M. (1987): Mol. Cell. Endocr. 51: 41-50.
21. Gonzales, G.F., Risbridger, G.P. & de Kretser, D.M. (1988): Mol. Cell. Endocrinol. (submitted).
22. Hasegawa, Y., Miyamoto, K., Igarashi, M., Yanaka, T., Sasaki, K. & Iwamura, S. (1987): In: Inhibin-Non-steroidal regulation of follicle stimulation hormone secretion. edited by H.G. Burger, D.M. de Kretser, J.K. Findlay & Igarashi, M. Serono Symposium, Raven Press, New York. 42: 119-133.
23. Hsueh, A.J., Dahl, K.D., Vaughan, J., Tucker, E., Rivier, J., Bardin,C.W. & Vale, W. (1987): Proc. Natl. Acad. Sci. USA, 84: 5082-5086.
24. Jackson, A.E., O'Leary, P., Ayers, M. & de Kretser, D.M. (1986): Biol. Reprod. 35: 425-437.
25. Jackson, C.M. & Morris, I.D. (1977) Andrologia, 9: 29-32.
26. Lee, P.A., Jaffe, R.B., Midgeley, A., Rees, Jr, Kohen, F. & Niswender, G.D. (1972): J. Clin. Endocrinol. Metab. 35: 636-641.
27. Le Gac, F. & de Kretser, D.M. (1982) Mol. Cell. Endocrinol. 28: 487-498.
28. Ling, N., Ying, S.Y., Ueno, N., Esch, F., Denorary, L. & Guillemin, R. (1985): Proc. Natl. Acad. Sci. USA. 82: 7217-7221.
29. Ling, N., Ying, S.Y., Ueno, N., Shimasaki, S., Esch, F., Hotta, M. & Guillemin, R. (1986): Nature, 321: 779-782.
30. Main, S.J., Davies, R.V. & Setchell, B.P. (1980): J. Endocrinol. 86: 135-146.
31. Mason, A.J., Hayflick, J.S., Esch, F., Ueno, N., Ying, S.Y., Guillemin, R.,

Niall, H. & Seeburg, P.H. (1985): Nature, 318: 659-663.

32. Mason, A.J., Niall, H.D. & Seeburg, P.H. (1986): Biochem. Biophys. Res. Commun. 135: 957-964.
33. McCullagh, D.R. (1932): Science. 76: 19-20.
34. McLachlan, R.I., Robertson, D.M., Healy, D.L., de Kretser, D.M. & Burger, H.G. (1986): Lancet i, 1233-1234.
35. McLachlan, R.I., Robertson, D.M., Burger, H.G. & de Kretser, D.M. (1986): Mol. Cell. Endocrinol., 46: 175-185.
36. McLachlan, R.I., Robertson, D.M., Healy, D.L., Burger, H.G. & de Kretser, D.M. (1987): J. Clin. Endocrinol. Metab. 65: 954-961.
37. McLachlan, R.I., Matsumoto, A.M., de Kretser, D.M., Burger, H.G. & Bremner, W.J. (1988): J. Clin. Invest. (submitted).
38. Mercer, J.E., Clements, J.A., Funder, J.W. & Clarke, I.J. (1987): Mol. Cell. Endocr. 53: 251-254.
39. Merchenthaler, I. Cullen, M.D., Petrusz, P. & Negros-Vilar, A. (1987): Mol. Cell. Endocrinol., 54: 239-242.
40. Miyamoto, K., Hasegawa, Y., Fukuda, M., Nomura, M., Igarashi, M., Kangawa, K. & Matsuo, H. (1985): Biochem. Biophys. Res. Commun., 129: 396-403.
41. O'Leary, P., Jackson, A.E., Averill, S. & de Kretser, D.M. (1986): Mol. Cell. Endocrinol., 45: 183-190.
42. Rivier, C. & Vale, W. (1987): Endocrinology. 120: 1688-1690.
43. Rivier, J., Spiess, J., McClintock, R., Vaughan, J. & Vale, W. (1985): Biochem. Biophys. Res. Commun. 133: 120-127.
44. Robertson, D.M., Foulds, L.M., Leversha, L., Morgan, F.J., Hearn, M.T.W., Burger, H.G., Wettenhall, R.E.H. & de Kretser, D.M. (1985): Biochem. Biophys. Res. Commun. 126: 220-226.
45. Robertson, D.M., Klein, R., de Vos, F.L., McLachlan, R.I., Wettenhall, R.E.H., Hearn, M.T.W., Burger, H.G. & de Kretser, D.M. (1987): Biochem. Biophys. Res. Commun., 149: 744-749.
46. Robertson, D.M., Tsonis, C.G., McLachlan, R.I., Handlesman, D.J., Leask, R., Baird, D.T., McNeilly, A.S., Hayward, S., Healy, D.L., Findlay, J.K., Burger, H.G. & de Kretser, D.M. (1988): J. Clin. Endocrinol. Metab. (in press).
47. Robertson, D.M., Hayward, S., Irby, D.C., Jacobsen, J.V., Clarke, L.J., McLachlan, R.I. & de Kretser, D.M. (1988): Mol. Cell. Endocrinol. (in press).
48. Scott, R.S., Burger, H.G. & Quigg, H. (1980): Endocrinology, 107: 1536-1542.
49. Steinberger, A. & Steinberger, E. (1978): Endocrinology, 99: 918-921.
50. Steinberger, A., Janecki, A. & Jakubowiak, A. (1987): In: Inhibin, non-steroidal regultion of follicle stimulating hormone secretion, edited by H.G. Burger, D.M. de Kretser, J.K. Findlay, M. Igarashi. Serono Symposium, Raven Press, New York, USA 42: 163-177.
51. Stewart, A.G., Milborrow, H.M., Ring, J.M., Crowther, C.E. & Forage, R.G. (1986): FEBS 206: 329-333.
52. Tenover, J.S., McLachlan, R.I., Burger, H.G., de Kretser, D.M. & Bremner, W.,J. (1988): J. Clin. Endocrinol. & Metab. (submitted).
53. Ultee-van Gessel, A.M., Leemborg, F.G., de Jong, F.H. & van der Molen, H.J. (1986): J. Endocr. 109: 411-418.
54. Vale, W., Rivier, J., Vaughan, J., McClintock, R., Corrigan, A., Woo, W., Karr, D. & Spiess, J. (1986): Nature, 321: 776-779.

55. Verhoeven, G. & Franchimont, P. (1983): Acta Endocr. 102: 136-143.
56. Ying, S.Y., Becker, A., Swanson, G., Tan, P., Ling, N., Esch, F., Ueno, N., Shimasaki, S. & Guillemin, R. (1987): Biochem. Biophys. Res. Commun. 149: 133-139.
57. Wang, Q.F., Farnworth, P.G., Findlay, J.K. & Burger, H.G. (1988): Endocrinology. (submitted).

Interstitial Cell Cultures Secrete an Activity with Characteristics of the Inhibin β - β Homodimer, Activin

W. Lee, R. Schwall, A.R. Mason and J.P. Mather

Genentech, Inc. South San Francisco, USA

INTRODUCTION:

Inhibin is a protein secreted by testis and ovary which decreases FSH, but not LH, secretion from pituitary cells *in vitro* (1). Inhibin is a heterodimer composed of an α and one of two possible β chains (β$_A$ or β$_B$) (2). During the purification of inhibin, proteins were found in porcine follicular fluid which have FSH-stimulating activity and are, in fact, the homodimers of the inhibin β (β$_A$β$_A$ or β$_A$β$_B$) subunits (3,4). It has been suggested that these molecules be called activin (4) and the terminology activin-A, activin-AB, etc. be used to designate their composition. It is not known which cell type in the ovary or testis may secrete activin, or how it's secretion may be regulated compared to that of inhibin.

The results presented in this communication confirm that inhibin is secreted by rat Sertoli cells in vitro, and extend these observations to porcine Sertoli cell cultures. In addition, we show that both rat and pig interstitial cell cultures secrete an activity which has the characteristics of activin. This observation suggests that previously unsuspected modes of endocrine, paracrine and autocrine control may operate in the reproductive system utilizing the activin/inhibin peptides.

EXPERIMENTAL DESIGN:

Sertoli-enriched and Leydig-enriched cultures were prepared from 17-22 day old rats or 3-4 week old piglets using the collagenase (for interstitial) or glycine (for Sertoli) methods previously described (5). Some rat cultures were prepared by gentle mechanical dissociation of the interstitial tissue from the tubules with minimum disruption of the tubular tissue. This method gives a low yield of interstitial tissue but provides cultures with minimal contamination by tubular cells. Minimizing the contamination by Sertoli cells is essential in order to observe activin bioactivity in the conditioned medium since inhibin from the Sertoli cells may mask the activin activity in the assay. Removing the contaminating Sertoli cells is especially difficult in the porcine Leydig cell preparations since the anatomy of the porcine testis requires prolonged enzymatic digestion to obtain single cell suspensions which, particularly at the early stage of development used, will result in contamination by single Sertoli and peritubular cells. The preparations reported here were estimated to contain 10-20% tubular cell contaminants.

Cells were plated in F12/DME (1:1) supplemented with porcine insulin (10 ug/ml), human transferrin (10 ug/ml), mouse EGF (5 ng/ml), α -tocopherol (5 ug/ml) and aprotinin (100 ug/ml) (5F). Medium was changed on day 1 of culture and replaced with fresh 5F medium, or 5F + pregnant mare's serum gonadotropin (PMSG,2ug/ml) or forskolin (FOR, 2uM). Medium was collected at 3 or 4 day intervals thereafter and held at -20 °C prior to assay. The medium was assayed for the ability to stimulate or inhibit the acute release of FSH from gonadotrophs using primary pituitary cell cultures as previously described (6). Control cultures were run using medium supplemented with the same hormones as the experimental medium and incubated at 37°C for the same period of time but without cells. These controls were run in several assays. None of the media had any affect on FSH or LH secretion by the pituitary cell cultures except that containing forskolin which stimulated the release of both FSH and LH.

Conditioned medium collected from the cultures described above was loaded directly onto 10% SDS gels either with or without reduction by ß-mercaptoethanol. The proteins were transferred to nitrocellulose paper for an immune blot. The proteins were visualized using a rabbit antisera raised to the partially purified 32 kd form of recombinant human inhibin. The antisera recognizes epitopes in both the α and ß subunits of inhibin. The second antibody was an anti-rabbit IgG antiserum conjugated to alkaline phosphatase (Sigma Co.).

RESULTS AND DISCUSSION:

Conditioned medium from Sertoli cell cultures prepared from 17-day old rat testis caused a decrease in FSH release from rat pituitary cell cultures (figure1) . The decrease seen was greater when the Sertoli cells were cultured in the presence of PMSG or forskolin (a stimulator of adenylate cyclase). The addition of testosterone and 2% fetal bovine serum to the Sertoli cultures had no effect on FSH release by the pituitary cultures. The cell free controls (see above) were subtracted from the test medium values to obtain the values reported. These controls did not significantly differ from the baseline except for the forskolin-containing medium. This effect of forskolin on the release of FSH and LH by pituitary cell cultures has been reported elsewhere (7). The level of LH in the pituitary cultures was not significantly affected by the conditioned media (again excepting the forskolin condition where the subtraction of the cell- free control values resulted in LH levels significantly below control values). Similar results were obtained using conditioned medium from Sertoli cell cultures from 20 and 22-day old rats.

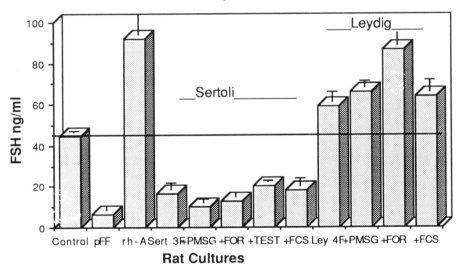

FIG. 1.

Conditioned medium from Sertoli-enriched cultures prepared from 2-4 week old piglets also decreased FSH secretion from pituitary cell cultures without affecting LH release (figure 2).Similar results were seen in three separate Sertoli cell-enriched preparations.

Conditioned media from rat interstitial cell cultures, however, significantly stimulated FSH secretion from the pituitary cell cultures without affecting LH secretion (figure 1). The addition of both PMSG and FBS to the interstitial cultures slightly stimulated subsequent FSH production by pituitary cultures while a strong stimulation was seen with forskolin (after subtraction of the value obtained from the cell-free control). This activin-like activity could be seen in cell culture media after three to four changes of medium (two weeks in culture). Similar results were seen using cells from animals at all three ages.

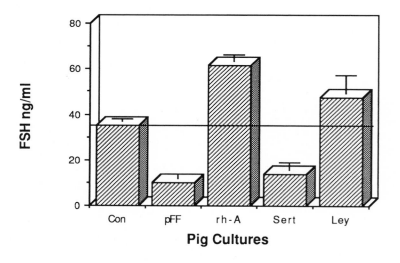

FIG. 2.

Conditioned medium from porcine interstitial cells cultured in the 5F supplements described above also caused an increase in FSH release by pituitary cells (figure 2). Parallel dose response curves were run on pituitary cultures to compare the response to conditioned medium from rat Leydig cell cultures and from cultures producing recombinant human activin (β_A-β_A, rh-activin).   There was a parallel increase in FSH secretion in cultures incubated with rat Leydig cell medium and with rh-activin (data not shown).

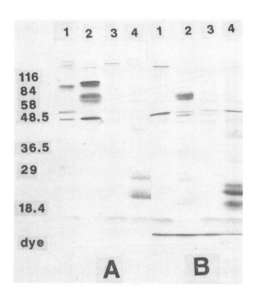

FIG. 3.   Immunoblot of testicular cell culture media conditioned by: 1. rat interstitial cells, 2. rat Sertoli cells, 3. pig interstitial cells, or 4. pig Sertoli cells.   Samples were either: A. non-reduced or B. reduced.   Molecular weight markers are shown at left.

The rat and porcine cultures both produced multiple immunoreactive bands on the Western gels.   The pattern of the bands of the immunoreactive material is different for interstitial cell and Sertoli cultures in both the pig and the rat (figure 3).   In addition, the Sertoli cell- produced material from the pig and rat have quite distinct patterns, as do the interstitial cell cultures from the two species.   Culture medium from rat peritubular cells prepared from the same animals as the interstitial cultures, and early passage rat lung epithelial cell culture medium both show only two faint bands at >100 kd MW   (not shown) suggesting that the majority of the bands visualized in the Western are related to inhibin, activin, their precursors, or products.   Work is in progress to determine the nature of these immunoreactive bands.

The hypothesis that Leydig cells are a source of testicular activin is further supported by results from the TM3 mouse Leydig cell line.   These cells secrete an activin-like activity as measured in the bioassay.   In addition, they contain mRNA of the correct size on Northern blot analysis which hybridizes with both the β_A and β_B, but not the α , subunit human cDNA probes (submitted for publication).   Since this is a clonal cell line, it would suggest that at least one source of activin in the interstitial cultures of the rat and pig cells is the Leydig cell.

The above data shows the presence of both immunoreactivity and bioactivity produced by interstitial cell cultures of the rat and pig which are distinct from inhibin and consistent with the presence of activin in the   culture medium of interstitial cells.   The presence of both activin-like bioactivity and mRNA which hybridizes with a cDNA probe for the ß subunit of inhibin, but not the α subunit, in the clonal mouse Leydig cell line (TM3) further supports the hypothesis that activin is produced by Leydig cells in the testis while inhibin is produced by the Sertoli cells.   The data presented above from rat, pig and the mouse cell line suggest that this is widespread and not limited to a single species.

CONCLUSIONS:

The data presented above confirm earlier reports of inhibin production by rat Sertoli cells in vitro and expand this observation to porcine Sertoli cell cultures.   In addition the data support the novel   hypothesis that the FSH-stimulating activity found in the testis is not produced by differential association of α and B subunits produced in the Sertoli cell, but rather is produced by an entirely different cell in the interstitial tissue, probably the Leydig cell.   By analogy, it is possible that the activin and inhibin found in follicular fluid are produced by different cell types in the ovary.   This production could be continuous or activin could be expressed by non-granulosa cells in the ovary at different times of the cycle or during ovarian development.

The fact that inhibin and activin seem to be secreted by different cells in the testis suggests novel possibilities for the endocrine, paracrine and autocrine regulation of these two factors. Results concerning the effects of unpurified conditioned medium from testis cultures containing both Leydig and Sertoli cells, and results from experiments where the effects of inhibin and activin are studied on such mixed cultures should be interpreted with caution in light of the known antagonistic effects of these two factors (4,8).

REFERENCES:
1). McLachlan, et al. (1987) Bailier's Clin. Endo. & Metab. vol.1 p.89.
2). Mason, et. al. (1985) Nature. 318:659.
3). Vale, et al. (1986) Nature. 321:776.
4). Ling, et al. (1986) Nature. 321:779.
5). Mather & Phillips (1984) in: Cell Culture Meth. for Cell and Molec. Biol., Barnes et. al. (eds.) p. 29.
6). Ling, et. al. (1985) Proc. Natl. Acad. Sci. USA, 82:7217.
7). Cronin, et. al. (1984) Am. J. Physiol. 246 (Endocrinol. and Metab. 9) E44-E51.
8). Hsueh, et al. (1987) Proc. Natl. Acad. Sci. USA 84:5082.

Effects of FSH and Testosterone on Inhibin mRNA Levels and Inhibin Synthesis in Highly Purified Rat Sertoli Cells

A.M.W. Toebosch, D.M. Robertson[1], J. Trapman[2],
F.H. de Jong and J.A. Grootegoed

*Departments of Biochemistry II and [2]Pathological Anatomy I,
Erasmus University Rotterdam, P.O. Box 1738, 3000 DR Rotterdam,
The Netherlands and [1]Department of Anatomy, Monash University,
Wellington Road, Clayton, Victoria, Australia*

INTRODUCTION

Inhibin is a glycoprotein consisting of two partially homologous subunits, α and β, which are products of separate genes. Inhibin acts on the pituitary to preferentially suppress the production and secretion of FSH. In addition to the αβ-dimer, ββ-dimers, termed activins, have been identified and shown to have a stimulatory effect on FSH release from pituitary cells (6,18).

In the testis, Sertoli cells are the source of inhibin production (15). We previously reported that FSH stimulates α-subunit mRNA expression in Sertoli cells isolated from immature rats (16), whereas FSH also stimulates inhibin synthesis in these cells (4,16,17). Reports on the regulation of inhibin production by testosterone are contradictory (see review by de Jong (1)).

The aim of the present study was to further investigate the in vitro effects of FSH and testosterone on inhibin α- and β_B-subunit mRNA expression, and on the synthesis of immunoreactive and bioactive inhibin in Sertoli cells from immature rats. Highly purified Sertoli cell preparations were used to try to exclude indirect effects of hormones on Sertoli cells via other testicular cell types and also effects of those other cell types on the regulation of inhibin production by Sertoli cells. For example, some effects of testosterone on Sertoli cells could be mediated by peritubular myoid cells (13), and germ cells may influence androgen binding protein production by Sertoli cells (3).

METHODS

Highly purified Sertoli cells were isolated from testes of 21-23-day-old rats using a modification of the method described by Skinner and Fritz (14). In brief, the testes were decapsulated, chopped and the tissue fragments were subjected to sequential treatments with trypsin, collagenase, vigorous mechanical agitation and hyaluronidase. The cells were incubated for 48h at 37°C in Eagle's minimum essential medium (MEM) containing 1% fetal calf serum (FCS). Subsequently, most of the remaining spermatogenic cells were removed by hypotonic shock treatment (10% MEM in water for 2.5 min), and the culture was continued for another 24h in MEM supplemented with 0.1% bovine serum albumin (BSA). This isolation and incubation procedure resulted in a Sertoli cell preparation in which the germ cell contamination was 1-3% and the peritubular cell contamination was less than 0.5%. At the end of the 3-day preincubation period, the cells were incubated for different time periods in MEM with 0.1% BSA, in the presence or absence of ovine FSH (NIH S16) and testosterone.

Total RNA from the Sertoli cell preparations was isolated using a guanidinium thiocyanate-phenol extraction procedure. The RNA samples were electrophoresed and analysed by Northern transfer using a 480 bp cDNA fragment corresponding to the α-subunit of bovine inhibin and a 920 bp cDNA fragment corresponding to the β_B-subunit of human inhibin, as described previously (16).

Inhibin immuno- and bioactivity were measured in lyophilised Sertoli cell media and Triton-lysed cells using a radioimmunoassay (RIA) (11) and an in vitro bioassay (media only) as described by Scott et al. (12). The RIA consisted of a rabbit antiserum raised against purified bovine 31 KDa inhibin and iodinated 31 KDa bovine inhibin as tracer and showed minimal cross-reactivity with activin and isolated α- and β-subunits following reduction and alkylation of inhibin. In both RIA and bioassay, a rat ovarian extract obtained from PMSG-treated immature rats was used as standard which was calibrated in terms of an ovine testicular lymph standard preparation with an arbitrary unitage of 1 unit per mg protein. Sertoli cell protein was measured according to Lowry et al. (7) using BSA as standard.

RESULTS AND DISCUSSION

Previous results have shown that one α-subunit mRNA species of 1.6 kb and two β_B-subunit mRNA species of 4.2 kb and 3.5 kb can be detected in immature rat testes and cultured Sertoli cells (16). FSH stimulated the expression of α-subunit mRNA in cultured Sertoli cells within 24h in a dose dependent manner (ED_{50} of 5-50 ng/ml). There was no effect of FSH on the β_B-subunit mRNA levels (16).

In the present experiments, the expression of the inhibin mRNAs in highly purified Sertoli cell preparations was estimated 6h and 24h after addition of FSH. The results were similar to those obtained previously using Sertoli cell preparations with higher contaminations of peritubular and germinal cells, showing FSH stimulation of inhibin α-subunit mRNA and no effect of FSH on β_B-subunit mRNA.

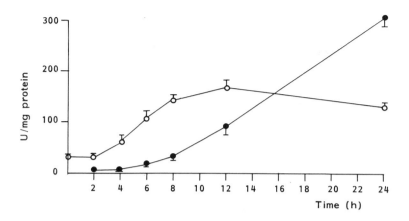

Figure 1. Amounts of immunoreactive inhibin secreted by (●—●) or present in (o—o) Sertoli cells, after incubation with 500 ng/ml FSH for different time periods.

The amounts of immunoreactive inhibin, present in or secreted by cultured Sertoli cells, were increased by FSH in a dose-dependent manner with an ED_{50} between 5 and 50 ng/ml and a maximally stimulating dose of 500 ng/ml (data not shown). Using a maximally stimulating dose of FSH, it was observed that intracellular immunoreactive inhibin levels reached a plateau of approximately 100-125 U/mg protein after 6-8 h of incubation. Concomitantly, the rate of secretion of inhibin was low from 0-6h and became maximal after 6-8h (Fig. 1). The relatively high intracellular inhibin concentration during 0-8h indicates that there was a delay of the secretion of immunoreactive inhibin, which could be associated with posttranslational processing of the protein.

The present results indicate that there was a correlation between FSH stimulation of inhibin α-subunit mRNA expression and inhibin immunoreactivity. All immunoreactive samples were bioactive. The amount of bioactive inhibin secreted by the Sertoli cells was also increased by FSH. However, a decrease in the ratio of bioactive and immunoreactive inhibin levels (B/I ratio) was observed after stimulation with high doses of FSH (Fig. 2). At low doses of FSH (<5 ng/ml) a B/I ratio of approximately 1 was observed, whereas at higher doses (50-5000 ng/ml) the B/I ratio was approximately 0.5 (results not shown).

Addition of testosterone (1 µM) to the highly purified Sertoli cells in culture did not affect the expression of inhibin α- or $β_B$-subunit mRNAs (data not shown). Moreover, incubation of the

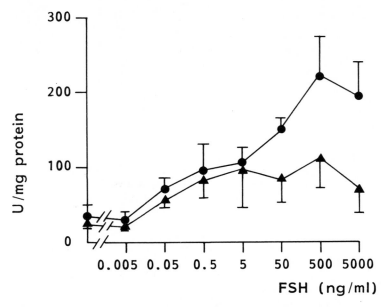

Figure 2. Amounts of immunoreactive inhibin (●——●) or bioactive inhibin (▲——▲) secreted by Sertoli cells, after incubation with different doses of FSH.

Sertoli cells with testosterone, or with testosterone in combination with FSH, did not affect the levels of immunoreactive inhibin present in or secreted by the cells (Fig. 3). As yet the effect of testosterone on bioactive inhibin has not been assessed owing to the possible interference of testosterone in the <u>in vitro</u> bioassay. On the other hand, Ultee-van Gessel et al. (17) detected suppression of levels of secreted bioactive inhibin after addition of testosterone in medium of cultured Sertoli cells.

The observed change of B/I ratios following FSH stimulation may be caused by the production of activin which could lead to an underestimation of inhibin bioactivity. However, it seems likely that activins are not produced in large amounts by Sertoli cells of 21-23 day old rats. Until now, two forms of activin, $\beta_A \beta_A$ and $\beta_A \beta_B$ dimers, have been isolated whereas a β_B subunit activin has not yet been reported. We have previously reported that β_A mRNA could not be detected in testes of 21-23 day old rats (16). This is in agreement with data from Esch et al. and Meunier et al. (2,8). Other possible explanations for a B/I ratio lower than 1 include the production of larger (58 kDa) forms of inhibin (2,5,10), and the presence of isoforms of inhibin which are detected in the RIA but may have intrinsically different bioactivities (9).

From the present data it is concluded that FSH can stimulate inhibin α-subunit mRNA expression, immunoreactivity and bioactivity, whereas testosterone has no effect on mRNA levels and inhibin immunoreactivity. There is a correlation between inhibin α-subunit mRNA expression and immunoreactivity, whereas the relationship between bio- and immunoactive inhibin changes with FSH stimulation. It is suggested that complex hormonal regulation of post-transcriptional events involved in processing of the protein moieties and glycosylation play an important role in the production of bioactive inhibin.

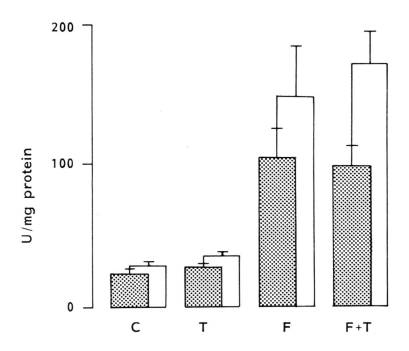

Figure 3. Amounts of immunoreactive inhibin secreted by (open bars) or present in (dotted bars) Sertoli cells, after incubation without (C) or with FSH (F)(500 ng/ml) and/or testosterone (T)(1 µM) for 24h.

ACKNOWLEDGEMENTS

We thank Miss M. Giacometti, Mrs. J. Jacobsen and Miss L. Iarke for the inhibin assays. This work was financially supported by the Dutch Foundation for Medical Research (Medigon) and the National Health and Medical Research council of Australia. We thank Biotechnology, Australia Pty.Ltd. for providing us with the cDNA probes used in the present experiments.

1. de Jong F.H. (1988): Physiological Reviews, 68 (in press).
2. Esch F.S., Shimasaki, S., Cooksey, K., Mercado, M., Mason, A.J., Ying, S-Y., Ueno, N., and Ling, N. (1987): Mol. Endocr., 1:388-396.
3. Galdieri M., Monaco, L., Stefanini, M. (1984): J. Androl., 5:409-415.
4. Le Gac, F., and de Kretser, D.M. (1982): Mol. Cell. Endocr., 28:487-498.
5. Leversha L.J., Robertson, D.M., de Vos, F.L., Morgan, F.J., Hearn, M.T.W., Wettenhall, R.E.H., Burger, H.G., and de Kretser, D.M. (1987): J. Endocr.,113:213-221.
6. Ling N., Ying, S-Y., Ueno, N., Shimasaki, S., Esch, F., Hotta, M., and Guillemin, R. (1986): Nature, 321:779-782.
7. Lowry O.H., Rosebrough, N.J., Farr, A.L., and Randall, R.J. (1951): J. Biol. Chem., 193:265-275.
8. Meunier H., Rivier, C., Evans, R.M., and Vale, W. (1988): Proc. Natl. Acad. Sci. USA, 85:247-251.
9. Robertson, D.M., de Vos, F.L., McLachlan, R.I., Salamonson, L.A., Hearn, M.T.W., Morgan, F.J., Findlay, J.K., Burger, H.G., and de Kretser, D.M. (1988): In: Inhibin - non steroidal regulation of FSH secretion, edited by H.G. Burger, D.M. de Kretser, and J.K. Findlay, Ares Serono Symposium, 42:17-33.
10. Robertson D.M., Foulds, L.M., Leversha, L.J., Morgan, F.J., Hearn, M.T.W., Burger, H.G., Wettenhall, R.E.H., and de Kretser, D.M. (1985): Biochem. Biophyp. Res. Comm., 126:220-226.
11. Robertson, D.M., Hayward, S., Irby, D.C., Jacobson, J.B., Clarke, L.J., McLachlan, R.I., and de Kretser, D.M. (1988): Mol. Cell. Endocr., in the press.
12. Scott R.S., Burger, H.G., Quigg, H. (1980): Endocr., 107:1536-1541.
13. Skinner M.K., and Fritz, I.B. (1985): Proc. Natl. Acad. Sci. USA, 82:114-118.
14. Skinner M.K., and Fritz, I.B. (1985): Mol. Cell. Endocr., 40:115-122.
15. Steinberger A., and Steinberger, E. (1976): Endocr., 99:918-921.
16. Toebosch A.M.W., Robertson, D.M., Trapman, J., Klaassen, P., de Paus, R.A., de Jong, F.H., and Grootegoed, J.A. (1988): Mol. Cell. Endocr., 55:101-105.
17. Ultee-van Gessel A.M., Leemborg, F.G., de Jong, F.H., and van der Molen, H.J. (1986): J. Endocr., 109:411-418.
18. Vale W., Rivier, J., Vaughan, J., McClintock, R., Corrigan, A., Woo, W., Karr, D., and Spiess, J. (1986): Nature, 321:776-779.

Signal Transduction by G Proteins. Regulation of Ion Channels as Seen with Native and Recombinant Subunits and Multiplicity of Intramembrane Transduction Pathways

L. Birnbaumer[1,2], A. Yatani[2], J. Codina[1], R. Mattera[1],
R. Graf[1], G.-F. Liao[1], A. Themmen[1], J. Sanford[1],
H.E. Hamm[3], R. Iyengar[4], M. Birnbaumer[1] and A.M. Brown[2]

*Department of [1]Cell Biology and [2]Physiology and Molecular Biophysics,
Baylor College of Medicine, Houston, TX 77030,
[3]Physiology and Biophysics, University of Illinois School of Medicine,
Chicago, IL 60680, and [4]Pharmacology, Mount Sinai School of Medicine,
New York, NY 10029*

INTRODUCTION[1]/

About 80% of all known hormones and neurotransmitters, as well as many neuromodulators and auto- and paracrine factors that regulate cellular interactions, termed **primary messengers**, are now known to elicit cellular responses by combining to specific receptors which are coupled to effector functions by G proteins. Yet, even though the primary messengers are many, the number of distinct receptors that mediate their action is even larger. This is well exemplified by the existence of at least four types of adrenergic receptors ($\beta1$, $\beta2$, $\alpha1$ and $\alpha2$) , of at least five types of muscarinic acetylcholine receptors (M1 through M5), two types of dopamine receptors (D1 and D2), and several types each of adenosine, purinergic and light (rhodopsin) receptors. Multiplicity of receptors is not restricted to neurotransmitters. There are at least three types of vasopressin receptors (V1a, V1b and V2 and vasoactive intestinal peptide interacts with receptors that either stimulate adenylyl cyclase or phosphoinositide turnover. At this time about 75 distinct receptors can be identified that recognize 30 hormones and neurotransmitters. It seems reasonable to assume that the total number of distinct receptors coupled by G proteins will be around 100 (Figure 1)

In contrast, both the final effector functions regulated by these receptors and the G proteins that provide for receptor-effector coupling are much fewer, probably not much more than 10 each.

---

[1]/ Several minireviews, reviews and updates on G proteins and their functions have appeared within the last 12 months with more or less extensive referencing to the original contributions (4,5, 8,13,17,23,30). Because of space limitations, only selected work is referenced. We apologize for omissions that had to occur.

Figure 1 Flow of information through G protein-dependent signal transduction systems as found in vertebrates.

	input	transduction		output
Loca-tion	Extra-cellular Milieu	Plasma Membrane		Intracellular Milieu or Plasma Membrane
		G-Protein Coupled Receptor	G-Protein Regulated Effector	
Func-tional Ele-ments	Primary Messen-ger ⟧ —> R	—> G Protein	—> E —>	⟦Secondary Messenger; Membrane Potential

Molecular Diversity					
					cAMP, IP's,
# known	ca.30	75	12	6	DAG, Ca^{2+},
# estimated	?	ca.100	up to 15	ca. 12	cGMP, AA

Thus, at this time we know of about 8 to 10 classes of G proteins, including G_s, several G_i's, a G_o and two transducins and of about as many effector functions, including adenylyl cyclase, the "original" effector system, the cG MP-specific phosphodiesterase of photoreceptor cells, polyphosphoinositide-specific phospholipase C, a phospholipase of the A_2-type that releases arachidonic acid, and two classes of ionic channels, one specific for K^+ and relatively independent of membrane potential for its activity, the other specific for Ca^{2+} and strongly dependent on membrane potential for its activity. Based on this, the responses elicited through occupancy of G protein-coupled receptors by primary messengers include not only changes of intracellular second messenger levels -- cyclic nucleotides, inositol phosphates, diacylglycerol, arachidonic acid and Ca^{2+} -- but also of the cell membrane potential, which itself is a potent regulator of cellular function.

Of the three elements that constitute signal transduction units, i.e., receptors, G proteins and effectors, the effectors are presently the least understood in molecular terms. Only two have been purified to close to homogeneity -- adenylyl cyclase and the camp-specific phosphodiesterase regulated by transducin in rod photoreceptor cells (ROS PDE)-- and studies at the molecular level are just beginning. In contrast, the other elements of the signal transduction machinery, the G proteins and the receptors coupled by them, are much better known.

Several of the receptors have been purified and cloned. These include the rhodopsins, the β- and α-adrenergic receptors, five types of muscarinic receptors and the receptor for substance K, a neuropeptide. The structural analysis afforded through the cloning revealed that they all belong to a family of homologous opsin-like proteins that on grounds of homology to crystalline bacteriorhodopsin are predicted to span the plasma membrane seven times as

<u>Figure 2</u> Typical transmembrane arrangement of G protein-coupled receptors as deduced from hydropathy plots of the cloned molecules

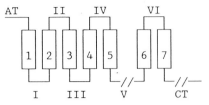

Hydropathy plot of the amino acid composition deduced from the cDNA's of the eight G protein-coupled receptors cloned thus far -- rhodopsin, the β_1-, β_2- and α_2-adrenergic receptors, five muscarinic acetylcholine receptors and the substance K receptor -- revealed that they have a common structural background and predicts that they are formed of seven transmembrane (**tm**) α helices (numbered 1 through **7**), each composed of 19-24 amino acids, connected by intra- and extracellular loops (numbered I through VI), an extracellular amino terminal end (**AT**) and an intracellular carboxyl end (**CT**). Loops and termini vary in length from receptor to receptor, with **loop V** and the **CT** segments showing the biggest variations thus far. A search for amino acid sequence conservation among these receptors shows the highest stretch of identity to include the end of **loop I** and the beginning of **tm 2** segment. This area may be involved in interaction with a common element of G proteins, such as the β and/or γ subunits. β and γ subunits are common to all G proteins and are required for the interaction of the different α subunits with the receptors. The site of interaction of retinal with opsin to give photosensitive rhodopsin is a lysine in **tm 7** segment. On the other hand, an aspartic acid present in **tm 2** segment is involved in binding of the catecholamine to the β-adrenergic receptor. The determination of the actual points of contact between ligand and receptor and G protein and receptor will be subjects of intense and independent investigation for each of the 100 or so receptors engaged in this type of signal transduction.

---

illustrated in Figure 2.

    G proteins, the central theme of this article, are heterotrimers formed of α, β and γ subunits. The α subunits, of Mr between 39,000 and 50,000, bind and hydrolyze GTP, define the receptor and effector specificity of a G protein and differ from G protein to G protein. By purification and molecular cloning there are now ten distinct vertebrate α subunits known, i.e., as many as G proteins, and there may be more. In addition, two homologous α subunits have been cloned from yeast and one from dictyostelium. By purification and molecular cloning there appear to be only two β subunits with approximate Mr values of 35,000 and there seem to exist between two and three γ subunits with Mr values between 6,000 and 10,000 of which only the one associated with transducin has

<u>Figure 3</u> SDS-PAGE analysis of G_s and G_k (G_i-3) purified from human erythrocyte membranes.

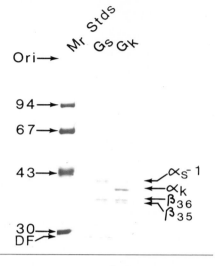

Ori→

94→
67→
43→
30→
DF→

$\propto_s^- 1$
$\propto_k$
$\beta 36$
$\beta 35$

Note that each of the proteins has its share of $\beta\gamma$ dimers. High resolution urea gradient/SDS-PAGE analysis and immunoblotting with α subunit-specific antibodies of these protein preparations, revealed G_k to be G_i-3, with less than 5% of either G_i-1, G_i-2 or G_o as well as being essentially free of G_s. Likewise, G_s is essentially free of any PTX substrate.

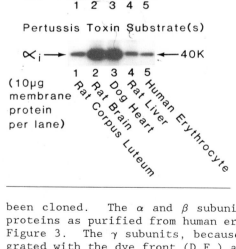

Cholera Toxin Substrates

$\propto_{S2}$→
$\propto_{S1}$→
←50K
←42K
1 2 3 4 5

Pertussis Toxin Substrate(s)

$\propto_i$→
←40K
1 2 3 4 5

(10µg
membrane
protein
per lane)

Rat Corpus Luteum
Rat Brain
Dog Heart
Rat Liver
Human Erythrocyte

<u>Figure 4</u>   CTX and PTX label α subunits of G proteins in membranes. Top panel, 21-hour autoradiogram; bottom panel, 4-hour autoradiogram.

been cloned. The α and β subunit composition of two typical G proteins as purified from human erythrocyte membranes is shown in Figure 3. The γ subunits, because of their small size, have migrated with the dye front (D.F.) and are not visible as such.
    The α subunits of all G proteins (for exception see below) are substrates of one or both of two ADP-ribosyltransferases, the toxin of <u>Vibrio</u> <u>cholera</u> (cholera toxin or CTX) which requires a proteic cofactor for its action which depends on GTP for its activity and the toxin of <u>Bordetella</u> <u>pertussis</u> (pertussis toxin or PTX) which depends on ATP for its action. Figure 4 presents a

Figure 5   Schematic representation of α subunit mRNA molecules of vertebrate animals as deduced from cDNA cloning.

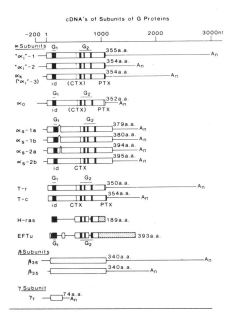

Open boxes represent the open reading frames or coding sequences and lines represent 5' and 3' untranslated sequences which may be incomplete. Black boxes within the open reading frames of α subunits denote sequences highly homologous to those known in bacterial elongation factor TU to be involved in GTP binding and hydrolysis. Sequences homologous to these are present also in the <u>ras</u> molecules. The mRNA molecules encoding the β_{36}, β_{35}, and γ_T are shown for comparison. The position of amino acids ADP-ribosylated by CTX and PTX are indicated. i.d., location of the identity box. The scale is in nucleotides.

typical autoradiogram obtained on ADP-ribosylating the α subunits of membrane bound G proteins with ^{32}P-labeled NAD and separating the reaction products by standard 12.5% sodium dodecylsulfate polyacrylamide gel electrophoresis (SDS-PAGE).

STRUCTURE OF THE α SUBUNITS AS DEDUCED BY MOLECULAR CLONING

Ten vertebrate and three lower eukaryotic α subunits have been cloned and their amino acid sequence has been predicted. The cloning of an eleventh α subunit structurally homologous to the α_i molecules but lacking a cysteine that is ADP-ribosylated by PTX has been announced. The intron/exon splice junctions of the human α_s gene have been established as well (22). All α subunits contain sets of sequences highly homologous to sequences known in bacterial elongation factor TU to be involved in GTP binding and hydrolysis. Among these there is a stretch of 18 amino acids that is invariable in all ten cloned vertebrate α subunits and serves as an identifying signature or identity box flanked on both sides by either Lys (K) or Arg (R). Interestingly, the exon 1/exon 2 splice junction of α_s lies within this identity box separating ...LLLL from GAGS... Figure 5 presents the structures of cDNA's coding for α, β and γ subunits as they are known at this time. An expanded version of the three-dimensional arrangement of the guanine nucleotide binding sequences, as deduced from x-ray crystallographic studies, and the predicted likelihood of α helix and β pleated sheet formation

<u>Figure 6</u> Predicted secondary structure of an α_{avg} subunit as proposed by   Masters et al. (25) on the basis of X-ray crystallographic analysis of bacterial elongation factor TU and amphipatic analysis of the primary amino acid sequence of α_s, α_i, α_o, α_t-c and α_t-r.

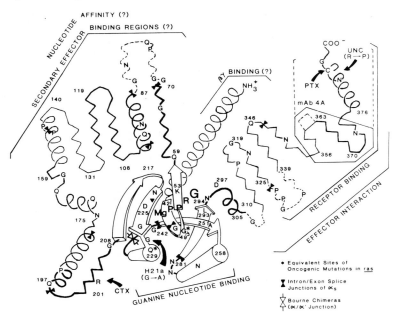

Some of the amino acids present in at least four of the five α subunits are highlighted, numbers refer to numbering of α_{avg} (25). <u>Symbols.</u> <u>Cylinders and ribbons</u>, guanine nucleotide binding regions as deduced from X-ray diffraction of EF-TU (19); <u>thick lines</u>, regions in which the amino acid sequence of the five chains is greater than 90% homologous; <u>middle thick lines</u>, 70 to 89% homo-homology; <u>thin lines</u>, less than 60% homology; <u>dashed lined</u>, sequences unique to α_s. The molecule is shown with Mg-GDP bound to it. G^{49} and Q^{229} (marked by asterisks) correspond to the oncogenic mutation sites of Gly^{12} and Glu^{61} of p21 <u>ras</u> proteins. The location of the antigenic epitope of monoclonal antibody 4A (<u>mab 4A</u>) as deduced on the basis of proteolytic and peptide competition studies (12,15) is indicated. <u>Heavy arrows</u>: sites of ADP-ribosylation by CTX and PTX and molecular nature of the UNC (Arg to Pro; ref. 31) and H21a (Gly to Ala; Bourne, personal communication) mutations. Regions thought most likely to be responsible for interaction with receptors (C terminal end) and $\beta\gamma$ dimers (N-terminal end) are shown. Studies with α/α' chimaera by Bourne and collaborators (26, personal communication), spliced at α_{avg} position 223 (<u>opposing double arrow</u> on the figure), have shown that the terminal 40% of the molecules carry receptor and effector specificity information. Thus, the region responsible

<u>Fig. 6 legend (cont'd):</u>
for interaction with effectors includes at least partially the
one "seen" also by receptors, and may include the remainder of
the molecule as indicated. <u>Opposing solid arrows</u>, exon/exon splice
junctions of α_s (22).

---

by the remainder of a G protein α subunit are shown in Figure 6,
adapted from Masters <u>et al.</u>(25). The figure incorporates locations
of ADP-ribosylation by toxins (35,36), of intron/exon splice junctions of α_s (22), of the antigenic epitope recognized by monoclonal antibody 4A (12, 15), mutations responsible for UNC (31) and
H21a (Bourne, personal communication) S49 cell phenotypes, and
splice junction of α/α' chimaeras constructed by Bourne and collaborators (26) showing that the COOH-terminal 40% of α_s specifies
specificity for both, interaction with receptor and in-teraction
with effector.
   Figure 7 (next page) depicts the complete predicted amino acid
sequences of cloned α subunits of G proteins.

   <u>The Turnover Cycle.</u>   G proteins are activated by GTP and
deactivate on hydrolyzing GTP. With non-hydrolyzable GTP analogs,
activation is associated with subunit dissociation giving α-GTP
analog complexes plus $\beta\gamma$ dimer. Although not yet proven, the same
is thought to occur also with GTP. This gives rise to a disso-
ciation/reassociation GTPase-driven turnover cycle in which
reassociation of $\beta\gamma$ dimers to the α subunits occurs after GTP is
hydrolyzed to GDP to give inactive α-GDP subunits with increased
affinity for $\beta\gamma$ (Figure 8).

<u>Figure 8</u>   Turnover cycle of a G protein.

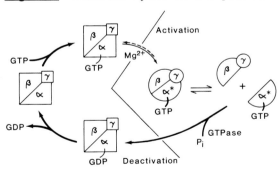

Squares and semi-squares
represent inactive
conformations as they
relate to modulation of
effector functions.
Circular and semi-
circular shapes represent
activated forms of the
G protein. Activation
is both GTP- and Mg^{2+}-
dependent and stabilized
by subunit dissociation
to give an activated α-
GTP complex plus the
$\beta\gamma$ dimer. Hydrolysis of GTP by the α subunit deactivates it,
increases its affinity for $\beta\gamma$ and leads to reassociation to give
an inactive holo-G protein with GDP bound to it. Re-initiation
of the activation cycle requires release of GDP and renewed
binding of GTP.

Figure 7

DIRECT REGULATION OF IONIC CHANNELS BY G PROTEINS

One of the new discoveries made during the last one and one half years is that in addition to enzymes, G proteins regulate ion channels (5 and references therein; 38, 39). The first such channel discovered was the heart inwardly rectifying "muscarinic" K^+ channel, the second was the dihydropyridine sensitive Ca^{2+} channels of heart and skeletal muscle.

The G Protein-gated K^+ Channel

Regulation of K^+ channels by a G protein, designated G_k was established in patch clamp-experiments (Figure 9) on addition of GTPγS-activated G_k or α_k (G_k^* and α_k^*) to inside-out membrane patches as illustrated for regulation of the G protein K^+ channel of the rat pituitary GH_3 cell line in Figure 10. These and other experiments showed that G protein regulation of K^+ channels by receptors is critically dependent on GTP, that activation of G_k by GTP requires the participation of agonist occupied receptor, that G_k is uncoupled from regulation by receptor by PTX and that a PTX-uncoupled system is readily reconstituted by addition of

---

Figure 9 Three typical configurations of the patch clamp technique for the study of single channel and whole cell currents as developed at the University of Goettingen by Neher, Sakmann, Sigworth and collaborators.

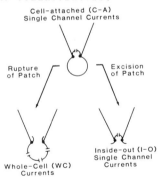

Cell-attached (C-A)
Single Channel Currents

Rupture of Patch

Excision of Patch

Inside-out (I-O)
Single Channel Currents

Whole-Cell (WC)
Currents

In this technique a small heat-polished glass pipette is pressed against the plasma membrane of a cell and a seal with a resistance in the order 10-100 gigaohm is caused to form by suction. The seal isolates the membrane patch at the pipette tip electrically, physically and structurally. This permits the membrane patch to be voltage clamped without the use of microelectrodes, prevents lateral diffusion of membrane components into and out of the patch, and allows both excision of the membrane to give a cell free patch that spans the tip of the pipette, or disruption of the membrane patch keeping the pipette attached to the cell. In this manner ionic channels can be voltage clamped and single channel currents recorded in the cell-attached (C-A)mode before patch excision, and in the inside-out (I-O) mode after patch excision. In addition, after patch dis- ruption, the direct electrical and physical access to the interior of cells allowing for recording of whole cell currents under voltage clamp conditions (W-C mode) and, since in the process the cellular cytoplasm equilibrates with the pipette solution, for introduction of test agents. Adapted from Hamill et al. (14).

exogenous unactivated G_k, provided GTP is present in the bath. Further, since resolved GTPγS-activated α subunits of G_k (α_k^*) mimic the actions of GTPγS-activated G_k (G_k^*) and do so with comparable potency (not shown), which resolved βγ dimers do not, the experiments also indicate that the most plausible signal transduction pathway used by muscarinic receptors to stimulate K^+ channels of the inwardly rectifying type is catalysis of the activation of G_k by GTP and formation of activated free α_k^* which in turn acts as mediator to stimulate the K^+ channel.

Figure 10 Properties of G_k-mediated regulation of G protein sensitive K^+ channels as seen in inside-out membrane patches of GH_3 rat pituitary tumor cells.

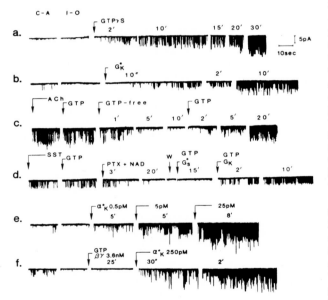

Each line represents a separate experiment in which single channel K^+ currents were recorded before (cell-attached or C-A) and after membrane patch excision to the inside out configuration (C-F or I-O). Records were obtained at holding potentials that varied between -80 and -100 mV and using symmetrical 130 to 140 mM KCl or K-methanesulfonate solutions in 5 mM Hepes pH 7.5, containing in addition either 1.8 mM $CaCl_2$ in the pipette, or 5 mM EGTA and 2 mM $MgCl_2$ in the 100-μl bathing chamber. Other additions are shown or described for each experiment . Numbers above the records denote time elapsed between the indicated additions and the beginning of the segment of record shown. Routinely, the first addition was made between 5 and 10 min after patch excision and subsequent additions were at 5 to 25 min intervals, depending on the purpose of the experiments. 5-min intervals were used when dose-response relationships were studied; 25-min intervals were used when substances added had no apparent effect. In some instances the bathing solutions were exchanged by perfusion at 1 to 2 ml/min. Cells were grown as monolayers on cover slips and membrane patches excised from their upper membrane surface. **Experiment a**: effect of GTPγS added to the bathing medium. **Experiment b**: Representative time course of activation

Fig. 10 legend (cont'd):
of GH_3 cell K^+ channel by a saturating concentration (2 nM) of
GTPγS-activated human erythrocyte G_k (G_k^*). **Experiment c**: Dependence on GTP and reversibility of receptor-mediated stimulation
of the G_k-sensitive K^+ channel. Acetylcholine (ACh) was present
in the pipette solution throughout. 100 μM GTP was present in the
bathing medium, removed and re-added as shown. **Experiment d**:
Stimulation of GH_3 cell G_k-sensitive K^+ channels by somatostatin
(SST): demonstration of PTX sensitivity of the GH_3 G_k protein and
reconstitution of the signal transduction pathway by addition of
unactivated native human erythrocyte G_k in the presence of GTP.
Experiments e and f: Mimicry of the effects of GTPγS-activated G_k
by resolved GTPγS-activated α subunit of human erythrocyte G_k and
lack of effect of resolved βγ dimers free of α subunits. (Adapted
from refs. 9,37)

Inhibition of G_k action by anti-α subunit mAb 4A. F u r t h e r
support for the contention that $α_k$ subunits and not the βγ dimers
are the mediators of receptor stimulation, came from studies with
a monoclonal antibody mAb 4A prepared against the α subunit of
transducin. Part of the epitope for which it is specific (trans
ducin 311-328), is present on the α subunit of G_k (Figures 6 and
7). When added to inside-out guinea pig atrial membrane patches
stimulated by carbachol and GTP, mAb 4A blocks muscarinic activation of atrial K^+ channels in an irreversible manner. mAb 4A
also immunoneutralizes K^+ channel activation by GTPγS-preactivated
G_k or GTPγS-preactivated $α_k$. Interestingly, it was found that
for development of a persistent block, mAb 4A needed to be added
to membranes in which G_k was being activated. No persistent block
of muscarinic activation was obtained when membrane patches were
incubated with saturating concentrations of mAb 4A under conditions
where G_k remained inactive such as when the muscarinic ligand was
omitted from the pipette solution or when in spite of presence of
muscarinic ligand in the pipette its activation of G_k was prevented
by omitting GTP from the medium bathing the cytosolic aspect of
the membrane patch. If, as is commonly assumed, G protein
activation is accompanied by subunit dissociation, the mAb 4A block
of muscarinic stimulation proves that physiologically formed βγ
dimers do not stimulate the K^+ channel. Figure 11 summarizes key
findings in this regard.
    Among the receptors that catalyze activation of G_k by GTP are
the heart atrial muscarinic, adenosine and neuropetide Y receptors,
hippocampal 5HT1a and $GABA_B$ receptors and endocrine cell somatostatin and muscarinic receptors. The list is bound to grow.

Figure 11 Monoclonal anti-transducin antibody 4A (mAb 4A)
interacts with $α_k$, blocks irreversibly carbachol-stimulated K^+
currents but does not interact with unactivated G_k: Evidence
against a stimulatory effect of naturally formed βγ dimers.

Top experiment: A persistent block results on exposing the cyto-

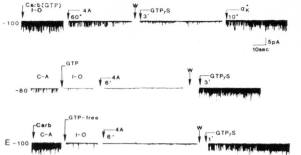

plasmic side of a membrane patch stimulated by carbachol (pipette) and GTP (bath) to mAb 4A. **Middle and bottom experiments:** Exposure of the membrane patch to mAb 4A under conditions that do not lead to G_k activation, does not lead to a persistent block to activation by GTPγS after mAb 4A washout. Other experiments showed that the block is specific for mAb 4A, neither non-specific IgG nor another antitransducin α monoclonal antibody with a different epitope specificity had any effect.

Figure 12 Strategy of incorporation of dihydropyridine-sensitive Ca^{2+} channels into planar phospholipid bilayers to study their direct regulation by a G protein (c.f., refs. 1 and 27).

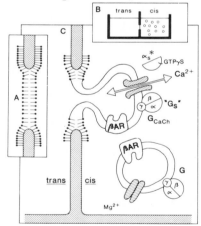

Phosphatidylcholine and phosphatidylethanolamine in decane are painted onto a hole of 0.1 to 0.3 mm in diameter in a partition separating two chambers of 0.15 to 0.5 ml referred to as **cis** and **trans**, with respect to the side from which membranes are forced to be fused with the lipid bilayer. Prior to membrane addition the **trans** chamber is filled with buffer A (50 mM NaCl, 2 mM $MgCl_2$ and 5 mM Hepes, pH 7.0) and the **cis** chamber with buffer A containing 100 mM $BaCl_2$. Incorporation of ionic channels into the lipid bilayer is obtained after addition of membrane vesicles in 10 to 20 μl aliquots to the **cis** chamber. After incorporation has occurred and to prevent further incorporations from occurring during the course of the experiments, one of two protocols are followed. In one, the liquid in the **cis** chamber is extensively exchanged with the same solution, buffer A plus 100 mM $BaCl_2$, free of membranes. In the other, the liquids of the chambers are exchanged, the **trans** chamber receiving the original **cis** solution (buffer A plus 100 mM $BaCl_2$), and the **cis** chamber receiving buffer A. In both cases Ba^{2+} is used as the charge carrier, the difference being that single channel currents are in the **cis** to **trans** direction in the first and in the **trans** to **cis**

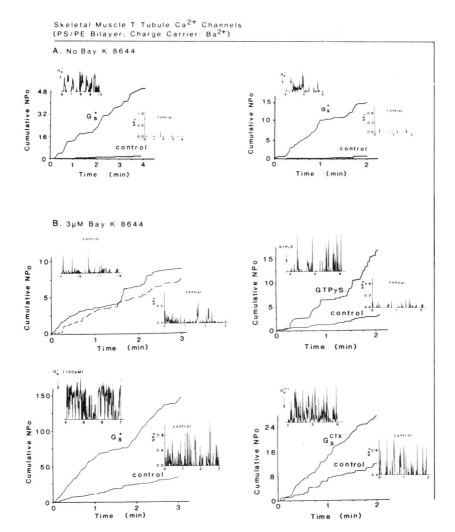

Skeletal Muscle T Tubule Ca^{2+} Channels
(PS/PE Bilayer; Charge Carrier: Ba^{2+})

Fig. 13 legend (cont'd):
ding cumulative NPo curves. The holding potentials were either 0
or +20 mV, and all experiments were done with BaCl$_2$ in the cis
chamber. Average stimulations of activity were between 10- and
20-fold in the absence and 2- to 3-fold in the presence of 3 μM
Bay K 8644. Note that the Ca^{2+} channels incorporated into the
bilayers can be stimulated either by exogenously activated G$_s$, or
by activation of an endogenous T tubule G protein, presumably also G$_s$, co-incorporated with the Ca^{2+} channel. In other experiments it was established that to be effective GTPγS had to be added
to the cis chamber, confirming the sidedness of the T tubule membranes.

Fig. 12 legend (cont'd): direction in the second of these protocols. The figure depicts a membrane vesicle that is inside-out
with respect to the orientation of its cytoplasmic side before
and after its fusion to the lipid bilayer, and illustrates the
sidedness of skeletal muscle T tubule membranes.

The dihydropyridine-sensitive, Voltage-gated Ca^{2+} Channel

Although initial data were obtained with inside-out membrane
patches of guinea pig ventricles (38), conclusive data were
obtained on incorporation of Ca^{2+} channels from skeletal muscle T
tubules into planar lipid bilayers (black lipid membranes) following procedures (1, 27) summarized in Figure 12. Of particular
interest was the finding that the G protein active in stimulating
these Ca^{2+} channels is none other than G_s (Figure 13), or if not
G_s, then a very closely related G protein that comigrates with G_s
throughout extensive purification.

The above results on ionic channel regulation by G proteins were
all obtained in the absence of ATP and hence not mediated by channel phosphorylation. This indicated that under the assay conditions used, the channels are indeed under direct control of the G
protein or its α subunit, as opposed to being regulated in a manner
secondary to activation (or deactivation) of a kinase and/or phosphatase.

Dual regulation of Ca^{2+} channels by G protein and phosphorylation. In agreement with data from whole cell recordings obtained
by others, addition to the cis chamber of catalytic unit of protein
kinase A and ATP or ATPγS also stimulates single Ca^{2+} channel
currents by increasing their opening probability (NPo values on
the figures). In a series of 4 experiments in the presence of Bay
K 8644 such stimulation averaged 2-fold (not shown), and bilayers
stimulated in this way were still responsive to G_s, which increased
opening probability by another 2-fold.

Figure 14 presents a diagram that summarizes our current concept as to how G proteins are involved in regulation of membrane
functions, and the fact that direct regulation of a given effector
function does not rule out indirect regulation as would occur upon
phosphorylation by a G protein dependent protein kinase.

Figure 13 (facing page) Representative experiments showing direct
regulation of the skeletal muscle T tubule dihydropyridine-
sensitive Ca^{2+} channel by purified human erythrocyte G_s (adapted
form ref. 39).

Experiments were carried out both in the absence (panel A) and
the presence of the dihydropyridine agonist Bay K 8644 in the cis
chamber (panel B). Shown are the NPo diaries priorto and after
addition of GTPγS-activated G_s, GTPγS-activated α_s, CTX-treated
G_s (in the presence of GTP) or GTPγS (insets) and the correspon-

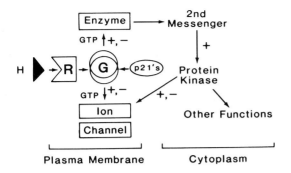

Figure 14   Effector functions may be under dual control:

1. directly by a G protein;

2. indirectly by a G protein-regulated phosphorylation event.

UNCERTAINTIES IN ASSIGNMENT OF FUNCTION:
USE OF BACTERIAL SYNTHESIS OF α SUBUNITS

One set of problems raised implicitly in the previous paragraphs, is how pure are purified G proteins made by the biochemist and how reliable are functional assignments.

For example, is it indeed G_s that stimulates the Ca^{2+} channel or a contaminant?; and, which of the cloned G proteins is the G_k?. G proteins are so similar, that even though the purified preparations appear to have no significant contaminants, comigration of unexpected α subunits cannot be excluded. This applies particularly, but not necessarily only, to PTX-sensitive G proteins. Assigning a specific function to a specific α subunit is under such circumstances difficult if not impossible.

It is standard practice in the field of organic chemistry that structures of purified active principles deduced by analytical methods need confirmation by de novo synthesis. Although with proteins this was impossible in the past, the advent of recombinant DNA techniques and bacterial expression vectors opened the possibility to test and/or confirm the assignment of function to purified polypeptides. A search for an adequate bacterial expression vector to synthesize α subunits encoded in their respective cDNA molecules led to the use of pT7-plasmids developed by Tabor and Richardson at Harvard (32,33). α-Subunits made in this way were then tested for function: α_s for reconstitution of the cyc⁻ adenylyl cyclase system and stimulation of skeletal muscle Ca^{2+} channels in lipid bilayers, and one of the α_i molecules (α_i-3), suspected of being an α_k, for stimulation of single channel K^+ currents in inside-out atrial membrane patches.

Experiments to be published shortly elsewhere (Yatani, Codina, Mattera, Brown and Birnbaumer, submitted) and summarized in Figures 15 and 16, showed that indeed biologically active subunits can be made this way and that bacterially made α_i-3 (recombinant α_i-3), but not bacterially made α_s, stimulates atrial K^+ channels and

<u>Figure 15</u> Stimulation of the atrial G protein-gated K^+ channel by recombinant α_i-3.

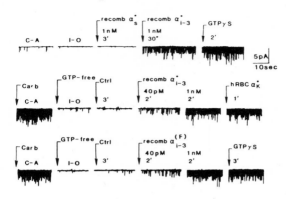

Recombinant α subunits inserted into pT7-7 vector were expressed in E coli by the one plasmid/one phage method of Tabor and Richardson (32, 33). E. coli K238 cells, transformed with pT7-α_i-3 plasmid, were grown, infected with phage mGP1-2 in the presence of rifampicin and IPTG, harvested 60 min later, shocked with 2.4 M sucrose and lysed lysozyme in the cold. The lysed cells were diluted, treated with disopropylfluorophosphate in the cold and GTPγS plus Mg, or AlF$_4^-$ plus Mg and GDP at 32°C and centrifuged at 100,000 xg to obtain a soluble extract containing GTPγS-activated (recomb α_{i-3}^*) or Fluoride activated (recomb $\alpha_{i-3}^{(F)}$) recombinant α_i-3 subunits. These were partially purified by ion exchange chromatography over DEAE-Sephacel, and concentrated by ultrafiltration. The same was done to prepare GTPγS-activated recombinant α_s (recomb α_s^*). The activated and partially purified forms were added to inside-out membrane patches of guinea pig atria as described in the legend to Figure 4, to test for possible K^+ channel stimulatory effects. **Experiment a**: recombinant α does not but recombinant α-3 does stimulate the atrial K^+ channel. **Experiments b and c**: Effects of two different doses of GTPγS-activated or fluoride-activated recombinant α_i-3. In these and repeat experiments recombinant α_i-3 was about 3 to 10 % as active as purified human erythrocyte GTPγS-activated G_k.

---

that bacterially made α_s, but not α_i-3, stimulates the skeletal muscle and bovine cardiac dihydropyridine sensitive Ca^{2+} channels.

These findings not only confirmed that Ca^{2+} channels are controlled directly by G_s, but also that G_s, and potentially any other G protein may interact with more than a single effector function.

INTERMOLECULAR SPECIFICITIES: HOW ARE THE DIFFERENT SIGNAL TRANSDUCTION PATHWAYS BUILT? QUESTIONS THAT EMERGE

Ever since the discoveries in the late 1960's that up to five different hormone receptors can activate a single adenylyl cyclase system in an isolated membrane, and, in the early and mid 1970's, that receptors can be transferred from one cell to another and that there are no species and/or tissue specificity restrictions as to the source of G_s for reconstitution of a hormonally stimulable adenylyl cyclase system in <u>cyc</u>⁻ membranes,

<u>Figure 16</u> Stimulation of skeletal muscle T tubule dihydropyridine-sensitive Ca^{2+} channel incorporated into lipid bilayers by the short form of recombinant α_s.

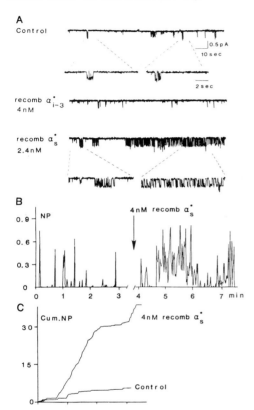

Recombinant α_s (Asp[71], Ser[72] version) and recombinant α_i-3 were prepared in their GTPγS-activated form and partially purified by DEAE-Sephacel chromatography as described in the legend of Figure 16, except that the two plasmid approach was used to express the recombinant proteins (for strategy see Figure 13). **Panel A:** single channel Ba^{2+} currents (**trans to cis**) before and after addition first of GTPγS-activated recombinant α_i-3 and then of GTPγS-activated recombinant α_s. **Panel B and C:** NPo diaries of Ca^{2+} channel activities before and after addition of GTPγS-activated recombinant α_s to the **cis** chamber (**B**) and cumulative NPo values as a function of time of the same experiment (**C**).

it has been clear that single G proteins are designed to interact with classes of receptors as opposed to single receptor subtypes. The quantitative considerations mentioned at the beginning of this article, indicating that not more than about ten G proteins receive the input of probably as many as 100 different receptors, actually require this to be so.

Several problems need resolution. The first is to define the functions of PTX substrates. Experiments are therefore ongoing to determine whether only α_i-3 has K^+ channel stimulatory activity or whether perhaps α_i-1 or/and α_i-2 have similar activities and if so how potent they are. Further, since all agonists that stimulate K^+ channels also inhibit adenylyl cyclase, one or the other of the α_i molecules should have G_i activity. Tests with G_i-3, which as mentioned has G_k activity, have thus far failed to show G_i effects on adenylyl cyclase, while preparations of brain

G_i, probably mostly G_i-1, show some G_i activity. Further, since G_i-2 is quite abundant in HL-60 cells, it may be a this cell's PTX-sensitive stimulator of phospholipase C, i.e., a G_p. Recent immunoblotting studies with antibodies that distinguish between the three forms of α_i, showed that all three α_i molecules can be expressed in a single cell type, the human erythrocyte (unpublished).   Yet the relative abundance of the three α_i molecules varies widely among cells. Resolution as to their true functional significance has to await the testing of their individual properties as can be done after bacterial expression.

The second question that needs to be raised relates to the effector specificity of G proteins. The studies on the regulation of ionic channels by G proteins has led to the surprising discovery that one and the same G protein may affect more than one effector function.   Presently the example is only one, but it is likely that more such cases may be found once they are searched for.

Another question is with how many different G proteins may any given receptor interact? Although the intuitive answer to this question might be <u>one</u>, indirect data from several different systems and a direct test in which a cloned receptor was transfected into a receptor-negative recipient cell, indicate that receptors are likely to interact with more than one of the G proteins present in the membrane. Some examples stand out. Thrombin receptors in human platelets stimulate primarily phospholipase C activity, i.e., a G_p, but also inhibit adenylyl cyclase when tested in isolated membranes, i.e., couple to G_i (11,18,20). The same is true for TRH receptors of GH_4C_1 cells (29,34) and angiotensin II receptors in liver (28) and adrenal glomerulosa cells (21) which activate both G_p (PTX insensitive) and G_i (PTX sensitive).   For all three, thrombin, TRH and angiotensin II, activation of G_p appears to be the physiologically relevant response, because manipulations of the intact cells, e.g., incubation with phorbol esters and/or ionophores, which mimic phospholipase C activation, mimic the effects of the receptor ligands (2,21). With muscarinic ACh receptors of chick and mouse heart, the situation is reversed. ACh stimulates primarily G_i, causing a decrease in cAMP levels, but at higher concentrations also increases phosphoinositide turnover, indicative of G_p stimulation (6; Figure 17A).   On the other hand, while thrombin stimulates both G_p and G_i in the human platelet, α_2-adrenergic stimulation of platelets seems to be restricted to G_i, there being no evidence for a G_p stimulatory action, as seen through mobilization of intracellular Ca^{2+} (11). But there is also evidence that receptors of the α_2-adrenergic type, such as somatostatin and "cardiac" or M2-type muscarinic ACH receptors, affect more than one function. Thus, in all cases thus far measured, receptors that either stimulate K^+ channels acting through a G_k (e.g., somatostatin in pituitary cells, muscarinic in heart and pituitary cells) or inhibit Ca^{2+} currents (e.g., α_2-adrenergic in dorsal root ganglia, opioid in neuroblastoma X glioma cells), also inhibit adenylyl cyclase via stimula-

Figure 17   A single receptor may interact with more than one G protein.

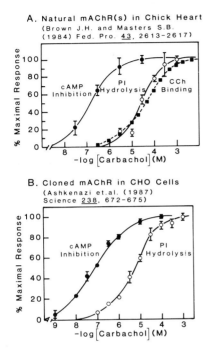

A. Natural mAChR(s) in Chick Heart
(Brown J.H. and Masters S.B. (1984) Fed. Pro. 43, 2613-2617)

B. Cloned mAChR in CHO Cells
(Ashkenazi et.al. (1987) Science 238, 672-675)

Dual effect of muscarinic agonist on intact chick atrial cell cAMP metabolism and phosphoinositde metabolism (Panel A) and of occupancy by agonist of a single M2-subtype of muscarinic receptor on the same parameters in an artificially constructed cell line (Panel B). Panel A is from Heller Brown et al.(6). Panel B is from Capon and collaborators (3).

tion of a PTX-sensitive G_i. The finding in FRTL-5 cells that α_1-adrenergic stimulation activates independently both a PhL C-specific and a PhL A_2-specific G_p (7) provides yet another example of the possibility that single receptors may interact with more than one G protein.

However, in none of the above examples of one agonist eliciting activation of more than one G protein, can the involvement of more than one receptor subtype be ruled out. Single cells can express multiple subtypes of the same receptor as determined by Bockaert and collaborators for β_1- and β_2-adrenergic receptors in cultured cells..

The potential ability of a single receptor to interact unequivocally with more than one G protein was first observed in in vitro reconstitution experiments, in which purified G proteins were co-incorporated with purified receptors into phospholipid vesicles, and the ability of the receptors to drive the G proteins through their GTP-dependent regulatory cycle (Figure 8) was assessed by measurement of GTP hydrolysis. Notably, rhodopsin was found to stimulate not only the GTP hydrolysis by transducin, the G protein with which it normally interacts, but also of a mixture of human erythrocyte G_i-2 and G_i-3, of which the latter is now known to have G_k activity (10, Figure 15). That a single receptor may indeed interact with more than one type of with more than one type of G protein in the normal setting of intact cell membranes was more recently shown with a cloned cardiac, M2-type muscarinic acetylcholine receptor (Figure 17B). On transfection into recipient cells, occupancy of the M2 receptor by ACh was found to cause in a dose-dependent manner both inhibition of adenylyl cyclase, i.e., activation of G_i, and stimulation of phosphatidyl-inositol bis-phosphate hydrolysis, i.e., activation of a G_p (3). Interestingly, the agonist dose-response curves differ for the two effects, ACh or carbachol being more potent in inhibiting adenylyl cyclase than in promoting phosphoinositide hydrolysis. Since the same difference in potencies for these two effects had previously been found on stimulation of intact tissue with muscarinic agonists (6), it is likely that at least in this case the two muscarinic effects were due to the action of a single receptor rather than the independent effects of two separate receptor subtypes.

Thus, one receptor can couple to more than one G protein and one G protein can regulate more than one effector function.

A final question is with how many different types of G protein does any given effector interact? In the case of adenylyl cyclase the answer is at present ambiguous because clearly both the short and the long α_s molecules can activate this enzyme. However, since to date no functional differences have been found for the various α_s molecules and they are all derived from a single gene, it is possible to argue honestly that to date only one G protein, G_s, has been found to stimulate the catalytic unit of the adenylyl cyclase system.

Given that receptor types far exceed the number of G proteins, yet effector systems are about as many as G proteins (Figure 1); given too that many receptors interact with a single G protein, that a single receptor may interact with more than one G protein, that one G protein may interact with more than one effector system, that indeed several G proteins may interact with a single effector system and that each cell type has a separate complement of receptors, G proteins and effector systems, it is no longer possible to speak of single or simple signal transduction pathway where a given receptor triggers a single effect. Figure 18 is a modification of Figure 1 that includes these complexities.

It is very likely that the norm is going to be that receptor stimulation leads to a complex set of G protein stimulations and effector modulations, of which one or the other will dominate and vary from cell to cell depending on the presence or absence of given G proteins and/or effector systems. It will also depend on the specificity of receptor-G protein and G protein-effector interactions and since specificity does not appear to be absolute on selectivity parameters governing these interactions. As applied to any particular biological system the unravelling of its G pro-

Figure 18 Flow of information through G protein-dependent signal transduction systems of a cell with $\underline{n}$ receptors (R_1 through R_n), three G proteins (G_a through G_c) and three effector systems (Effector-I through Effector-III), each having separate and different selectivity for mutual interaction.

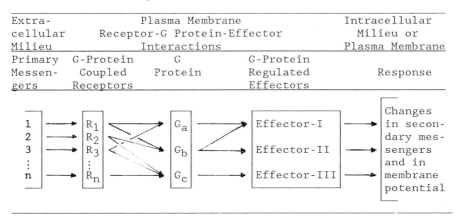

Extra-cellular Milieu	Plasma Membrane Receptor-G Protein-Effector Interactions			Intracellular Milieu or Plasma Membrane
Primary Messengers	G-Protein Coupled Receptors	G Protein	G-Protein Regulated Effectors	Response

tein-dependent signal transductions, ultimately responsible for final cellular responses to agonists, be they stimulatory or inhibitory, will require first of all qualitative and then quantitative analyses of which receptors, which G proteins and which effector systems are present in the cell systems under study, e.g., liver, heart, muscle, pancreatic β-cells, neurons, testicular Leydig cells, etc. Tools for nucleic acid hybridization and protein immunoblotting are becoming available to accomplish these goals. Finally, as indicated in the schemes of Figures 14 and 18, superimposed onto these primary receptor-G protein-effector connections is the fact that effector systems, G proteins and receptors are themselves real or potential substrates for phosphorylation reactions triggered by the homologous activating pathway (feed back effect) or an heterologous activating pathway (pathway crosstalk). These possibilities for feedback and crosstalk surely make for further difficulties in separating primary from secondary regulations of signal transductions, and also for new and by definition unexpected discoveries.

Acknowledgements: Supported in part by United States Public Health Service research grants DK-19318, HD-09581, HL-31164 and HL-37044 to LB; HL-39262 to AMB; EY-06062 to HEH and DK-38761 and CA-44998 to RI, the Baylor College of Medicine Diabetes and Endocrinology Research Center grant DK-27685 (Dr. James B. Field, Director), and grant Q1075 from the Welch Foundation.

REFERENCES

1. Affolter, H., and Coronado, R. (1985): <u>Biophys. J.</u>, 48:341-347.
2. Albert, P.R., Wolfson, G., and Tashjian, A.H., Jr. (1987): <u>J. Biol. Chem.</u>, **262**:6577-6581.
3. Ashkenazi, A., Winslow, J.W., Peralta, E.G., Peterson, G.L., Schimerlik, M.I., Capon, D.J., and Ramachamdran, J. (1988): <u>Science</u>, **238**:672-675.
4. Birnbaumer, L., Codina, J., Mattera, R., Yatani, A. Scherer, N., Toro, J.-M., and Brown, A.M. (1987): <u>Kidney International</u>, **32 (Suppl.23)**: S14-S32.
5. Brown, A.M., and Birnbaumer, L. (1987): <u>Am. J. Physiol.</u>
6. Brown, J.H., and Masters, S.B. (1984): <u>Fed. Proc.</u>, **43**:2613-2617.
7. Burch, R.M., Luini, A., and Axelrod, J. (1986): <u>Proc. Natl. Acad. Sci. USA</u>, **83**:7201-7205.
8. Casey, P.J., and Gilman, A.G. (1988): <u>J. Biol. Chem.</u>, **269**:2577-2580.
9. Codina, J., Grenet, D., Yatani, A., Birnbaumer, L., and Brown, A.M. (1987): <u>FEBS Letters</u>, **216**:104-106.
10. Codina, J., Olate, J., Abramowitz, J., Mattera, R., Cook, R.G., and Birnbaumer, L. (1988): <u>J. Biol. Chem.</u>, **263**: in press.
11. Crouch, M.F., and Lapetina, E.G. (1988): <u>J. Biol. Chem.</u>, **263**: 3363-3371.
12. Deretic, D., and Hamm, H.E. (1987): <u>J. Biol.Chem.</u>, **262**:10839-10847.
13. Gilman, A.G. (1987): <u>Annu. Rev. Biochem.</u>, **56**:615-649.
14. Hamill, O.P., Marty, A., Neher, E., Sakmann, B., and Sigworth, F.J. (1981): <u>Pf uegers Archiv (Eur. J. Physiol.)</u>, **391**:85-100.
15. Hamm, H.E., Deretic, D., Hofmann, K.P., Schleicher, A., and Kohl, B. (1987): <u>J. Biol. Chem.</u>, **262**:10831-10838.
16. Hausdorff, W.P., Sekura, R.D., Aguilera, G., and Catt, K.J. (1987): <u>Endocrinol.</u>, **120**:1668-1678.
17. Iyengar, R., and Birnbaumer, L. (1987): <u>ISI Atlas Science (Pharmacology)</u>, **1**:
18. Jakobs, K.H., Bauer, S., and Watanabe, Y. (1985): <u>Eur. J. Biochem.</u>, **151**:425-431.
19. Jurnak, F. (1985): <u>Science</u>, **230**:32-36.
20. Katada, T., Gilman, A.G., Watanabe, Y., Bauer, S., Jakobs, K.H. (1985): <u>Eur. J. Biochem.</u>, **151**:431-437.
21. Kojima, I., Kojima, K., and Rasmussen (1985): <u>J. Biol. Chem.</u>, **260**:4248-4256.
22. Kozasa, T., Itoh, H., Tsukamoto, T, Kaziro, Y. (1988): <u>Proc. Natl. Acad. Sci. USA</u>, **85**:2081-2085.
23. Lefkowitz, R.J., and Caron, M.C. (1988): <u>J. Biol. Chem.</u>, **263**: 4993-4996.
24. Litosch, I., Wallis, C., and Fain, J.N. (1985): <u>J. Biol. Chem.</u>, **260**:5464-5471.
25. Masters, S.B., Stroud, R.M., and Bourne, H.R. (1987): <u>Prot. Engineering</u>, **1**:47-54.

26. Masters, S.B., Sullivan, K.A., Miller, R.T., Beiderman, B, Lopez, N.G., Ramachandran, J, and Bourne, H.R. (1988): <u>Science</u> in press.

27. Mueller, P., Rudin, D., Tien, T.H., and Wescott, W.C. (1962) <u>Circulation</u>, **26**:1167-1171.

28. Pobiner, B.F., Hewlett, E.L., and Garrison, J.C. (1985): <u>J. Biol. Chem.</u>, **260**:16200-16209.

29. Straub, R.E., and Gershengorn, M.C. (1986): <u>J. Biol. Chem.</u>, **261**:2712-2717.

30. Stryer, L, and Bourne, H.R. (1986): <u>Annu. Rev. Cell Biol.</u>, **2**:391-419.

31. Sullivan, K.A., Miller, R.T., Masters, S.B., Beiderman, B., Heideman, W., and Bourne, H.R. (1988): <u>Nature</u>, **330**:758-760.

32. Tabor, S., Huber, H.E., and Richardson, C.C. (1987): <u>J. Bio l. Chem.</u>, **262**:16212-16223.

33. Tabor, S., and Richardson, C.C. (1985): <u>Proc. Natl. Acad. Sci. USA</u>, **82**:1074-1078.

34. Toro, J-.M., and Birnbaumer, L. (1986): <u>Endocrinology</u>, **118** (**Supplement 1**): abstract 415.

35. VanDop, C. Tsubokawa, M., Bourne, H.R.and Ramachandran, J. (1984): <u>J. Biol. Chem.</u>, **259**:696-699.

36. West, R.E., Jr., Moss, J., Vaughan, M., Liu, T., and Liu, T.-Y. (1985): <u>J. Biol. Chem.</u>, **260**:14428-14430.

37. Yatani, A., Codina, J., Sekura, R.D., Birnbaumer, L., and Brown, A.M. (1987): <u>Mol. Endocrinol.</u>, **1**:283-289.

38. Yatani, A., Codina, J., Imoto, Y., Reeves, J.P., Birnbaumer, L., and Brown, A.M. (1987): <u>Science</u>, **238**:1288-1292.

39. Yatani, A., Imoto, Y., Codina, J., Hamilton, S.L., Brown, A.M., and Birnbaumer, L. (1988): <u>J. Biol. Chem.</u>, **263**: in press.

The effect of Deglycosylated and Native LH upon Rat Testis Leydig Cells; Evidence for Activation of More than One Transduction Mechanism

E.A. Platts, M.R. Sairam[1], D. Schulster[2] and B.A. Cooke

*Department of Biocheministry, Royal Free Hospital Medical School,
University of London, Rowland Hill St., London, UK;
[1]Clinical Research Institute of Montreal, Montreal, Canada;
[2]Endocrinology Division, National Institute for Biological Standards and Control,
Blanche Lane, South Mimms, Potters Bar, Herts., UK.*

INTRODUCTION

Previously it was found that deglycosylated LH (dGLH) had little effect upon cyclic AMP and testosterone production in testis interstitial cells, but rather functioned as a competitive antagonist, inhibiting the effect of LH (3). LH itself increases both cyclic AMP and Ca^{2+} levels in Leydig cells (4) and also desensitises Leydig cell adenylate cyclase (1). This desensitisation is not cyclic AMP dependent and can be mimicked by compounds that activate protein kinase C. dGLH was used in the present study to investigate further the mechanisms whereby signal transduction and desensitisation are affected in Leydig cells.

METHODS

Rat testis Leydig cells were purified (>95%) by centrifugal elutriation followed by Percoll density gradient centrifugation (2). The cells were incubated at 32°C for 1 hour prior to addition of stimulants and then incubated for 1 hour with dGLH and/or LH. Desensitisation experiments were carried out by pre-treating the cells for 1 hour with LH, dGLH, 8-Br cyclic AMP or medium alone. The cells were then washed 3x with glycine buffered saline at pH 7.4 or at pH 3 to remove receptor bound hormone. After being replaced in fresh media, the cells were incubated for a further hour in the presence or absence of LH. Cyclic AMP and testosterone were assayed by RIA.

RESULTS

LH gave a dose dependent increase in cyclic AMP production which had not reached a maximum with 10ng/ml. (fig 1). Although dGLH was far less potent than LH it also gave a dose-dependent stimulation of cyclic AMP production (fig 1). When dGLH was added with LH the effects of the latter were decreased until with 1000ng/ml dGLH, no effect of LH could be detected on cyclic AMP production.

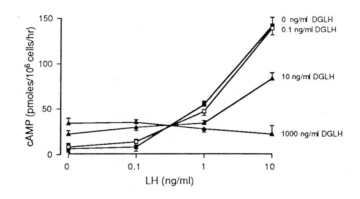

FIG 1   The effect of different concentrations of dGLH on cyclic AMP production in Leydig cells in the presence of different concentrations of LH

LH gave a dose-dependent increase in testosterone production which reached a maximum with 1 ng/ml LH. dGLH was equipotent as LH in the stimulation of testosterone production (fig 2). In similarity with the responses in terms of cyclic AMP production, dGLH inhibited the effects of LH on testosterone production when these two compounds were added together (fig 2). Again with 1000 ng/ml dGLH little of no stimulation of testosterone production could be observed in the presence of 10ng/ml LH.

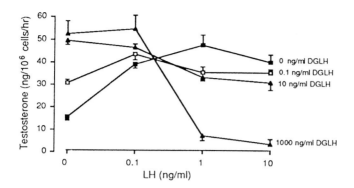

FIG. 2   The effect of different concentrations
of dGLH on testosterone production in
Leydig cells in the presence of
different concentrations of LH

Pretreatment of the cells with dGLH or LH inhibited
cyclic AMP production in response to a further dose
of LH (fig 3).   It was thought that the effect of
dGLH might be due to residual hormone bound to the
LH receptor, thus blocking the effect of LH.
However, acid washing the cells to remove receptor
bound hormone did not alter the ability of either LH
or dGLH to desensitize cyclic AMP production (fig
3).

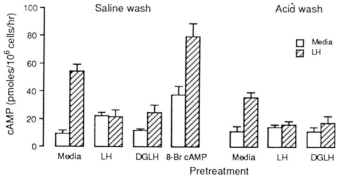

FIG. 3   The effect of pretreating Leydig cells
with LH, dGLH and 8 BrcAMP on the
subsequent response to LH.

The results of the present study demonstrate that in agreement with previous work (3) dGLH antagonizes the action of LH on cyclic AMP and testosterone production. In addition we have shown that dGLH will give a small increase in cyclic AMP production and fully stimulates testosterone production. This is different from the previous study (1) where no increases in cyclic AMP were observed and only a submaximal testosterone response was obtained. This may be due to the impure Leydig cell preparation previously used because in the present study >95% pure Leydig cells were incubated; we have shown that this increases the sensitivity to LH (unpublished results).

Also in disagreement with work on granulosa cells (5) we have shown that dGLH is equally as effective as LH in desensitizing the cyclic AMP response to subsequent challenges with LH. This was shown not to be due to binding of residual dGLH to the LH receptor because acid washed cells were still unresponsive to LH. In granulosa cells dGLH partially prevented desensitization. One explanation for these differences may be the different incubation times used because in the latter study the cells were incubated for 20hr compared with 2hr in the present study.

The mechanisms of the inhibitory effects of dGLH are not known. One possible mechanism may be that dGLH stimulates protein kinase C. This may cause phosphorylation and uncoupling of the receptor from the stimulatory GTP binding protein which couples to the adenylate cyclase. Preliminary data from our studies indicate that inhibition of protein kinase C and/or inhibition of calcium entry into the Leydig cell increases the cyclic AMP response to dGLH. We have also proposed that LH causes desensitisation by activation of protein kinase C (1). It may be that while both LH and dGLH activate protein kinase A and protein kinase C, dGLH is more effective upon the latter.

SUMMARY

The effects of deglycosylated LH (dGLH) and LH on cyclic AMP and testosterone production in highly purified Leydig cells have been compared. dGLH itself was found to give a small increase in cyclic

AMP and to stimulate maximally testosterone production. However it gave a dose-dependent inhibition of LH-stimulated cyclic AMP and testosterone production. dGLH was equally as effective as LH in desensitising the cells to subsequent challenges with LH. It is suggested that the mechanism of action of dGLH is via activation of protein kinase C.

ACKNOWLEDGEMENTS

We are grateful to the Science and Engineering Research Council for financial support.

REFERENCES

1) Dix, C.J., Habberfield, A.D. & Cooke, B.A. (1987): Biochem. J. **262:** 373-377
2) Platts, E.A., Schulster, D. & Cooke B.A. Biochem. J. (1988): **253:** (in press)
3) Sairam, M.R. & Fleshner, P. (1981): Molec. Cell. Endocrinol **22:** 41-54
4) Sullivan, M.H.F. & Cooke, B.A. (1986): Biochem. J. 236: 45-51 J. Biol. Chem. **262:** 6093-6100 (1985): J. Endocrinol. **105:** (supplement) abs. 49
5) Zor, U., Shentzer, P., Azrad, A., Sairam, M.R. & Amsterdam, A. (1984): Endocrinology **114:** 2143-2147

Hormonal Regulation of mRNA for Cyclic AMP-Dependent Protein Kinases and Steroid Biosynthesis in Mouse Tumor Leydig Cells

A. Frøysa[1], M. Ascoli[2], D. Segaloff[2], S. Beebe[1,3], T. Jahnsen[1,3] and V. Hansson[1]

[1]Institute of Medical Biochemistry, University of Oslo, 0317 Oslo, Norway;
[2]The Population Council, New York 10021, USA;
[3]Institute of Pathology, University of Oslo, Rikshospitalet, 0027 Oslo 1, Norway

INTRODUCTION

A cell line derived from a mouse Leydig cell tumor (MA-10 cells) responds to LH/hCG by increased cAMP and progesterone production (1,4). Cyclic AMP is known to act via cAMP-dependent protein kinases. The cAMP-dependent protein kinase holoenzyme, consisting of two regulatory (R) and two catalytic (C) subunits, dissociates on binding of two cAMP molecules to each of the R subunits. [for a review see ref. (2)]. The activated C subunits then phosphorylate specific substrate proteins on serine and threonine and thereby alter the activity or function of these proteins. Alternatively, cellular effects might be mediated by free R subunits, independent of phosphorylation (7). However, conclusive evidence supporting this possibility is lacking.

Type I and Type II cAMP-dependent protein kinases are distinguished by their regulatory subunits (RI and RII, respectively). Four different regulatory subunits RI_α (6), RI_β (3), RII_α (RII_{54}) (8) and RII_β (RII_{51}) (5) and two different catalytic subunits C_α (10) and C_β (9,11) for cAMP-dependent protein kinases have now been identified at the gene/mRNA level.

Studies on the cellular localization of mRNA for cAMP-dependent protein kinase subunits in rat testis have shown that RII_β is predominantly localized in Leydig cells and cAMP stimulated Sertoli cells (12). In the present study we have examined the effect of LH/hCG, 8-Br-cAMP, and agents that increase endogenous cAMP (cholera toxin and forskolin) on the mRNA levels for subunits of cAMP-dependent protein kinases as well as on steroid biosynthesis in mouse tumor Leydig cells.

EXPERIMENTAL PROCEDURES

Cells

Mouse tumor Leydig cells (MA-10 cells) were handled as described by Ascoli (1). Cells were plated at a density of $2 \cdot 10^6$ cells/dish and used 3 days later when the cell density was $2 \cdot 10^7$ cell/dish.

Incubation of the cells.

Experiments were performed with cells plated in 10 cm dishes. The cells were washed twice with 5 ml of Waymouth's MB752/1 medium pretreated to $37^\circ C$ and modified to contain 1.1 g/litre $NaHCO_3$, 20 mM Hepes, (pH 7.4). Luteinizing hormone (LH), human chorion gonadotropin (hCG), and cholera toxin were dissolved in 0.15 M NaCl/ 20 mM Hepes containing 1 mg/ml of albumin (pH 7.4). 8-Bromo-cAMP was dissolved in the same buffer devoid of albumin. Forskolin was dissolved in 95% ethanol. Cells were incubated at $37^\circ C$ in a total volume of 5 ml medium in a humidified atmosphere containing 5% CO_2 in air.

Extraction of total RNA.

At the end of incubation, the dishes were placed on ice and washed three times with ice-cold Hanks Balanced Salt Solution and thereafter scraped with a rubber policeman in 3 ml 5 M guanidinium iso-thio-cyanate solution (GTC). The cells were transferred to a Dounce homogenizer and homogenized by 15 strokes with a tightly fitting pestle. The homogenate was centrifuged at 2800 g for 5 min. The supernatant was layered on top of 5.7 M caesium chloride and then centrifuged at 36,000 g for 15h at $20^\circ C$. The RNA pellet was resuspended in 300 ul Tris-HCl (10 mM,pH 7.4)/EDTA (5 mM)/SDS (1%) and phenol/chloroform extracted. The RNA was ethanol precipitated overnight at $-20^\circ C$ and thereafter centrifuged at 13,000 g for 30 min at $4^\circ C$. The RNA pellet was resuspended in auto-claved destilled water and stored at $-70^\circ C$.

Northern Analysis

Total RNA (20 µg) was denatured at $50^\circ C$ for 15 min in 50% formamid, 6% formaldehyde and thereafter placed on ice for 15 min. The RNA samples were electrophoresed on a 1.5% agarose gel containing 6.7% formaldehyde, 20 mM sodium phosphate, pH 7.0 and then transferred to BioTrans nylon filter (ICN) by capillary blotting technique using 20XSSC. The nylon filter was baked at $80^\circ C$ for 1h and prehybridized at $42^\circ C$ for 2h in 50% formamide containing denatured salmon sperm DNA. The filter was hybridized under the same conditions with the nick-translated probe for an additional 16h at 42°C. After hybridization the filter was washed four times in 2XSSC and 0.1% SDS for 5 min at 20°C and then washed twice in 0.1XSSC and 0.1% SDS at 50°C for 20 min. The filter was then placed with Hyperfilm MP (Amersham) and Kodak intensifying screens at -70°C. The mRNA bands were scanned using a Vitatron (TLD 100) densitometer and the intensities were estimated by a Hewlett Packard (HP 3390A) integrator.

Nick translation

The cDNA were nick translated by using α-^{32}P-labeled dCTP and a standard nick translation kit (N.5000, Amersham). The labeled cDNA had a final specific activity of 1-$5\cdot10^8$ cpm/µg DNA.

Complementary DNA probes.

The probe used for rat skeletal muscle RII$_\alpha$ was a 0.7 kb SalI-BglII fragment (8). The cDNA for C$_\alpha$ (2.2kb) and the cDNA for RII$_\beta$ (3.3kb) were isolated from a human testis lamda gt11 expression cDNA library.

Determination of progesterone levels.

At the end of the incubation, the medium was saved, and progesterone, the major steroid produced by the MA-10 cells, was measured by radioimmunoassay (1).

Materials

Purified hCG and LH was obtained from the National Institute of Health. Cholera toxin, forskolin, 8-Br-cAMP were purchased from Sigma. $(1,2,6,7$-^{3}H)Progesterone (90-100 Ci/mmol) was obtained from DuPont-NEN. Cell culture supplies were purchased from GIBCO, and cell culture plastic ware was from Falcon.

RESULTS

Effects of LH/hCG, cholera toxin, and forskolin on mRNA levels of cAMP-dependent protein kinases.

Incubation of the mouse tumor Leydig cells for 6h with LH (20 ng/ml), hCG (20 ng/ml), cholera toxin (20 ng/ml) and forskolin (75 µM) resulted in an increase in the level of the 3.2 kb mRNA for RII$_\beta$ compared to control. In contrast the 2.4 kb mRNA for C$_\alpha$ and the 6.0 kb for RII$_\alpha$ remained relatively constant under these treatments (Fig. 1).

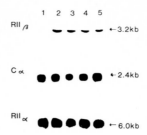

FIG. 1.   Distribution of mRNA for RII$_\beta$, C$_\alpha$, and RIIα
of cAMP-dependent protein kinases in mouse
tumor Leydig cells incubated with cholera
toxin, forskolin, LH or hCG.
Lane 1. Control, lane 2. Cholera toxin
(20 ng/ml), lane 3. Forskolin (75 µM), lane
4. LH (20 ng/ml), lane 5. hCG (20 ng/ml).

Effects of cholera toxin,   forskolin,   and   LH/hCG on steroid accumulation.

Progesterone measured in the medium from the same
experiment as described in Fig. 1 shows that LH, hCG,
cholera toxin, and forskolin all increased progesterone
accumulation (Fig. 2).

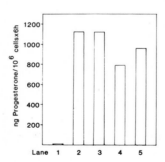

FIG. 2. Progesterone levels in the medium after 6h
incubation at   37°C with cholera toxin,
forskolin, LH or hCG.
Lane 1. control, lane 2. cholera toxin
(20 ng/ml), lane 3. forskolin (75 µM), lane
4. LH (20 ng/ml), lane 5. hCG (20 ng/ml).

Effects of 8-Br-cAMP on mRNAs for cAMP-dependent protein kinase subunits.
The results presented in Fig. 3 show that low concentrations (50-200 µM) of 8-Br-cAMP for 6h., induced an 4 to 5 fold increase in mRNA levels for RII_β and a slight increase in RII_α and C_α. However, higher concentrations of 8-Br-cAMP (500-1000 µM) caused a concentration dependent decrease in mRNA levels for all the subunits.

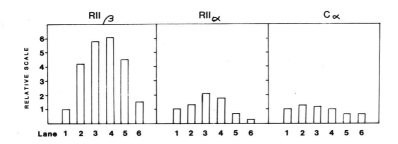

FIG. 3. Densitometric scanning of a Northern blot. Cells incubated for 6h, with various concentrations of 8-Br-cAMP, were RNA extracted. The RNA was then blotted onto a nylon filter and probed with cDNAs for RII_β, RII_α and C_α.
Lane 1. Control, lane 2. 50 µM, lane 3. 100 µM, lane 4. 200 µM, lane 5. 500 µM, lane 6. 1000 µM.

Effects of 8-Br-cAMP on progesterone accumulation.
Progesterone measured in the medium in the same experiment as described in Fig. 3 showed that 8-Br-cAMP in concentrations ranging from 50-1000 µM caused a dose dependent increase in progesterone accumulation (Fig. 4).

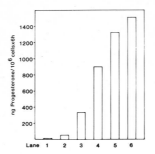

FIG. 4   Progesterone levels in the medium after 6h
          incubation at 37°C with various concentra-
          tions of 8-Br-cAMP.
          Lane 1. Control, lane 2. 50 µM, lane 3.
          100 µM, lane 4. 200 µM, lane 5. 500 µM,   lane
          6. 1000 µM.

DISCUSSION

The present study documents changes in the levels of
mRNA for various subunits of cAMP-dependent protein
kinases in   tumor Leydig cells incubated in the
presence of agents that increase intracellular cAMP
levels and steroid biosynthesis.
The increase in RII_β mRNA in tumor Leydig cells after
LH/hCG treatment is associated with an increase in
biosynthesis of progesterone. However, the mRNA level
for the RII_α and C_α remained relatively constant under
these various treatments of the cells. The results
obtained with other agents that increase endogenous
cAMP levels (cholera toxin, forskolin) show that these
agents also coincidently increase mRNA levels for RII_β
and progesterone biosynthesis. These data indicate
that the gene coding for RII_β is positively regulated
by cAMP. Whether some of the effect of cAMP on mRNA
levels for RII_β may be due to changes in rates of mRNA
degradation/turnover has not been determined. The
finding that cAMP stimulates mRNA levels for RII_β as
well as steroid production, does not necessarily
indicate a cause effect relationship. It is still not
known whether the steroid response of cAMP is mediated
via one or several of the existing regulatory subunits
of cAMP-dependent protein kinases. The existence of
multiple regulatory subunits of cAMP-dependent protein
kinases opens for the possibility that different cell
functions may be mediated via different subunits.

Results from the dose-response study with the cAMP analog 8-Br-cAMP showed that 8-Br-cAMP stimulate RII_β in a concentration dependent manner. Maximal stimulation of RII_β was found with 200 μM 8-Br-cAMP. Employing this cAMP analog, we also observed a small increase (2 fold) in the 6.0 kb mRNA for RII_α. In addition 6h incubation of these cells with higher concentrations (500-1000 μM) of 8-Br-cAMP gave a concentration dependent inhibition of mRNA levels for RII_α, RII_β. The functional consequences of the bimodal effects of 8-Br-cAMP on mRNA for RII is not known. The increase in mRNA`s for the subunits of cAMP-dependent protein kinase in mouse tumor Leydig cells by cAMP, and especially in mRNA for RII_β, raises an interesting question: Will corresponding increases in the protein cause signal amplification? (more protein kinase holoenzyme gives more response). Such questions can not be properly answered until the isomeric forms of RI, RII and C can be separated at the protein level. If the increases in mRNA levels for subunits of cAMP-dependent protein kinase, demonstrated by this study, give rise to signal amplification, this may represent an important self-amplifying mechanism for LH/hCG and cAMP action on Leydig cells. Alternatively the cAMP-stimulated increase in mRNA for RII subunits could attenuate the cAMP response by producing more R subunits which could increase the amount of cAMP required to activate the kinase. The subsequent decrease in mRNA levels for cAMP-dependent protein kinase subunits at high concentrations of 8-Br-cAMP may represent a general, negative feedback type of regulation occurring at the level of cAMP-dependent protein kinase.
The possible functions of RII_β and the mechanism by which hormones and 8-Br-cAMP regulates the regulatory subunits of cAMP dependent protein kinases in Leydig cells remain to be further investigated.

REFERENCES

1. Ascoli, M. (1981): Endocrinology 108:88-95
2. Beebe, S. and Corbin, J.B. (1986) In: Enzymes edited by P.D. Boyer and E.G. Krebs Vol 17 pp. 43-111 Academic press Orlando Florida.
3. Clegg, C., Cadd, G., McKnight, G.S. In preparation.
4. Freeman, D.A., and Ascoli, M. (1981): Proc. Natl. Acad. Sci. U.S.A. 78:6309-6313

5. Jahnsen, T., Hedin, L., Kidd, V.J., Beattie, W.G., Lohmann, S.M., Walter, U., Durica, J., Schulz, T.Z., Schiltz, E., Browner, M., Law rence, C.B., Goldman, D., Ratoosh, S.L., and Richards, J.S., (1986): J. Biol. Chem., 261:12352-12361

6. Lee, D.C., Carmichael, D.F., Krebs, E.G., and McKnight, G.S. (1983): Proc. Natl. Acad. Sci. U.S.A. 80:3605-3612

7. Lohmann, S.M., DeCamilli, P., Einig, I. and Walter, U. (1984): Proc. Natl. Acad. Sci. U.S.A. 81:6723-6727

8. Scott, J.D., Glaccum, M.B., Zoller, M.J., Uhler, M.D., Helfman, D.M., McKnight, G.S., and Krebs, E.G. (1987): Proc. Natl. Acad. Sci. U.S.A. 84:5192-5186

9. Showers, M.O., and Maurer, R.A. (1986): J. Biol. Chem. 261:16288-16291.

10. Uhler, M.D., Carmichael, D.F., Lee, D.C., Chrivia, J.C., Krebs, E.G., and McKnight G.S. (1986): Proc. Natl. Acad. Sci. U.S.A., 83:1300-1304

11. Uhler, M.D. Chirivia, J.C., and McKnight, G.S. (1986) J. Biol. Chem. 261:15360-15363

12. Øyen, O., Frøysa, A., Sandberg, M., Eskild, W., Joseph, D., Hansson, V., and Jahnsen, T. (1987): Biol. Reprod., 37:947-956

Use of Recombinant DNA Technology to Study the Enzymes Involved in Steroid Hormone Biosynthesis

E.R. Simpson, J.I. Mason, C.R. Mendelson, R.W. Estabrook
and M.R. Waterman

*Departments of Obstetrics & Gynecology & Biochemistry and
The Cecil H. & Ida Green Center for Reproductive Biology Sciences,
University of Texas Southwestern Medical Center, Dallas, TX 75235*

INTRODUCTION

The enzymes involved in catalyzing the various steps in steroid hormone biosynthesis can be divided into two categories; a) mixed function oxidases or hydroxylases, and b) dehydrogenases. The mixed function oxidases involved in the steroidogenic pathways are all members of the enzyme family known collectively as cytochrome P-450. As shown in Fig. 1, various members of this superfamily of genes catalyze most of the reactions involved in steroid hormone biosynthesis including the major regulatory steps, namely cholesterol side-chain cleavage, the first step in the overall biosynthetic pathway from cholesterol; 17α-hydroxylation, the branch point reaction leading on the one hand to glucocorticoids, and on the other hand to androgens; and aromatization, the reaction which results in the conversion of androgens to estrogens. Each of these reactions, along with 11β-hydroxylation and 21-hydroxylation, is catalyzed by a separate and distinct member of the cytochrome P-450 superfamily of genes. Thus, the conversion of cholesterol to pregnenolone is catalyzed by cholesterol side-chain cleavage cytochrome P-450, or P-450$_{scc}$; 17α-hydroxylation and the removal of the remaining two carbons from the side-chain of C_{21} steroids to give the corresponding C_{19} steroids, namely the 17,20-lyase reaction, are both catalyzed by the one enzyme, namely 17α-hydroxylase cytochrome P-450 (P-450$_{17\alpha}$; 20). The conversion of androgens to estrogens, a multi-step reaction involving loss of the C_{19} angular methyl group and aromatization of the A-ring to give the corresponding phenolic A-ring, is catalyzed by another member of this family, namely aromatase cytochrome P-450 (P-450$_{AROM}$). In the adrenal cortex, 11β-hydroxylation and 21-hydroxylation are catalyzed by 11β-hydroxylase (P-450$_{11\beta}$), and 21-hydroxylase cytochrome P-450 (P-450$_{C21}$), respectively. In addition to these cytochrome P-450- catalyzed reactions, two dehydrogenase steps are required in the overall steroidogenic pathway. The conversion of Δ^5-3β-hydroxysteroids to the corresponding Δ^4-3-one-steroids is catalyzed by the 3β-hydroxysteroid dehydrogenase/Δ$^{4-5}$ isomerase, and the interconversion of steroids with a 17β-hydroxy group and those with a 17-keto group, is catalyzed by the 17β-hydroxysteroid dehydrogenase.

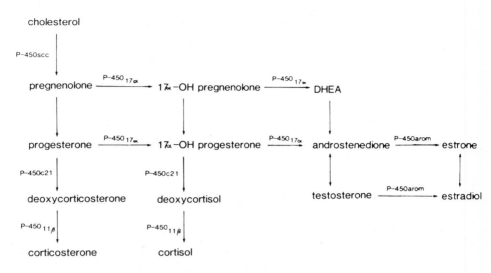

FIG. 1. Pathways of steroid hormone biosynthesis in the zona fasciculata of the adrenal cortex, ovaries and testes. The cytochrome P-450 species involved in several of the steps in the pathway are indicated:- P-450$_{SCC}$, cholesterol side-chain cleavage cytochrome P-450; P-450$_{17\alpha}$, 17α-hydroxylase cytochrome P-450; P-450$_{AROM}$, aromatase cytochrome P-450; P-450$_{C21}$, 21- hydroxylase cytochrome P-450; P-450$_{11\beta}$, 11β-hydroxylase cytochrome P-450.

Study of the steroidogenic forms of cytochrome P-450 is important for several reasons. In the first place, the reactions which these enzymes catalyze are of great interest from a physicochemical point of view, not only in terms of understanding how a molecule of oxygen is split and one of the atoms is reacted with a saturated carbon atom to form a hydroxyl group, but also because many of these enzymes catalyze multi-step reactions, frequently involving insertion of oxygen at different sites in the steroid molecule. A second important reason to study these enzymes is to understand the mechanisms of regulation of their expression in the steroidogenic tissues in which they occur. Both these goals have been greatly facilitated by the application of recombinant DNA technology to the study of these enzymes. In the first place, this has provided important sequence information about the enzymes, which was difficult to obtain by classical protein purification and sequencing methods, due to their intractability to solubilization and purification. Secondly, expression of cDNA sequences complementary to mRNA encoding these enzymes has allowed for definitive characterization of the reactions catalyzed by each of them, and site-specific mutagenesis will permit detailed analysis of the structure-function relationships underlying this specificity. Furthermore, the future holds promise that large scale synthesis of these enzymes might be possible using bacteria containing recombinant DNA, thus allowing the individual P-450 hemoproteins to be crystallized and subjected to x-ray crystallography. Finally, analysis of the genes for the steroidogenic forms of cytochrome P-450 permits definition of the regulatory sequences by which the various stimulatory and inhibitory factors cause differential expression of these genes. Genetic analysis also permits definition of the mutations underlying the various genetic diseases with which these reactions are associated, such as the various forms of congenital adrenal hyperplasia.

Our work has focussed primarily on three of these steroidogenic forms of cytochrome P-450, namely, cytochrome P-450$_{scc}$ along with its companion iron sulphur protein, adrenodoxin; cytochrome P-450$_{17\alpha}$; and cytochrome P-450$_{AROM}$.

STRUCTURAL FEATURES OF THE STEROIDOGENIC CYTOCHROME P-450 SPECIES

Because of the relatively facile nature of DNA sequencing, knowledge of the primary sequence of the steroidogenic cytochrome P-450 species has come about almost entirely due to the isolation and cloning of cDNA inserts complementary to mRNA encoding these enzymes, and the sequencing of such cDNAs. The first of the steroid hydroxylase cytochrome P-450 species to be cloned was bovine P-450$_{scc}$ (18,12). Subsequent to this, cDNA clones specific for bovine P-450$_{17\alpha}$ (39), P-450$_{11\beta}$ (13,6), P-450$_{C21}$ (35,38,14), and adrenodoxin (22,25) have been characterized as have cDNA clones for human P-450$_{scc}$ (8), human P-450$_{17\alpha}$ (9,2), and mouse P-450$_{C21}$, as well as human P-450$_{AROM}$ (28,5). The sequence of one of these cDNAs, namely that of bovine P-450$_{17\alpha}$, is shown in Fig. 2. The overall sequence homology of one steroidogenic cytochrome P-450 compared to another is generally less than 33%. This implies, then, that these steroidogenic forms of cytochrome P-450 evolved one from another more than 600 Myr ago. On this basis, each of these has been placed into a separate gene family within the overall superfamily of genes known collectively as cytochrome P-450 (21). In spite of this, within the sequence there are several regions of high homology which have been conserved throughout evolution. Most notable is that indicated in the box in Fig. 2 towards the carboxy terminal end of the protein. This is a sequence of high homology which has been conserved in all forms of cytochrome P-450 thus studied, as illustrated in Fig. 3. This is known to be the region of the proteins which is in proximity to the heme prosthetic group. The cysteine in the middle of the sequence, which is common to all of the cytochrome P-450's, is believed to be the 5th coordinating ligand of the heme ion. It is the presence of a thiolate-iron complex which is believed to give cytochrome P-450 species their unique spectrophotometric properties.

Cytochrome P-450 17alpha   LIMITS: 49   1578

```
                    AAGCCACTCCACAGCTCTTTGTCCTGACTGCTGCCACCCAGACACA      46
ATG TGG CTG CTC CTG GCT GTC TTT CTG CTC ACC CTC GCC TAT TTA TTT TGG CCC AAG ACC   106
Met Trp Leu Leu Leu Ala Val Phe Leu Leu Thr Leu Ala Tyr Leu Phe Trp Pro Lys Thr    20

AAG CAC TCT GGT GCC AAG TAC CCC AGG AGC CTC CCA TCC CTG CCC CTG GTG GGC AGC CTG   166
Lys His Ser Gly Ala Lys Tyr Pro Arg Ser Leu Pro Ser Leu Pro Leu Val Gly Ser Leu    40

CCG TTC CTC CCC AGA CGT GGC CAG CAG CAC AAG AAC TTC TTC AAG GTC CAG GAA AAA TAT   226
Pro Phe Leu Pro Arg Arg Gly Gln Gln His Lys Asn Phe Phe Lys Val Gln Glu Lys Tyr    60

GGC CCL ATC TAT TCC TTT CGT TTG GGT TCC AAG ACG ACT GTG ATG ATT GGA CAC CAC CAG   286
Gly Pro Ile Tyr Ser Phe Arg Leu Gly Ser Lys Thr Thr Val Met Ile Gly His His Gln    80

TTG GCC AGG GAG GTG CTT CTC AAG AAG GGC AAG GAA TTC TCT GGG CGT CCC AAA GTG GCC   346
Leu Ala Arg Glu Val Leu Leu Lys Lys Gly Lys Glu Phe Ser Gly Arg Pro Lys Val Ala   100

ACT CTA GAC ATC CTG TCA GAC AAC CAA AAG GGC ATT GCC TTT GCC GAC CAT GGT GCC CAC   406
Thr Leu Asp Ile Leu Ser Asp Asn Gln Lys Gly Ile Ala Phe Ala Asp His Gly Ala His   120

TGG CAG CTG CAT CGG AAG CTG GCA CTG AAT GCC TTT GCC CTG TTC AAG GAT GGC AAC CTG   466
Trp Gln Leu His Arg Lys Leu Ala Leu Asn Ala Phe Ala Leu Phe Lys Asp Gly Asn Leu   140

AAG TTA GAG AAG ATC ATT AAT CAG GAA GCC AAT GTG CTC TGT GAT TTC CTG GCC ACC CAG   526
Lys Leu Glu Lys Ile Ile Asn Gln Glu Ala Asn Val Leu Cys Asp Phe Leu Ala Thr Gln   160

CAT GGA GAG GCC ATA GAT CTG TCC GAG CCT CTC TCT CTG GCG GTG ACC AAC ATA ATC AGC   586
His Gly Glu Ala Ile Asp Leu Ser Glu Pro Leu Ser Leu Ala Val Thr Asn Ile Ile Ser   180

TTT ATC TGC TTC AAC TTC TCC TTC AAG AAT GAG GAT CCT GCC CTG AAG GCC ATA CAA AAT   646
Phe Ile Cys Phe Asn Phe Ser Phe Lys Asn Glu Asp Pro Ala Leu Lys Ala Ile Gln Asn   200

GTC AAT GAT GGC ATC CTG GTG GTT CTG AGC AAG GAA GTT CTG TTA GAC ATA TTC CCT GTG   706
Val Asn Asp Gly Ile Leu Val Val Leu Ser Lys Glu Val Leu Leu Asp Ile Phe Pro Val   220

CTG AAG ATT TTC CCC AGC AAA GCC ATG GAA AAG ATG AAG GGT TGT GTT CAA ACG CGA AAT   766
Leu Lys Ile Phe Pro Ser Lys Ala Met Glu Lys Met Lys Gly Cys Val Gln Thr Arg Asn   240

GAA TTG CTG AAT GAA ATC CTT GAA AAA TGT CAG GAG AAC TTC AGC AGT GAT TCC ATC ACT   826
Glu Leu Leu Asn Glu Ile Leu Glu Lys Cys Gln Glu Asn Phe Ser Ser Asp Ser Ile Thr   260

AAC TTG CTG CAC ATA CTG ATC CAA GCC AAG GTG AAT GCA GAC AAT AAC AAT GCT GGC CCA   886
Asn Leu Leu His Ile Leu Ile Gln Ala Lys Val Asn Ala Asp Asn Asn Asn Ala Gly Pro   280

GAC CAG GAT TCA AAG CTG CTT TCA AAT AGA CAC ATG CTC GCT ACT ATA GGG GAC ATC TTC   946
Asp Gln Asp Ser Lys Leu Leu Ser Asn Arg His Met Leu Ala Thr Ile Gly Asp Ile Phe   300

GGG GCT GGT GTG GAG ACC ACG TCT GTG ATA AAG TGG ATC GTG GCC TAC CTG CTA CAC  1006
Gly Ala Gly Val Glu Thr Thr Thr Ser Val Ile Lys Trp Ile Val Ala Tyr Leu Leu His   320

CAT CCT TCG TTG AAG AAG AGG ATC CAG GAT GAC ATT GAC GAG ATT ATA GGT TTC AAT CGC  1066
His Pro Ser Leu Lys Lys Arg Ile Gln Asp Asp Ile Asp Glu Ile Ile Gly Phe Asn Arg   340

ACC CCA ACC ATC AGT GAC CGG AAC CGC CTT GTC CTG CTG GAG GCG ACC ATC AGA GAA GTG  1126
Thr Pro Thr Ile Ser Asp Arg Asn Arg Leu Val Leu Leu Glu Ala Thr Ile Arg Glu Val   360

CTC CGA ATC AGG CCT GTG GCC CCT ACG CTG ATC CCC CAC AAG GCT GTC ATT GAC TCC AGC  1186
Leu Arg Ile Arg Pro Val Ala Pro Thr Leu Ile Pro His Lys Ala Val Ile Asp Ser Ser   380

ATT GGC GAC CTT ACC ATT GAC AAA GGC ACA GAC GTT GTG GTC AAC CTG TGG GCA CTG CAT  1246
Ile Gly Asp Leu Thr Ile Asp Lys Gly Thr Asp Val Val Val Asn Leu Trp Ala Leu His   400

CAC AGT GAG AAG GAG TGG CAG CAT CCC GAC CTG TTC ATG CCC GAG CGC TTC TTG GAC CCC  1306
His Ser Glu Lys Glu Trp Gln His Pro Asp Leu Phe Met Pro Glu Arg Phe Leu Asp Pro   420

ACG GGG ACG CAA CTC ATC TCG CCA TCA TTA AGC TAC TTG CCC TTT GGA GCA GGA CCC CGC  1366
Thr Gly Thr Gln Leu Ile Ser Pro Ser Tyr Leu Pro Phe Gly Ala Gly Pro Arg   440

TCC TGC GTA GGT GAG ATG CTA GCC CGC CAG GAG CTC TTC CTC TTC ATG TCC CGG CTG CTG  1426
Ser Cys Val Gly Met Leu Ala Arg Gln Glu Leu Phe Leu Phe Met Ser Arg Leu Leu   460
        442
CAG AGG TTC AAC CTC GAG ATC CCG GAT GAT GGG AAG CTA CCT TCT CTG GAG GGC CAT GCC  1486
Gln Arg Phe Asn Leu Glu Ile Pro Asp Asp Gly Lys Leu Pro Ser Leu Glu Gly His Ala   480

AGT CTC GTC TTG CAG ATC AAA CCT TTC AAG GTG AAG ATC GTG CGC CAG GCC TGG AAG  1546
Ser Leu Val Leu Gln Ile Lys Pro Phe Lys Val Lys Ile Val Arg Gln Ala Trp Lys   500

GAA GCC CAG GCT GAG GGT AGC ACC CCA TGA CTCCACCCTATGTGACCCCCACCGCACAGAATTAGAGGAG  1616
Glu Ala Gln Ala Glu Gly Ser Thr Pro End   509

CTCCCCCACCCTCTCCCACCATTCCTTCTTCCTCCCCGCLCACTCTGCCTTCTTTCCCAGCCTGCAGCCCTGGCAGTGAT  1696

GTGCATTAAACAGTTTCTTTCTCCAAAACAAAAA...
```

FIG. 2. Nucleotide sequence, and derived amino-acid sequence, of a cDNA insert encoding bovine cytochrome P-450$_{17\alpha}$. The boxed sequence near the N-terminal of the protein is believed to be the leader sequence anchoring the protein to the endoplasmic reticulum. The boxed sequence near the carboxy-terminal is believed to be the heme-binding region (From: 39).

AMINO ACID HOMOLOGIES OF THE HEME-BINDING REGION
OF STEROIDOGENIC FORMS OF CYTOCHROME P-450

Human Cytochrome P-450$_{AROM}$	F G F G P R G $\underline{C}$ A G K Y I A
Human Cytochrome P-450$_{C21}$	F G C G A R V $\underline{C}$ L G E P V A
Bovine Cytochrome P-450$_{C21}$	F G C G A R V $\underline{C}$ L G E C L A
Human Cytochrome P-450$_{17\alpha}$	F G A G P R S $\underline{C}$ I G E I L A
Bovine Cytochrome P-450$_{17\alpha}$	F G A G P R S $\underline{C}$ V G E M L A
Bovine Cytochrome P-450$_{scc}$	F G W G V R Q $\underline{C}$ V G R R I A

FIG. 3. Comparison of the derived amino-acid sequence of the presumptive heme-binding region of several steroidogenic forms of cytochrome P-450.

Isolation and characterization of full-length cDNAs encoding these proteins has, in turn, allowed for their expression in cells which normally do not have steroidogenic capacity. For these studies we have utilized SV-40 transformed COS-1 monkey kidney tumor cells which can readily be transfected with suitable expression vectors containing the cDNA inserts of interest. Results of such a study are shown in Table 1, in which the COS-1 cells were triple transfected with vectors containing full-length cDNAs encoding P-450$_{scc}$, adrenodoxin, and P-450$_{17\alpha}$ (41). Presentation to these cells of 22-hydroxycholesterol as steroidogenic substrate allowed for its conversion to pregnenolone, 17α-hydroxypregnenolone, and thence to dehydroepiandrosterone. Thus, it was possible in these cells that do not normally have steroidogenic capacity to reconstitute a steroidogenic phenotype, thereby allowing the conversion of a C_{27} sterol to a C_{19} steroid. To do this, these cells had to have the capacity not only to transcribe the transfected DNA, but also to translate the corresponding mRNA, and insert the apoprotein into the appropriate membrane compartment. In the case of the mitochondrial enzymes, P-450$_{scc}$ and adrenodoxin, this involved removal of the N-terminal precursor fragment during the insertion of the protein into the mitochondria. In addition, the appropriate prosthetic group had to be inserted, namely the iron-containing heme in the case of the P-450's, and the iron-sulphur center in the case of adrenodoxin.

Table 1

Steroids Produced in Triple Transfected COS-1 Cells

Adx[a]	SCC[b]	17α[c]	pmol steroid/ml/24h[d]		
μg DNA	μg DNA	μg DNA	Preg	17αOH-Preg	DHEA
--	--	--	21	<6	<1.6
10	10	--	550	<6	<1.6
--	10	30	53	21	19
10	10	30	190	136	54

[a] μg adrenodoxin plasmid DNA used in transfection
[b] μg P-450$_{scc}$ plasmid DNA used in transfection
[c] μg P-450$_{17\alpha}$ plasmid DNA used in transfection
[d] produced from 2 nmol/ml 22R-hydroxycholesterol; each no. is an average of 2 determinations on each sample of medium

It should also be noted that COS-1 cells transfected only with P-450$_{17\alpha}$ had the capacity to convert pregnenolone to dehydroepiandrosterone (40), thus providing formal proof of the claim by Hall and colleagues (20) that P-450$_{17\alpha}$ does indeed catalyze not only 17α-hydroxylation, but also the 17,20-lyase reaction.

REGULATION OF EXPRESSION OF STEROIDOGENIC CYTOCHROME P-450 SPECIES

Effects of ACTH on Levels of mRNA Encoding Steroidogenic Enzymes in the Adrenal Cortex

We have utilized cDNA inserts as hybridization probes to determine mRNA levels in bovine adrenocortical cells in primary culture. It was established that ACTH treatment leads to accumulation of mRNA species specific for each of these enzymes, namely P-450$_{scc}$ (12), P-450$_{17\alpha}$ (39), P-450$_{11\beta}$ (13), P-450$_{C21}$ (14), and adrenodoxin (22). In cases where a time-course was determined, it was found that an increase in the levels of mRNA could be detected in as little as 4 hours after initiation of ACTH treatment. Once again, the actions of ACTH could be mimicked by dibutyryl cAMP, indicative that cAMP mediates these actions of ACTH. Similar results have been found in the case of the action of ACTH on human fetal adrenal cells in culture (15,34). Such an action of ACTH to increase the levels of mRNA species encoding these enzymes could be the result of increases in the rates of transcription of the respective genes, increases in the half-life of the mRNA, or both of these. The half-lives of mRNA species encoding P-450$_{C21}$, P-450$_{17\alpha}$, P-450$_{11\beta}$, and adrenodoxin were determined to be unchanged in bovine adrenal cortical cells upon addition of ACTH. However, it was found that ACTH did lead to a 5-fold increase in the half-life of P-450$_{scc}$ mRNA (Boggaram, V., unpublished observation).

It would appear that a major action of ACTH to regulate the levels of mRNA species encoding these enzymes might be at the level of expression of these genes. In order to establish that this indeed is the case, nuclear run-on assays have been conducted utilizing nuclei isolated from bovine adrenal cortical cells maintained in the absence or presence of ACTH (16). In this manner, it has been demonstrated that ACTH causes an increase in the number of transcripts encoding the various steroidogenic enzymes. We may conclude, therefore, that the accumulation of mRNA species encoding these various steroid hydroxylase enzymes is the result of increased transcription of the genes encoding these proteins. Thus, it is apparent that the principal mechanism whereby ACTH exerts its long-term action in the adrenal cortex via the mediation of cAMP, is by regulating the transcription of the genes encoding the various steroidogenic enzymes. This pathway, therefore, provides another example of cAMP-mediated gene expression, the mechanism of which is still not understood.

An important question which arises from these studies, therefore, is whether this action of cAMP is a direct one or whether it requires ongoing protein synthesis, indicative of a mediatory role of short-lived protein factors. To address this issue, we have investigated the action of cycloheximide, an inhibitor of RNA translation, on the increase in steroid hydroxylase mRNA levels induced by ACTH (16). It has been found in the case of each of the steroidogenic cytochrome P-450's, as well as adrenodoxin, that cycloheximide inhibits the accumulation of these RNA species induced by ACTH under conditions where total mRNA levels are unaffected. This result is indicative that the action of cAMP to regulate the expression of the steroidogenic genes requires the mediation of some short-lived protein factor(s).

Regulation of Steroidogenic Enzyme Expression in the Ovary

In contrast to the adrenal, steroidogenesis in the ovary is markedly episodic in nature, and occurs in a precisely coordinated fashion under the control of the gonadotropins, as well as other undefined factors. We have shown previously that the pattern of steroidogenesis by the ovary can be explained in terms of the pattern of synthesis of the various steroidogenic enzymes (26) and this, in turn, is explicable in terms of the expression of the mRNAs encoding these proteins (27). Thus, the levels of mRNA encoding P-450$_{scc}$ and adrenodoxin are high in corpus luteum, but are low in follicles prior to ovulation. Interestingly, the expression of the LDL receptor and of HMGCoA reductase, two proteins which are not directly involved in the steroidogenic pathway but rather are required to provide cholesterol precursors through this pathway, is also high in the corpus luteum and low in follicles prior to ovulation. In marked contrast, the expression of

P-450$_{17\alpha}$ is readily detectable in follicles, but drops to undetectable levels following ovulation.

In order to understand which factors are responsible for mediating these changes, as well as the molecular mechanisms which effect them, we have utilized rat and human granulosa cells in culture as model systems, and have observed that the gonadotropin FSH, as well as dibutyryl cAMP and forskolin, can induce the levels of mRNA encoding P-450$_{scc}$, adrenodoxin (31), as well as P-450$_{AROM}$ (29). Thus, FSH via cAMP acts on the granulosa cells in a similar fashion to ACTH in the adrenal cortex to alter the expression of the mRNA species encoding steroidogenic forms of cytochrome P-450.

Recently it has become apparent that many other factors can modify the expression of steroidogenic cytochrome P-450 species *in vitro*, most of which do not operate via increases in the levels of cAMP. This is particularly true in the case of the ovary in which, as stated previously, steroid hormone secretion is highly episodic in nature and clearly governed by a variety of factors. Thus, IGF-I can stimulate the expression both of P-450$_{scc}$ (33) and of P-450$_{AROM}$ in granulosa cells (30), whereas other growth factors such as EGF can stimulate the expression of P-450$_{scc}$ (32) but are inhibitory of the expression of P-450$_{AROM}$. Other agents such as phorbol esters are apparently inhibitory of cAMP-stimulated expression of both of these P-450 species (31). These factors act through various second messenger systems, for example, tyrosine kinase, phospholipid turnover, and calcium movement, as well as protein kinase C.

Tissue Specific Expression of Steroidogenic Cytochrome P-450 Species.

In addition to these factors, many of which act within the same cell, *e.g.* the ovarian granulosa cell, it is clear that tissue-specific regulation of the expression of these enzymes also exists. Thus, expression of P-450$_{11\beta}$ and P-450$_{C21}$ is confined to the adrenal cortex, whereas P-450$_{scc}$ is expressed in adrenal cortex, ovarian theca, ovarian corpus luteum, testicular Leydig cells, placenta and brain. P-450$_{17\alpha}$ is expressed in zona fasciculata of the adrenal cortex, ovarian theca and testicular Leydig cells, whereas P-450$_{AROM}$ is expressed in ovarian granulosa cells, testicular Sertoli and Leydig cells, placenta, as well as adipose tissue and brain.

STUDIES OF THE GENES ENCODING STEROIDOGENIC FORMS OF CYTOCHROME P-450

At the present time, the sequences of three genes encoding steroidogenic forms of cytochrome P-450 have been reported, namely P-450$_{C21}$ (7,37,10), P-450$_{17\alpha}$ (24,17), and P-450$_{scc}$ (19) (Fig. 4). Steroid 21-hydroxylase genes are associated with the HLA locus. The genes encoding this enzyme have been studied in mice, bovine and human species, and in each case two forms of the gene have been detected, one of which exists as a pseudogene. In the case of the mouse, this is due to the presence of a 215 nucleotide deletion spanning the second exon (4). Both the mouse and human genes lie within a duplicated portion of the class V region of the MHC (36,1). Deletion mutations of the functional gene have been implicated in some examples of steroid 21-hydroxylase deficiency, the most common cause of congenital adrenal hyperplasia. In addition, as indicated above, characterization of the gene encoding human cytochrome P-450$_{scc}$, as well as the genes encoding human and bovine P-450$_{17\alpha}$, have been reported. Thus, it can be expected that common structural features among these genes, including regulatory consensus sequences, will become apparent in the near future.

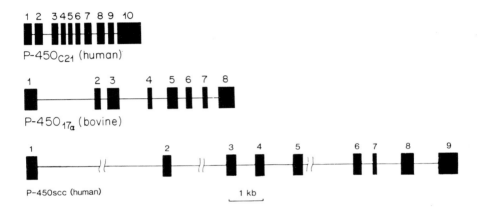

FIG. 4. Structures of the genes encoding human cytochromes P-450$_{C21}$, P-450$_{17\alpha}$ and P-450$_{SCC}$. The human P-450$_{C21}$ gene is approximately 3.2 kb in length (37); the human P-450$_{17\alpha}$ gene is approximately 6.7 kb in length (24), while the human P-450$_{SCC}$ gene is at least 20 kb in length (19).

In the case of a number of eukaryotic genes regulated by cAMP, consensus sequences have been established in the regulatory regions of these genes which are believed to mediate the action of cAMP. At present there is no clear indication as to whether a common functional cAMP consensus sequence exists in steroid hydroxylase genes. It is clearly pertinent in this context to determine whether such a consensus sequence, or indeed any other consensus sequence, does exist among the steroid hydroxylase genes regulated by this nucleotide. It has been shown that the 5'-end of the human P-450$_{scc}$ gene does confer cAMP sensitivity to a chimeric construct (11). In addition, a specific sequence has been established within the 5'-untranscribed region of the mouse gene encoding P-450$_{C21}$, which is believed to be important in the determination of the tissue-specific expression of this gene (23). Tissue- and cell-specific sequences associated with the other steroid hydroxylase genes will also be forthcoming in the near future..

As in the case of cAMP-mediated regulation of gene expression, the mechanisms whereby other regulatory pathways operate to alter the rates of expression of these genes will only be determined when various trans- and cis-acting elements associated with these genes, which mediate these diverse actions, are defined.

ACKNOWLEDGEMENTS

The authors wish to acknowledge their superb colleagues who were the ones responsible for the work, which was supported, in part, by USPHS Grants Nos. HD13234, AM28350, AG00306, CA30253 and AM31206. We also thank Dolly Tutton for skilled editorial assistance.

REFERENCES

1. Amore, M., Tosi, M., Cuponchel, C., Steinetz, M. and Meo, T. (1985): *Proc. Natl. Acad. Sci. U.S.A.*, 82:4455-4457.
2. Bradshaw, K.D., Waterman, M.R., Couch, R.T., Simpson, E.R. and Zuber, M.X. (1987): *Mol. Endocrinol.*, 1:348-354.
3. Carroll, M.C., Campbell, D. and Porter, K.R. (1985): *Proc. Natl. Acad. Sci. U.S.A.*, 82:521-525.
4. Chaplin, D.D., Galbraith, L.J., Seidman, J.G., White, P.C. and Parker, K.L. (1986): *Proc. Natl. Acad. Sci. U.S.A.*, 83:9601-9605.
5. Chen, S., Besman, M.J., Sparkes, R.S., Zollman, S., Klisak, I., Mohandas, T., Hall, P.F. and Shively, J.E. (1988) *DNA*, 7:27-38.
6. Chua, S.C., Szabo, P., Vitek, A., Grzeschik, K.H., John, M.E. and White, P.C. (1987) *Proc. Natl. Acad. Sci. U.S.A.*, 84:7193-7197.
7. Chung, B.C., Matteson, K.J. and Miller, W.L. (1986): *Proc. Natl. Acad. Sci. U.S.A.*, 83:4243-4247.
8. Chung, B.C., Matteson, K.J., Voutilainen, R., Mohandas, T.K., and Miller, W.L. (1986): *Proc. Natl. Acad. Sci. U.S.A.*, 83:8962-8966.
9. Chung, B.C., Picado-Leonard, J., Haniu, M., Bienkowski, M., Hall, P.F., Shiveley, J.E. and Miller, W.L. (1987): *Proc. Natl. Acad. Sci. U.S.A.*, 84:407-411.
10. Higashi, Y., Yoshioka, H., Vanane, M., Gotoh, O. and Fujii-Kuriyama, Y. (1986): *Proc. Natl. Acad. Sci. U.S.A.*, 83:2841-2845.
11. Inoue, H., Higashi, Y., Morohashi, K. and Fujii-Kuriyawa, Y. (1988) *Eur. J. Biochem.*, 171:435-440.
12. John, M.E., John, M.C., Ashley, P., MacDonald, R.J., Simpson, E.R. and Waterman, M.R. (1984): *Proc. Natl. Acad. Sci. U.S.A.*, 81:5628-5632.
13. John, M.E., John, M.C., Simpson, E.R. and Waterman, M.R. (1985): *J. Biol. Chem.*, 260:5760-5767.
14. John, M.E., Okamura, T., Dee, A., Adler, B., John, M.C., White, P.C., Simpson, E.R. and Waterman, M.R. (1986a): *Biochemistry*, 25:2846-2853.

15. John, M.E., Simpson, E.R., Waterman, M.R. and Mason, J.I. (1986b): *Mol. Cell. Endocrinol.*, 45:197-204.
16. John, M.E., John, M.C., Boggaram, V., Simpson, E.R., and Waterman, M.R. (1986c): *Proc. Natl. Acad. Sci. U.S.A.*, 83:4715-4719.
17. Kagimoto, M., Winter, J.S.D., Kagimoto, K., Simpson, E.R. and Waterman, M.R. (1988): *Mol. Endocrinol.*, (in press).
18. Morohashi, K., Fujii-Kuriyama, K., Okada, Y., Sagawa, Y., Hirose, T., Inayama, S., and Omura, T. (1984): *Proc. Natl. Acad. Sci. U.S.A.*, 81:4647-4651.
19. Morohashi, K., Sagawa, K., Omura, T. and Fujii-Kuriyama, Y. (1987): *J. Biochem.*, 101:879-887.
20. Nakajin, S. and Hall, P.F. (1981): *J. Biol. Chem.*, 256:3871-3876.
21. Nebert, D.W., Adesnik, M., Coon, M.J., Estabrook, R.W., Gonzalez, F.J., Guengerich, F.P., Gunzalus, I.C., Johnson, E.F., Kemper, B., Levin, W., Philips, I.R., Sato, R. and Waterman, M.R. (1987): *DNA*, 6:1-11.
22. Okamura, T., Kagimoto, M., Simpson, E.R. and Waterman, M.R. (1987) *J. Biol. Chem.*, 262:10335-10338.
23. Parker, K.L., Schimmer, B.P., Chaplin, D.D., Seidman, J.G. (1986): *J. Biol. Chem.*, 261:15353-15355.
24. Picado-Leonard, J. and Miller, W.L. (1987): *DNA*, 6:439-448.
25. Picado-Leonard, J., Voutilainen, R., Kao, L., Chung, B.C., Strauss, J.F. and Miller, W.L. (1988) *J. Biol. Chem.*, 263:3240-3244.
26. Rodgers, R.J., Waterman, M.R. and Simpson, E.R. (1986): *Endocrinology*, 118:1366-1374.
27. Rodgers, R.J., Simpson, E.R. and Waterman, M.R. (1987): *Mol. Endocrinol.*, 1:271-279.
28. Simpson, E.R., Evans, C.T., Corbin, C.J., Powell, F.E., Ledesma, D.B. and Mendelson, C.R. (1987): *Mol. Cell. Endocrinol.*, 52:267-272.
29. Steinkampf, M.P., Mendelson, C.R. and Simpson, E.R. (1987): *Mol. Endocrinol.*, 1:465-471.
30. Steinkampf, M.P., Mendelson, C.R. and Simpson, E.R. (1988): *Mol. Cell. Endocrinol.*, (in press)
31. Trzeciak, W.H., Duda, T., Waterman, M.R. and Simpson, E.R. (1987a): *J. Biol. Chem.*, 262:15246-15250.
32. Trzeciak, W.H., Duda, T., Waterman, M.R. and Simpson, E.R. (1987b): *Mol. Cell. Endocrinol.*, 52:43-50.
33. Veldhuis, J.D., Rodgers, R.J., Dee, A., and Simpson, E.R. (1986): *J. Biol. Chem.*, 261:2499-2502.
34. Voutilainen, R. and Miller, W.L. (1986): *J. Clin. Endocrinol. Metab.*, 63:1145-1150.
35. White, P.C., New, M.I. and DuPont, B. (1984): *Proc. Natl. Acad. Sci. U.S.A.*, 81:1986-1990.
36. White, P.C., Chaplin, D.D., Weis, J.H., DuPont, B., New, M.I., Seidman, J.C. (1984): *Nature*, 312:465-467.
37. White, P.C., New, M.I. and DuPont, B. (1986): *Proc. Natl. Acad. Sci. U.S.A.*, 83:511-515.

38. Yoshioka, H., Morohashi, K., Sagawa, K., Yamura, Y., Kominami, S., Takenoni, S., Okada, Y., Omura, T. and Fujii-Kuriyama, Y. (1986): *J. Biol. Chem.,* 261:4106-4109.
39. Zuber, M.X., John, M.E., Okamura, T., Simpson, E.R. and Waterman, M.R. (1986): *J. Biol. Chem.,* 26:2475-2482.
40. Zuber, M.X., Simpson, E.R. and Waterman, M.R. (1986): *Science,* 234:1258-1261.
41. Zuber, M.X., Mason, J.I., Simpson, E.R. and Waterman, M.R. (1988): *Proc. Natl. Acad. Sci. U.S.A.,* 85:699-705.

The Effect of Androgens on Adrenocortical Steroid Biosynthesis

S. Gallant, J. Alfano, L. Mertz, R.C. Pedersen
and A.C. Brownie

*Departments of Biochemistry and Pathology State University of New York at Buffalo
Buffalo, N.Y. 14214, USA*

INTRODUCTION

There are significant quantitative differences in adrenocortical function between male and female rats. The adrenal gland is larger in female rats than in male rats, with the difference due to an increase in cortical tissue. The levels of adrenal mitochondrial cytochromes P-450 are higher in female rats, as are activities of cholesterol side-chain cleavage (2). Also, circulating levels of corticosterone tend to be higher in female rats and there is a greater response to stress than found in males (20). Gonadectomy causes a reduction in the secretion of corticosterone by female or male rats and this effect is reversed by treatment with estradiol or testosterone, respectively (21). The mechanisms involved in these differences are not established. The work from Colby (12) suggests that changes in adrenocortical 5α-reductase activity induced by gonadal hormones is not involved. The finding of sex differences in the level of corticosteroids in humans (41) supports the concept that androgen effects on the function of the adrenal cortex may be relevant to human health and disease.

Our interest lies in the potential role of androgens in secondary hypertension. In humans, evidence that gonadal hormones may influence blood pressure comes from observations that increases in blood pressure occur at puberty (43) and that there are sex differences in mean blood pressures in adulthood (19). Most studies of androgen-induced hypertension in experimental animals are subsequent to the serendipitous finding by Skelton (45) that the anabolic androgen, 17α-methylandrostenediol (MAD), when used in an attempt to inhibit the severe nephrosclerosis brought about by 11-deoxycorticosterone acetate (DOCA) treatment in the rat, was hypertensinogenic in its own right. Confirmation of that finding by Salgado and Selye (40) and their finding that the adrenal cortex was essential for the development of MAD-induced hypertension focused subsequent research on the pathogenesis of androgen-induced hypertension on that gland.

Brownie and Skelton (5) found that MAD treatment altered steroid biosynthesis in adrenocortical tissue. Labeled progesterone incubated with adrenocortical homogenates from MAD-treated rats converted most of the substrate to 11-deoxycorticosterone (DOC) rather than the usual major products, corticosterone and 18-hydroxy-DOC. A role for DOC in the pathogenesis of androgen-induced hypertension was supported by findings that DOC secretion rates in MAD-treated rats (18) and plasma DOC levels in testosterone-treated rats (11) were both increased. McCall et al. (26) confirmed the finding of Hyde and Daigneault (18) that corticosterone secretion is lower in MAD-treated rats than in controls. They also found that 18-hydroxy-DOC secretion was lower and DOC secretion was higher in the MAD-treated animals.

The mechanism by which androgen treatment alters adrenocortical function at the molecular level has received some attention. Rembiesa et al. (39) showed that when MAD is incubated with rat adrenal tissue several products were formed, one of which was 17α-methyltestosterone (MT). Our studies have shown that MT but not MAD inhibited steroid 11β-hydroxylation of DOC when added directly to rat adrenal homogenates (46), an observation similar to that of Sharma et al. (42) with testosterone. This data suggests that a compound such as MAD, which is a Δ^5-3β-hydroxysteroid, would have to be converted to a Δ^4-3-ketosteroid in the target tissue (the adrenal cortex) in order to influence steroidogenesis. In our studies in which testosterone (11) and MT (31) were used to produce hypertension, we also found that DOC accumulated in adrenal incubates. However, several findings are incompatible with a mechanism that simply involves the production of a competitive inhibitor of steroid 11β-hydroxylase from MAD. First of all, we have observed consistently that MAD is more effective than either MT or testosterone in producing hypertension in rats. Secondly, there are obvious changes in the appearance of the gland which are not consistent with the hypertrophy that would be expected from increased ACTH secretion. The adrenal glands from androgen-treated rats are reduced in size and they are dark red as opposed to the pale amber appearance of normal rat adrenals. Thirdly, our studies indicate that very large decreases occur in the level of cytochrome P-450 in the adrenals of androgen-treated rats. Finally, some role for the pituitary in the pathogenesis of androgen-induced hypertension would be consistent with the finding that hypophysectomy prevents the development of MAD-induced hypertension (31).

We believe that these observations are in keeping with a more complex etiology for androgen-induced hypertension. At a minimum, changes are occurring in the function of the adrenal cortex and the pituitary (33). In this chapter we present some of our latest findings dealing with androgen effects on adrenocortical steroidogenic enzymes, pituitary-adrenal interactions, and the steroidogenesis activator peptide described by Pedersen and Brownie (36).

Effect of Androgen Treatment on Adrenal Steroidogenic Enzymes

After treatment of rats with androgen for several days or weeks there is a large fall in the level of adrenal mitochondrial cytochrome P-450 (7,8,10) and this correlates with lowered steroid 11β-hydroxylase activity. At the same time there is an increase in adrenal mitochondrial cytochrome oxidase levels. The resulting increase in activity of the classical electron transport chain (6) is in contrast to what happens to the electron transport chain supporting steroid hydroxylation. The alteration in adrenal mitochondrial cytochrome P-450 levels is associated with significant changes in the numbers of vesicular cristae in zona fasciculata-reticularis tissue (5), a change which is reversible after cessation of MAD treatment (34).

The studies mentioned above showed a correlation between the lowering by MAD treatment of adrenal steroid 11β-hydroxylase activity and low levels of adrenal mitochondrial cytochrome P-450. Steroid-induced absorption changes indicated that cytochrome P-450$_{11\beta}$ was decreased but information about cytochrome P-450$_{scc}$ was lacking in our initial studies. Fink *et al.* (14) addressed this question by measuring the rate-limiting cholesterol side-chain cleavage system following MAD treatment. Rats were treated for 2 or 4 weeks with MAD dissolved in corn oil (10 mg per day) or with vehicle alone. Blood was collected for assay of DOC and adrenocortical mitochondria were isolated for determination of enzyme activity and for measurement of DOC and cholesterol association with cytochromes P-450. Table 1 summarizes the findings in their study.

Cholesterol side-chain cleavage activity and the association of cholesterol with cytochrome P-450$_{scc}$ were increased to as much as 250 per cent of controls. In contrast, steroid 11β-hydroxylase activity and the association of DOC with cytochrome P-450$_{11\beta}$ were no more than 40 per cent of control values. The increase in cholesterol side-chain cleavage activity, coupled with a decrease in steroid 11β-hydroxylase, would serve to promote increased secretion of DOC following treatment with MAD. This was supported by a finding of elevated plasma levels of DOC in MAD-treated animals. Thus, the data from Fink *et al.* (14) are consistent with an etiology for MAD-induced hypertension whereby the major steroidogenic enzyme influenced by androgen treatment is steroid 11β-hydroxylase. This model of experimental hypertension has similarities to the 11β-hydroxylase form of congenital adrenal hyperplasia in humans, in which DOC is also implicated in the development of hypertension.

In order to more fully understand the selective change in cytochrome P-450$_{11\beta}$ following treatment with MAD, we have used Western blots with specific antibodies (23) to determine the levels of steroidogenic enzymes. When these measurements were

TABLE 1.   Effects of MAD Treatment on Adrenocortical Function

	Treatment	
	2 wks	4 wks
11β-Hydroxylase[a]	40	35
18-Hydroxylase[a]	35	33
Cholesterol SCC[a]	250	200
Cholesterol—P450 Association[b]	180	200
DOC—P450 Association[b]	45	48
Plasma DOC[c]	250	250

Rats were killed quiescently at 0600 h.   All data are expressed as per cent of the measurements obtained in control rats.
[a]Cholesterol side-chain cleavage (SCC), steroid 11β-hydroxylase, and 18-hydroxylase were measured according to Kramer *et al.* (22).
[b]Cholesterol association with cytochrome P-450$_{scc}$ was determined as the heat-generated Type I absorbance change (35) and DOC association with cytochrome P-450$_{11\beta}$ measured by adding saturating concentrations of DOC to adrenocortical mitochondria and measuring the observed Type I absorbance change (22).
[c]Plasma DOC was measured according to Bergon *et al.* (4).

carried out on female rats treated with MAD for 14 days, the sensitivity of adrenal cytochrome P-450$_{11\beta}$ to MAD treatment was confirmed (9).   Whereas adrenodoxin, cytochrome P-450$_{scc}$, cytochrome P-450$_{21}$ and cytochrome P-450 reductase were reduced by MAD treatment to 79, 86, 62 and 69 per cent of control values, respectively, cytochrome P-450$_{11\beta}$ levels were reduced to 34 per cent.   On the other hand, in untreated male rats, adrenal cytochrome P-450$_{11\beta}$, cytochrome P-450$_{scc}$, cytochrome P-450$_{21}$, and cytochrome P-450 reductase were each only 10 to 15 per cent lower as compared with untreated female controls.
   There are several possible explanations for the particular sensitivity of cytochrome P-450$_{11\beta}$ to MAD treatment.   Hornsby (16,17) has proposed a mechanism which involves damage to cytochrome P-450$_{11\beta}$ by the formation of pseudosubstrates from MAD.   The pseudosubstrate in this case would be 11β-hydroxy-MT derived from MT, a metabolite of MAD in adrenocortical tissue (39).   He has shown that 11β-hydroxylated androgens, as well as non-11β-hydroxylated androgens such as MT, are pseudosubstrates

for steroid 11β-hydroxylase (16). Studies from our laboratory have demonstrated a fall in adrenal mitochondrial cytochrome P-450 in rats treated with 11β-hydroxy-MT (8). However, the effects with MT or 11β-hydroxy-MT are always less than those seen with MAD. The lack of information on the levels of MAD, MT, and 11β-hydroxy-MT achieved following treatment of rats with MAD makes it difficult to interpret that observation. Also, the change that we observe in the level of steroid 21-hydroxylase is always much less than observed for steroid 11β-hydroxylase (9).

The proposal by Hornsby (17) that the steroid 11β-hydroxylase deficiency due to androgen treatment involves pseudosubstrates is an attractive one, though it is based upon studies using bovine adrenocortical cells in culture. He suggests (17) that in intact animals treated with androgen, the adrenocortical cytochromes P-450 are protected from damage by the high levels of antioxidants, especially ascorbate, present in the tissue. However, this does not in itself address the concurrent changes in cytochrome oxidase and electron transport chain activity in the adrenal cortex associated with androgen treatment. If pseudosubstrates damage cytochrome P-450 by means of superoxide generation, it may be that a resulting increase in heme could induce cytochrome oxidase transcription (29). However, adrenal regeneration is another example of altered adrenocortical function where steroid 11β-hydroxylase activity is decreased relative to cholesterol side-chain cleavage activity (3) and once again, there is an associated increase in adrenocortical cytochrome oxidase (15). As it is more difficult to impute a mechanism involving high concentrations of pseudosubstrates to explain the changes in adrenocortical cytochromes in regenerating tissue, we are inclined to seek other mechanisms to explain these changes in both experimental settings.

Pituitary-Adrenal Relationships in Androgen-Induced Hypertension

In order to better understand the mechanism by which MAD and related androgens produce such significant effects on cytochrome P-450$_{11\beta}$ — and therefore steroidogenesis — we have extended our studies to the pituitary. Our previous studies (47) had indicated that MAD effects on adrenocortical function are probably not due simply to a reduction in ACTH secretion because concurrent treatment with ACTH and MAD did not prevent the accumulation of DOC in adrenal incubates. Indeed, the severity of the hypertensive cardiovascular disease was enhanced by combined ACTH and MAD treatment (47).

Since 1969, when those studies were carried out, it has been shown that pro-γ-melanotropin — a peptide derived from the N-terminal portion of pro-opiomelanocortin (POMC) — synergizes with ACTH in stimulating glucocorticoid and aldosterone secretion by the rat and human adrenal (1,37) and may contain sequences that are adrenal growth factors (25). If MAD alters

the processing of POMC, this could effect the levels of steroidogenic enzymes.

In our initial studies reported here, we have taken a compre-
hensive approach by examining the adrenocorticotropic activity
of pituitary extracts produced by culturing pituitary cells in
the presence of MAD. In the design of these experiments, rat
adrenal (38,48) and pituitary (13) cells were established in
primary culture. Pituitary cultures were incubated with MAD,
corticotropin releasing factor (CRH), or a mixture of MAD and
CRH. Aliquots (20%) of the pituitary medium conditioned by
these treatments were added to replicate adrenal cell cultures.
After an additional 24 hours, adrenal cell media was removed for
the quantitation of corticosterone. Control studies involved
measuring the effect of MAD on the response to ACTH of adrenocortical cells in culture. Results from these experiments are
shown in Table 2. These preliminary data indicate that altered
pituitary function in response to MAD could be partially responsible for the altered adrenocortical function seen in
treated rats.

Effect of Androgen Treatment on Steroidogenic Activator Polypeptide

Recently we described the characterization of a steroidogenic
activator polypeptide (SAP) isolated from the rat H-540 Leydig
cell tumor (36). When added to adrenocortical mitochondria,
this factor stimulated cholesterol side-chain cleavage. The
peptide has 30 amino acid residues and has almost complete homology with the C-terminal portion of a minor heat shock protein,
78 kDa glucose-regulated protein (GRP78), present in liver endoplasmic reticulum (32). The synthesis of GRP78 is induced by
glucose starvation (44) and by a variety of other stressful conditions in vitro, including treatment with a calcium ionophore
(24).

The possibility existed that a putative adrenal GRP78 could be
the precursor of SAP. Mertz and Pedersen (27) reported that a
protein of similar size to GRP78 is present in rat adrenocortical extracts. They have developed methods for the quantitation of SAP production by isolated adrenocortical cells and have
used this approach to show that ACTH or cAMP increases the production of SAP (28). Although the addition of tumor-derived or
synthetic SAP to adrenocortical mitochondria increases the rate
of cholesterol side-chain cleavage (36), the mechanism by which
this occurs is unknown.

Because the studies by Fink et al. (14) had indicated that
cholesterol side-chain cleavage activity was increased in
adrenocortical mitochondria from MAD-treated rats, despite
levels of cytochrome P-450$_{scc}$ that were slightly lower than normal, it was of interest to examine both SAP and GRP78 in control
adrenals and adrenals from androgen-treated rats. We have carried out one study in which SAP production was measured in

TABLE 2.   Effect of MAD on the adrenocorticotropic activity
of pituitary culture media

Addition to Adrenal Cells	Corticosterone Production (μg/well/24 h)[a]
ACTH[c]	3.36 ± 0.06[b]
ACTH + MAD[d]	3.12 ± 0.30
ACTH + MAD[e]	2.48 ± 0.05
Pituitary medium/CRH[f]	15.34 ± 0.51
Pituitary medium/CRH + MAD[g]	11.37 ± 0.53
Pituitary medium/CRH + MAD[h]	8.30 ± 0.32

[a] 0.5×10^6 adrenal cells per well. The basal secretion of corticosterone was 1.01 μg/well/24 h.   [b] mean ± SEM
[c] Cells incubated with 10^{-10} M ACTH.
[d] Cells incubated with 10^{-10} M ACTH and 0.5×10^{-5} M MAD.
[e] Cells incubated with 10^{-10} M ACTH and 2.5×10^{-5} M MAD.
[f] Cells incubated with an aliquot (20%) of medium from pituitary cells exposed to 10^{-9} M CRH.
[g] Cells incubated with an aliquot (20%) of medium from pituitary cells exposed to 10^{-9} M CRH + 0.5×10^{-5} M MAD. The final concentration of MAD in the adrenal cell cultures was 0.1×10^{-5} M.
[h] Cells incubated with an aliquot (20%) of medium from pituitary cells exposed to 10^{-9} M CRH + 2.5×10^{-5} M MAD. The final concentration of MAD in the adrenal cell cultures was 0.5×10^{-5} M.

adrenocortical cells prepared from rats which had been treated for 2 weeks with MAD or testosterone at a dose of 10 mg/day. Cells were incubated in the presence and absence of 10^{-10} M ACTH and SAP was quantitated by RIA at 0, 4, 10, 15 and 30 minute intervals. In the absence of ACTH, adrenal cells from all three groups showed low levels of SAP.   ACTH stimulated a rise in intracellular SAP concentration that was of similar magnitude for control adrenocortical cells and for cells obtained from MAD- and from testosterone-treated animals.
In another experiment groups of 6 rats were treated for 2 weeks with MAD, testosterone, or 19-nortestosterone.   Control rats received vehicle only.   After 2 weeks adrenals were enucleated *in situ* and homogenized.   The homogenates were boiled in SDS buffer and subjected to electrophoresis on 12.5% polyacrylamide/SDS gels.   Gel proteins were electroblotted onto nitro-

cellulose and probed with an anti-GRP78 antiserum. Immunoreactive bands were visualized with a secondary alkaline phosphatase-linked antibody (Vectastain) and quantitated by laser densitometry. Adrenals from MAD, testosterone, and 19-nortestosterone treated groups had GRP78 levels which were 134%, 127%, and 118% of control levels, respectively.

CONCLUSIONS

Our recent studies have confirmed that adrenocortical 11β-hydroxylase activity is decreased by androgen treatment at a time when cholesterol side-chain cleavage activity is normal or increased. Normal production of steroidogenesis activator peptide in response to ACTH — coupled with normal levels of its putative precursor, GRP78 — are also consistent with an active cholesterol side-chain cleavage system in the adrenals of androgen-treated rats. The reason for this selective sensitivity of cytochrome P-450$_{11\beta}$ to androgen treatment is not fully apparent, but we provide evidence that altered pituitary function may play a role.

ACKNOWLEDGMENTS

The studies reported in this paper were supported by USPHS grants HL06975 and HL39390 to A.C.B., HL25256 to S.G. and DK18141 to R.C.P. R.C.P. is the recipient of Research Career Development Award HD00613. We thank L. Joseph, B. Buerger, and M.P. Russo for technical assistance.

REFERENCES

1. Al-Dujaili, E.A.S., Hope, J., Estavariz, F.E., Lowry, P.J., and Edwards, C.R.W. (1981): *Nature*, 291:156-159.
2. Alfano, J., Brownie, A.C., Orme-Johnson, W.H., and Beinert, H. (1973): *J. Biol. Chem.*, 248:7860-7864.
3. Bergon, L.L., Gallant, S., and Brownie, A.C. (1974): *Endocrinology*, 94:336-345.
4. Bergon, L.L., Gallant, S., and Brownie, A.C. (1975): *Steroids*, 25:323-342.
5. Brownie, A.C., and Skelton, F.R. (1968): In: *Functions of the Adrenal Cortex*, edited by K.W. McKerns, Volume 2, pp. 691-718. Appleton-Century-Crofts, New York.
6. Brownie, A.C., Skelton, F.R., Gallant, S., Nicholls, P., and Elliott, W.B. (1968): *Life Sciences*, 7:765-771.
7. Brownie, A.C., Simpson, E.R., Skelton, F.R., Elliott, W.B., and Estabrook, R.W. (1970): *Arch. Biochem. Biophys.*, 141:18-25.
8. Brownie, A.C., Colby, H.D., Gallant, S., and Skelton, F.R. (1970): *Endocrinology*, 86:1085-1092.
9. Brownie, A.C., Bhasker, C.R., and Waterman, M.R. (1988): *Mol. Cell. Endocrinol.*, 55:15-20.

10. Colby, H.D., and Brownie, A.C. (1971): *Biochem. Pharm.*, 20:803-813.
11. Colby, H.D., Skelton, F.R., and Brownie, A.C. (1970): *Endocrinology*, 86:1093-1111.
12. Colby, H.D. (1978): *J. Endocrinol.*, 77:271-2.
13. de Jong, F.H., Smith, S.D., and van der Molen, H.J. (1979): *J. Endocrinol.*, 80:91-102.
14. Fink, C., Gallant, S., and Brownie, A.C. (1980): *Hyper tension*, 2:617-622.
15. Gallant, S., and Brownie, A.C. (1969): *Arch. Biochem. Biophys.*, 131:441-448.
16. Hornsby, P.J. (1980): *J. Biol. Chem.*, 255:4020-4027.
17. Hornsby, P.J. (1986): *Endocrine Res.*, 12:469-494.
18. Hyde, P.M., and Daigneault, E.A. (1968): *Steroids*, 11:721-731.
19. Johnson, A.L., Coroni, J.C., Cassel, J.C., Tyroler, H.A., Heyden, S., and Hames, C.G. (1975): *Amer. J. Cardiol.*, 35:523-530.
20. Kitay, J.I. (1963): *Endocrinology*, 73:253-260.
21. Kitay, J.I. (1968): In: *Functions of the Adrenal Cortex*, edited by K.W. McKerns, volume 2, pp. 775-811. Appleton-Century-Crofts, New York.
22. Kramer, R.E., Gallant, S., and Brownie, A.C. (1979): *J. Biol. Chem.*, 254:3953-3958.
23. Kramer, R.E., DuBois, R.N., Simpson, E.R., Anderson, C.M., Kashiwagi, K., Lambeth, J.D., Jefcoate, C.R., and Waterman, M.R. (1982): *Arch. Biochem. Biophys.*, 215:478-485.
24. Lee, A.S. (1987): *Trends Biochem. Sci.*, 12:20-23.
25. Lowry, P.J., Estivariz, F.E., Silas, L., Linton, E.A., McLean, C., and Crocombe, K. (1985): *Endocrine Res.*, 10:243-258.
26. McCall, A.L., Stern, J., Dale, S.L., and Melby, J.C. (1978): *Endocrinology*, 103:1-5.
27. Mertz, L., and Pedersen, R.C. (1987): *Program of the Endocrine Society*, 1987.
28. Mertz, L., and Pedersen, R.C. (1988): *Program of the Endocrine Society*, 1988.
29. Meyers, A.M., Crivellone, M.D., Koerner, T.J., and Tzagoloff, A. (1987): *J. Biol. Chem.*, 262:16822-16829.
30. Molteni, A., Brownie, A.C., and Skelton, F.R. (1969): *Lab. Invest.*, 21:129-137.
31. Molteni A., Colby, H.D., Skelton, F.R., and Brownie, A.C. (1972): *Proc. Soc. Exper. Biol. Med.*, 141:936-939.
32. Munro, S., and Pelham, H.R.B. (1986): *Cell*, 46:291-300.
33. Nakayama, I., Nickerson, P.A., and Skelton, F.R. (1970): *Amer. J. Path.*, 58:377-401.
34. Nickerson, P.A., and Molteni, A. (1971): *Amer. J. Pathol.*, 64:31-44.
35. Paul, D.P., Gallant, S., Orme-Johnson, N.R., Orme-Johnson, W.H., and Brownie, A.C. (1976): *J. Biol. Chem.*,

251:7120-7126.

36. Pedersen, R.C., and Brownie, A.C. (1987): *Science*, 236:
    188-190.
37. Pedersen, R.C., Brownie, A.C., and Ling, N. (1980):
    Science, 208:1044-1045.
38. Rainey, W.E., Shay, J.W., and Mason, J.I. *J. Biol. Chem.*,
    (1986): 261:7322-7326.
39. Rembiesa, R., Holzbauer, M., Young, P.C.M., Birmingham,
    M.K., and Saffran, M. (1967): *Endocrinology*, 81:
    1278-1284.
40. Salgado, E., and Selye, H. (1954): *Arch. Int. Physiol.*,
    62:352-358.
41. Schoneshofer, M., and Wagner, G.G. (1977): *J. Clin.
    Endocrinol. Metab.*, 45:814-817.
42. Sharma, D.C., Forchielli, E., and Dorfman, R.I. (1963): *J.
    Biol. Chem.*, 238:572-575.
43. Shock, N.W. (1944): *Amer. J. Dis. Child.*, 68:16-22.
44. Shiu, R.P.C., Pouyssegur, J., and Pastan, I. (1977): *Proc.
    Natl. Acad. Sci. U.S.A.*, 74:3840-3844.
45. Skelton, F.R. (1953): *Endocrinology*, 53:492-505.
46. Skelton, F.R., and Brownie, A.C. (1968): In: *Endocrine
    Aspects of Disease Processes*, edited by G. Jasmin,
    pp. 271-301.
47. Skelton, F.R., Brownie, A.C., Nickerson, P.A., Molteni, A.,
    Gallant, S., and Colby, H.D. (1969): *Circ. Res.*,
    Suppl. I 24:I35-I57.
48. Trzeciak, W.H. (1987): Personal Communication.

HCG-Induced Regulatory Protein in the Mouse Leydig Cell: "To Be or Not To Be"

M. Schumacher and F.A. Leidenberger

*Institute for Hormone and Fertility Research,
Grandweg 64, 2000 Hamburg 54, Fed. Rep. Germany*

INTRODUCTION

From studies on the adrenal (11) and luteal cell (12) it is known that the rate limiting step in steroidhormone synthesis is the conversion of cholesterol to pregnenolone. This step is under the control of ACTH and lutropin, respectively, facilitating the availability of cholesterol to the mitochondrial cytochrome P450 side chain cleavage (P450scc) enzyme and/or the binding of cholesterol to its catalytic site (11,12). The hormone induced interaction of cholesterol with P450scc is rapidly blocked by protein synthesis inhibitors, like cycloheximide (CX), leading to the postulation of a hormone induced regulatory protein with a very short half-life (6). Similar conclusions were drawn from studies on rat Leydig cells, the steroidogenesis of which has been shown to be strictly dependent on protein synthesis (2,4). The fruitless search for such a hormone induced protein for nearly two decades recently succeeded in the isolation of an ACTH-induced peptide from rat adrenal cells, which stimulated pregnenolone production in isolated mitochondria (5) and which appeared to be present in rat tumour Leydig cells, too (7). Whether this candidate represents the postulated regulatory protein is not clear at present. The other possibility that a hormone induced regulatory protein/peptide does not exist, and that the presence of the CX-sensitive factor is independent of hormone stimulation, appears to be less attractive to scientists since no convincing studies in this direction have been reported.

The present study deals with the question of whether the CX-sensitive factor in the mouse Leydig cell is induced by hCG and is involved in the regulatory system, or whether it is a "permissive" factor being present all the time and keeping the steroidogenic machinery functioning. We are able to demonstrate

for   the   first   time   that   the   process   of   hCG-stimulation
(regulation) does not require protein synthesis,   indicating that
there   is no need for the search for a hormone-induced regulatory
protein!

METHODS

Mitochondria   and postmitochondrial supernatants were   prepared
from   mouse tumour Leydig cells (M5480 P,   (1))   preincubated   in
minimum   essential medium in the absence and presence of 10 IU/ml
hCG   and/or   36 μM cycloheximide (CX) for   90   min,   36° .   After
centrifugation   the medium was analyzed for cellular progesterone
production by RIA.   The tumour cells were homogenized in a dounce
homogenizer   (20   strokes)   in 10 mM Tris/HCl   (pH   7.4),   250   mM
sucrose   and   0.2   mM EDTA,   and mitochondria   were   isolated   by
differential centrifugation (1,500 g,   10 min / 8,000 g, 10 min).
Mitochondria   (50-100 μg protein) were incubated for 15 min (37°
in   250 μl buffer (pH 7.4) containing: 25 mM   Tris/HCl,   150   mM
sucrose,   20   mM   KCl,   5   mM MgCl$_2$,   10 mM KH$_2$PO$_4$,   10   mM   Na-
isocitrate,   0.1   % BSA,   1 μg/ml SU-10603,   1 μg/ml cyanoketone,
0.12   mM EDTA.   The incubation was stopped by the addition of 50 μl
1 M NaOH containing 0.14 %.   Tween 20 (freshly prepared) and   the
mixture   was left overnight at 6°.   On the next day samples   were
neutralized with 50 μl 0.6 M H$_3$PO$_4$ and aliquots were analyzed for
their   pregnenolone content   by   RIA   (antiserum Dr.   Rommerts,
Rotterdam). The assay was performed with a novel iodinated tracer
(3β-0-Succinyl-pregnenolone-glycyltyrosine-^{125}I), which increased
the sensitivity of the conventional ^{3}H-based assay several fold.
Cytosol   for   protein   fractionation was   obtained   from   solid
tumours   from mice treated with 100 IU hCG or saline for 2 hours.
The tumour tissue was homogenized in 3 volumes 1M acetic acid and
the   cytosolic   proteins   were   fractionated   by   Sephadex   G100
chromatography   in   the   presence of 0.2 M   acetic   acid.   Crude
peptides   were isolated by homogenization of the tumour tissue in
acidic peptide extraction mixture and ,   after delipidation .   by
absorption   to C$_{18}$-silica according to (5).   Protein and   peptide
fractions   were   freeze-dried and redissolved   in   buffer   before
addition   to the mitochondrial incubation.   For the study of   the
effect   of   CX   on basal and   hCG-stimulated   steroidogenesis   in
intact   cells and on protein synthesis,   Percoll purified native
Leydig   cells were used (8) and incubated as described previously
(10). For the comparison of protein synthesis and steroidogenesis
the   cell incubation was performed in the presence of   ^{3}H-leucine
(37   KBq/500 μl /10^5 cells) and stopped by the   addition of 500 μl
2M HClO$_4$.   After centrifugation testosterone was extracted from
the   supernatant with diethylether and measured by RIA.   and   the
washed pellet was analyzed for acid-precipitable radioactivity.

RESULTS AND DISCUSSION

FIG. 1 shows that in the purified mouse Leydig cell (as in other systems) steroidogenesis is dependent upon protein synthesis. Protein synthesis measured in terms of ^{3}H-leucine incorporation into protein and hCG (150 pg/ml) - induced testosterone production decreased nearly in parallel with increasing CX-concentrations, both showing halfmaximal inhibition around 0.3 µM CX. Basal testosterone production was inhibited by CX as sensitive as hCG-induced steroidogenesis although the degree of maximum inhibition was somewhat lower (65 % versus 95 %).

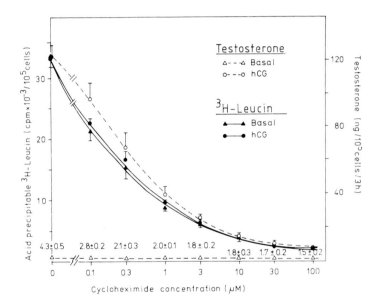

FIG.1. Effect of cycloheximide concentration on basal and hCG-induced testosterone production and on ^{3}H-leucine incorporation into acid precipitable protein

Pretreatment of tumour Leydig cells with hCG (10 IU/ml) for 90 min increased mitochondrial pregnenolone production 2-3-fold (Fig. 2). The presence of CX (36 µM) in the cell incubation prevented the hCG-induced increase (not shown). The addition of lipid free, crude peptide preparations (≙ 100 µg protein) from tumours treated with or without hCG in vivo (100 IU/mouse) to the mitochondrial incubation was without effect (Fig. 2). However, an over 10-fold increase in plasma progesterone level, had

indicated the in vivo stimulation of the tumours from which the
peptides have been isolated (not shown). The addition of
postmitochondrial supernatants (800 µg protein, from ⁻ hCG

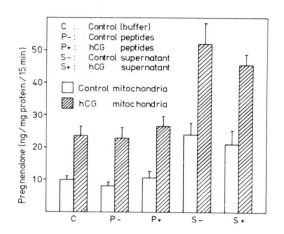

FIG.2. Effect of peptide preparations
and   postmitochondrial supernatants
on basal and hCG-stimulated mitochondrial pregnenolone production

treated Leydig cells (in vitro) caused about a two-fold increase
in basal as well as in hCG-induced pregnenolone production (Fig.
2). However, there was no effect of hCG on the stimulatory effect
of the supernatants. A similar increase in mitochondrial
pregnenolone production by postmitochondrial supernatants or
cytosols was observed, when mitochondria and/or the supernatants
were derived from CX (36 µM) or hCG + CX treated cells.
indicating a non-specific improvement of incubation conditions by
cellular factors independent of hCG or CX. Likewise. the
fractionation of peptides on Sephadex G 25 or of cytosolic
proteins on Sephadex G 100 under acid conditions, did not
result in the demonstration of stimulatory factors induced by hCG
or inhibited by CX (not shown).

Table 1 shows the effect of different CX-concentrations on the
dose-response relation of hCG-induced testosterone production. It
is evident from the table that all absolute levels of steroid

production were decreased by increasing concentrations of the inhibitor, whereas the dose response relationschip was preserved. E.g., under conditions where maximal steroidogenesis was inhibited by 96 % by 36 µM CX, hCG was able to stimulate testosterone production gradually from 1.5 ± 0.3 ng/10^5 cells (basal production) to 10.6 ± 1.4 ng/10^5 cells (maximum production). When basal levels are subtracted from hCG-induced levels and the latter are calculated as percentage of maximum for each CX-concentration, then it becomes evident that CX had no significant effect on the extent of stimulation (stimulation factor) (Fig. 3). The only effect of CX (aside from the reduction in absolute steroid production) was a dose-dependent and parallel shift of the response curves to the right increasing the ED_{50} values of hCG induced testosterone production; control: 185 ng hCG/ml; 0.36 µM CX: 240 ng hCG/ml; 1.44 µM CX: 480 ng hCG/ml; 36µM CX: 680 ng hCG/ml.

Table 1. Testosterone production by Percoll purified mouse Leydig cells under the influence of increasing hCG and/or cycloheximide concentrations

hCG (ng/ml)	Testosterone Production (ng/10^5cells)			
	without CX	0.36 µM CX	1.44 µM CX	36 µM CX
–	4.1 ± 0.4	2.3 ± 0.2	1.7 ± 0.1	1.5 ± 0.3
0.02	8.1 ± 2.0	3.8 ± 0.5	2.7 ± 0.3	1.7 ± 0.1
0.1	82 ± 17	43 ± 6	11 ± 2	2.1 ± 0.2
0.5	202 ± 29	115 ± 15	53 ± 10	5.3 ± 0.8
2.0	246 ± 20	156 ± 18	88 ± 4	8.8 ± 1.1
10.0	248 ± 17	166 ± 20	100 ± 5	10.6 ± 1.4

These results indicate that CX reduces the capacity of the steroidogenic machinery of the cell, but not the ability for hCG-stimulation. The smaller the capacity the higher the hormone concentration required to induce the same degree of stimulation.

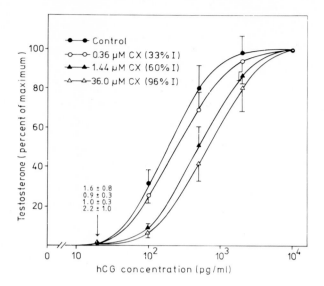

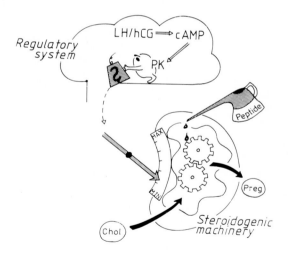

FIG.3. Effect of different cycloheximide concentrations on the dose-response curves of hCG-induced testosterone production

FIG.4. Our hypothesis: The labile peptide is an obligatory part of the steroidogenic machinery and is not involved in the hormone-dependent regulatory system.

The CX-sensitive protein appears to be less involved in the mediation of the hormonal signal than in receiving or transforming the signal at the steroidogenic site. It could also be a limiting co-factor in the conversion of cytoplasmic cholesterol to pregnenolone, whereby it is used up or inactivated, giving rise for its rapid hormone-independent resynthesis. Whatever the regulation of the synthesis of the labile protein may be, our data give strong evidence that its synthesis is not dependent on hormone concentration: Basal steroidogenesis is inhibited as sensitively as hormone-induced steroidogenesis and supramaximal hCG-concentrations (>1 ng/ml) leading to excessive cAMP-accumulation and protein kinase activation (9), are not able to overcome a partial CX- induced block.

In conclusion, we were unable to detect and isolate an hCG-induced proteinaceous factor in mouse Leydig cells, which stimulated pregnenolone production in isolated mitochondria, as has been reported for the adrenal (5) and rat tumour Leydig cell (7). This discrepancy is not explainable at present and differences in species or methods may be the reasons. However, our observation that the process of hCG stimulation is independent of protein synthesis indicates that there is no requirement for the existence of an hCG-induced regulatory protein in the mouse Leydig cell and our study is therefore internally consistent. Our conclusions also differ from those of Cooke et al. (3), who have postulated that in the rat Leydig cell lutropin induces the transformation of a stable and lutropin-independent protein into a labile form with regulatory properties. This postulation also presumes that lutropin increases the level of a regulatory protein which in turn stimulates the steroidogenic machinery. Our hypothesis, illustrated in Fig. 4, states that in the mouse Leydig cell the postulated hormone-induced regulatory protein does not exist. The CX-sensitive factor (obligatory for steroidogenesis) is part of the steroidogenic machinery, is not increased by gonadotropin and is not involved in intracellular signal transduction.

Acknowledgements: We thank Dr. Mario Ascoli, Nashville, for the supply of M5480P Tumour cells, Dr. Kevan Willey for caricaturing FIG. 4 and Petra Wahl for typing the manuscript

REFERENCES

1. Ascoli, M., Puett, D. (1978): Proc. Natl. Acad. Sci. USA, 75:99-102

2. Cooke, B.A., Janszen, T.H.A., Clotscher, W.F., van der Molen, H.J. (1975): Biochem. J., 150:413-418

3. Cooke, B.A., Lindh, L.M., van der Molen, H.J. (1979): Biochem. J., 184:33-38

4. Mendelson, C. Dufau, M.L., Catt, K.F. (1975): Biochem. Biophys. Acta, 411:222-230

5. Pedersen, R.C., Brownie, A.C. (1983): Proc. Natl. Acad. Sci. USA, 80;1882-1886

6. Pedersen, R.C. (1985): Endocrine Research, 10:533-561

7. Pedersen. R.C., Brownie, A.C. (1987): Science, 236:188-190

8. Schumacher, M., Schäfer, G., Holstein, A.F., Hilz, H. (1978): FEBS Lett., 91:333-338

9. Schumacher, M. Schwarz, M., Schäfer G., Lichtenberg, V., Hilz, H. (1979): FEBS Lett., 107:398-402

10. Schumacher, M. Schwarz, M., Leidenberger, F. (1985):Biol Reprod., 33:335-345

11. Simpson, E.R., Waterman, M.R. (1983): Can. J. Biochem. Cell. Biol. 61:692-707

12. Strauss, J.F. Schuler, L.A., Rosenbaum, M.F., Tanaka, T. (1981): Advances In Lipid Research, 18:99-157

On the Role of SCP_2 in Hormonal Regulation of Steroid Production in Leydig Cells

M. van Noort, F.F.G. Rommerts, A. van Amerongen[1] and K.W.A. Wirtz[1]

Department of Biochemistry (Division of Chemical Endocrinology),
Faculty of Medicine, Erasmus University Rotterdam,
P.O. Box 1738, 3000 DR Rotterdam,
and [1]Laboratory of Biochemistry, State University Utrecht, P.O. 80054,
3508 TB Utrecht, The Netherlands

INTRODUCTION

The mechanisms involved in the acute hormonal regulation of the cholesterol side-chain cleavage enzyme complex (CSCC) are still poorly understood. It appears from data in the literature that regulation of the availability of cholesterol for the CSCC enzyme is one of the control points and that SCP_2 may be involved in this process (1).

SCP_2, also designated non-specific lipid transfer protein (nsL-TP), accelerates the transfer of both phospholipids and cholesterol between membranes (2). Studies with adrenal mitochondria have shown that SCP_2 can increase the amount of cholesterol in the inner membrane as well as pregnenolone production (3-fold) (1).

In the rat testis SCP_2 is specifically localized in the Leydig cells (3) and the amount of SCP_2 in soluble fractions of Leydig cells is regulated by hormones and intracellular calcium levels (4). A maximal stimulatory dose of lutropin (LH) causes within 2 min a 2-fold increase in the level of SCP_2 in the soluble fraction of Leydig cells. This level is maintained for at least 24 h of incubation with LH (4).

These data indicate that the amount and properties of SCP_2 at the mitochondrial level may be an important factor for availability of cholesterol at the level of CSCC.

We have studied 1) effects of SCP_2 on steroid production by isolated Leydig cell mitochondria, 2) binding between sterols and SCP_2 and 3) possible mechanisms involved in regulation of the level of SCP_2 in the soluble fraction.

MATERIALS AND METHODS

1. Isolation and incubation of mitochondria

Tumour Leydig cells (150×10^6) were suspended in 7 ml buffer containing 10 mM Tris-Cl pH 7.4, 1 mM EDTA and 250 mM D-mannitol (5,6) and homogenized using a Dounce-Wheaton glass homogenizer (clearance 0.025-0.03 mm, 10 strokes). After differential centrifugation mitochondria were suspended in buffer containing 125 mM sucrose, 25 mM Tris-Cl (pH 7.4), 5 mM $MgCl_2$, 60 mM KCl to a final concentration of 1 mg protein/ml.

Incubation was started by addition of 100 µl of the mitochondrial suspension to 400 µl buffer at 37°C, containing 5 mM DL-isocitrate. Incubation was stopped after 10 minutes by cooling on ice and by addition of 2 volumes ethylacetate (p.a.). Pregnenolone production was determined as described previously (7). Where indicated cytosolic preparations (500 µg) were preincubated with anti-rat SCP_2 (50 µg) (8) or preimmune IgG antibody (150 µg) in a total volume of 200 µl for 18 h at 4°C. The mixtures were centrifuged at 10.000xg for 20 min and aliquots of the supernatant were used for experiments.

2. Equilibrium dialysis

Binding of 25-hydroxycholesterol to purified rat SCP_2 (8) was determined by equilibrium dialysis according to Fritz et al. (9). SCP_2 (3.4 nM) in 0.5 ml 0.9% NaCl was put into a dialysis bag and equilibrated for two days against a solution (40 ml 0.9% NaCl) of 25-hydroxy [26,27-^{3}H]-cholesterol (1 nM). Similar experiments were carried out with 1 mg/ml bovine serum albumin, poly-L-lysine and poly-L-aspartic acid. The binding of 25-hydroxycholesterol to the protein(s) was calculated from the increase of [^{3}H]-label in the dialysis bag relative to the medium.

3. Measurement of SCP₂ levels in different fractions of tumour Leydig cells

Leydig cells from the Leydig cell tumour H540 were isolated and incubated for 30 minutes with or without lutropin (LH, 1000 ng/ml) as described previously (10). Subcellular fractions were prepared and treated as described previously (11). In this treatment fractions are extracted with high salt to remove SCP_2 from membranes (12). The amount of SCP_2 released is measured using an enzyme immunoassay (EIA, 11).

RESULTS AND DISCUSSION

Addition of 0.7 µM purified rat liver SCP_2 to a suspension of mitochondria from tumour Leydig cells resulted in a 2- to 3-fold stimulation of pregnenolone production from endogenous cholesterol (Table 1). This steroidogenic response was dependent on a SCP_2

concentration between 10^{-7} and 10^{-5} M (data not shown).

TABLE 1. Steroid production by isolated mitochondria

Additions	pregnenolone pmol/100 mg protein/min
none	22.4 ± 2.7
cytosol	36.8 ± 1.4
cytosol and IgG	38.4 ± 1.4
cytosol and anti-SCP₂	21.6 ± 1.1
SCP₂	39.6 ± 1.6
SCP₂ and IgG	40.3 ± 2.3
SCP₂ and anti-SCP₂	12.8 ± 0.8
IgG	20.3 ± 1.6
anti-SCP₂	15.0 ± 2.1

Results are means ± SD (6) of 3 different mitochondrial preparations. For further details see Materials and Methods.

The stimulatory effect of SCP₂ was neutralized by pretreatment with anti-rat SCP₂ IgG (anti-SCP₂). The addition of this antibody to the mitochondria even inhibited pregnenolone production within the incubation period of 10 minutes. Addition of cytosolic preparations from Leydig tumour cells incubated with LH also stimulated the pregnenolone production 2-fold. After pretreatment with anti-SCP₂ this stimulatory effect was abolished, but rat serum IgG (IgG) had no effect.

These data indicate that SCP₂ stimulates steroid production in mitochondria of Leydig cells as has been reported earlier for adrenal mitochondria (1). Antibodies to SCP₂ can block the stimulatory effects of both pure SCP₂ and SCP₂ in cytosolic preparations. Anti-SCP₂ could even lower the basal production of pregnenolone by isolated mitochondria. This might be explained by binding of the antibody to SCP₂ located at the outer mitochondrial membrane.

This decrease in basal pregnenolone production was not observed in the presence of cytosolic preparations. This may be an indication for the presence of stimulatory peptides in the cytosolic preparations such as the 3.5 kDa peptide which could stimulate steroid production by mitochondria from Leydig tumor cells (13).

It has been proposed that SCP₂ carries cholesterol in a 1:1 molar soluble complex to the inner mitochondrial membrane and that this transfer is rate-limiting for steroidogenesis(1). However, actual binding of cholesterol to SCP₂ has never been shown. We have investigated binding of 25OH-cholesterol to SCP₂ using equilibrium dialysis at 4°C. Due to difficulties in dissolving cholesterol dialysis experiments with cholesterol were not possible.

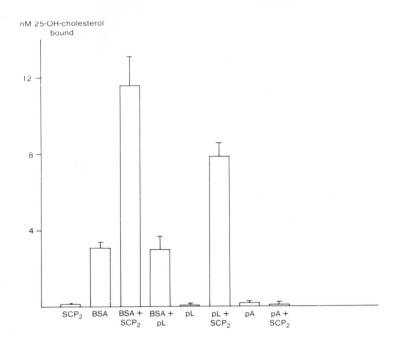

FIG. 1., binding of 25-hydroxycholesterol to SCP₂ (3.4 nM) and/or
1 mg/ml bovine serum (BSA) albumin poly-L-lysin (pL) and poly-L-
aspartic acid (pA). Binding is expressed as the increase of 25-
³H hydroxycholesterol in the dialysis bags over steady state
levels (1 nM). Values represent the means ± S.D.of 3 experiments.
For further details see Materials and Methods.

The data show that association between SCP₂ and 25OH-
cholesterol only occurs in the presence of other positively
charged peptides such as bovine serum albumin (BSA) or poly-L-lysine.
At neutral pH poly-L-aspartic acid is negatively charged and does
not affect binding of 25OH-cholesterol (Fig. 1). Since pure SCP₂
does not bind 25OH-cholesterol it seems unlikely that this protein
binds cholesterol and acts as a classical transport protein.
Interactions between SCP₂ and other cellular compounds seem to be
essential for transfer properties of SCP₂. As a dimer SCP₂ may
enable lipids to redistribute between close membranes (2).
    The rapid increase in SCP₂ levels in Leydig cell cytosol after
hormonal stimulation may contribute to rapid stimulation of
steroid production because the experiments with mitochondria have
shown that pregnenolone production can be regulated by SCP₂ (Table

1). Moreover, fusion of adrenocortical cells with liposomes containing anti-SCP$_2$ antibody reduced ACTH-stimulated steroidogenesis (14). However a correlation between SCP$_2$ levels in the membrane-free supernatant both in steroid production in Leydig cells (4) and cholesterol metabolism in liver cells (15) was not always observed. Thus the amount of SCP$_2$ in the cytosol seems not to be rate-limiting for steroidogenesis.

It is unlikely that SCP$_2$ is the labile intracellular protein postulated to mediate hormone action (16,17) because the half-life of SCP$_2$ in adrenal cells is 32 h (18). The half-life of SCP$_2$ in rat tumour Leydig cells is also high, since pretreatment of cells with cycloheximide for 18 h did not significantly influence the amount of SCP$_2$ detected in the supernatant fractions (4).

SCP$_2$ does not only occur in soluble fractions but also in membrane fractions (14,19). We have therefore investigated whether hormones may influence the transfer of SCP$_2$.

It was shown earlier that SCP$_2$ bound to rat liver mitochondria could be removed by washing with a high ionic strength buffer (23).

Using this high salt extraction procedure we investigated the hormonal regulation of SCP$_2$ levels in the 105,000xg supernatant (S) and particulate (P) fractions of rat tumour Leydig cells. After incubation of cells for 30 min with 1000 ng/ml LH, pregnenolone production was stimulated approximately 3-fold (basal: 90 ± 13 pmol/10^6 cells; stimulated: 275 ± 43 pmol/10^6 cells; mean ± SD, n=4). The subcellular distribution of SCP$_2$ is also influenced by LH (Fig. 2).

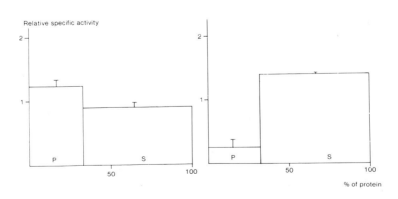

FIG. 2., Effect of LH on the distribution of SCP$_2$ between the 105,000xg particulate (P) and supernatant (S) fractions of isolated rat tumour cells. Cells were incubated for 30 min without LH (left panel) or with 1000 ng/ml LH (right panel). The total cellular amount of SCP$_2$ was not changed after incubation with LH.

SCP$_2$ levels in the particulate (P) fraction were decreased 4-fold whereas in the supernatant (S) fraction the levels increased 2-fold (from 238 ± 51 ng/mg protein to 406 ± 41 ng/mg protein, n=4). The total amount of SCP$_2$ was not influenced by incubation with LH (basal: 334 ± 45 ng/mg cellular protein; stimulated: 351 ± 55 ng/mg cellular protein; means ± SD, n=4).

The data show that LH can modify the interaction between SCP$_2$ and membranes. We have observed earlier that the influx of calcium ions is required for hormonal stimulation of SCP$_2$ levels in Leydig cell supernatant fractions (4). The cellular Ca^{2+} (20) concentrations could thus be important for the interaction between SCP$_2$ and membranes. It was suggested that this interaction is of an electrostatic nature (12). If release of SCP$_2$ from membrane fractions and the increase of SCP$_2$ in cytosol fractions also occurs in intact cells, this could explain part of the hormone effect on steroid production since SCP$_2$ added to mitochondria can stimulate steroid production.

Hormone effects on subcellular redistribution of other proteins have also been demonstrated. For instance phorbol esters cause redistribution of protein kinase C and it has been shown recently that translocation of this protein is coupled with activation (21). Hormones may thus regulate the subcellular aggregation of various proteins such as multi-enzyme complexes. More attention should be paid to this "topodynamic regulation" of proteins when studying mechanisms for regulation of cell function (22).

REFERENCES

1. Vahouny, G.V., Chanderbhan, R., Noland, B.J. and Scallen, T.J. (1984-1985): Endocrine Res., 10:473-505.
2. Van Amerongen, A., Teerlink, T., Van Heusden, G.P.H. and Wirtz, K.W.A. (1985): Chem. Phys. Lipids, 38:195-204.
3. Van Noort, M., Rommerts, F.F.G., Van Amerongen, A. and Wirtz, K.W.A. (1988): J. Endocrinol., 109:R13-R16.
4. Van Noort, M., Rommerts, F.F.G., Van Amerongen, A. and Wirtz, K.W.A. (1988): Mol. Cell. Endocrinol., 56:133-140.
5. Bakker, G.H., Hoogerbrugge, J.W., Rommerts, F.F.G. and Van der Molen, H.J. (1983): FEBS Lett., 161: 33-36.
6. Whipps, D.E. and Halestrap, A.P. (1984): Biochem. J., 221:147-152.
7. Van der Vusse, G.J., Kalkman, M.L. and Van der Molen, H.J. (1974): Biochim. Biophys. Acta 348:404-414.
8. Teerlink, T., Van der Krift, T.P., Van Heusden, G.P.H. and Wirtz, K.W.AA. (1984): Biochim. Biophys. Acta, 793:252-259.
9. Fritz, I.B., Rommerts, F.F.G., Louw, B.G. and Dorrington, J.H. (1976): J. Reprod. Fertil. 46:17-24.
10. Rommerts, F.F.G., Molenaar, R. and Van der Molen, H.J. (1985): Methods Enzymol. 109:275-288.

11. Van Amerongen, A., Van Noort, M., Rommerts, F.F.G., Orly, J. and Wirtz, K.W.A. (1988): Biochim. Biophys. Acta in press.

12. Megli, F.M., De Lisi, A., Van Amerongen, A., Wirtz, K.W.A. and Quagliariello, E. (1986): Biochim. Biophys. Acta, 861:463-470.

13. Pedersen, R.C., and Brownie, A.C. (1987): Science, 236:188-190.

14. Chanderbhan, R.F., Kharroubi, A.T., Noland, B.J., Scallen, T.J. and Vahouny, G.V. (1986): Endocr. Res., 12:351-370.

15. Van Heusden, G.P.H., Souren, J., Geelen, M.J.H. and Wirtz, K.W.A. (1985): Biochim. Biophys. Acta, 846:21-25.

16. Bakker, G.H., Hoogerbrugge, J.W., Rommerts, F.F.G. and Van der Molen, H.J. (1985): J. Steroid Biochem., 22:311-314.

17. Cooke, B.A., Lindh, L.M. and van der Molen, H.J. (1979): Biochem. J., 184:33-38.

18. Trzeciak, W.H., Simpson, E.R., Scallen, T.J., Vahouny, G.V. and Waterman, M.R. (1987): J. Biol. Chem., 262:3713-3717.

19. Van der Krift, T.P., Leunissen, J., Teerlink, T., Van Heusden, G.P.H., Verkleij, A.J. and Wirtz, K.W.A. (1985): Biochim. Biophys. Acta, 812:387-392.

20. Sullivan, M.H.F. and Cooke, B.A. (1986): Biochem. J., 236:45-51.

21. Munari-Silem, Y., Audebet, C. and Rousset, B. (1987): Mol. Cell. Endocrinol., 543:81-90.

22. Kaprelyants, A.S. (1988): Trends Biochem. Sci., 13:43-46.

Arachidonic Acid Metabolites and Leydig Cell Function

[1]M.H.F. Sullivan, D.R.E. Abayasekara and B.A. Cooke

*Department of Biochemistry, Royal Free Hospital School of Medicine,
Rowland Hill Street, London NW3 2PF, U.K.*
*[1]Present address: Institute of Obstetrics and Gynaecology, Royal Postgraduate
Medical School, Hammersmith Hospital, Du Cane Road, London W12 OHS, U.K.*

INTRODUCTION

It is well established that LH (luteinizing hormone) interacts with its plasma membrane receptor in testis Leydig cells which results in the activation of adenylate cyclase and formation of cyclic AMP. In addition it is now evident that other transducing mechanisms are involved in Leydig cells and other steroidogenic cells. For example, activation of phospholipase C may lead to the formation of inositol 1,4,5 trisphosphate (IP_3) and diacylglycerol and subsequently to the elevation of intracellular free calcium. Activation of phospholipase A_2 (PLA_2) leads to the release of arachidonic acid. Recently attention has focused on the lipoxygenase pathway of arachidonic acid metabolism which results in the formation of the leukotrienes. These compounds have high histamine-like activity in producing contraction of capillaries and permeabilization of capillary vessels (leading to oedema) and they are powerful chemotactic agents (9). Endocrine glands may also be regulated by leukotrienes, these include the pituitary (10), adrenal cortex (5) ovaries (7) and testes (3). These compounds may play a role in hormone synthesis and secretion and regulate blood and lymph flow in endocrine tissues.

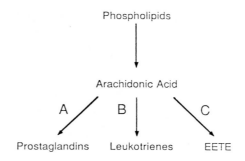

Phospholipids

Arachidonic Acid

A   B   C

Prostaglandins   Leukotrienes   EETE

Inhibitors A: ETYA, NDGA, BW755C, Indomethecin
B: ETYA, NDGA. BW755C, RG5901
C: ETYA

FIG 1.   Pathways of release and
metabolism of arachidonic acid.

Little is known about the mechanisms controlling
PLA_2 in endocrine cells. Recent evidence from other
cell types indicates that it might be a target for
protein kinase C as well as Ca^{2+} and lipocortin.
The further metabolism of arachidonic acid is via
three possible pathways catalyzed by
cyclooxygenases, lipoxygenases and cytochrome P_{450}
enzymes to the prostaglandins, leukotrienes and
epoxyeicosa-tetraenoic acids respectively (see Fig
1). The relative importance of these compounds in
controlling cellular processes can be assessed using
inhibitors (Fig 1). The available lipoxygenase
inhibitors (with the possible exception of RG5901)
inhibit both the lipoxygenase and cyclooxygenase
pathways. However the selective inhibition of the
latter can be achieved using aspirin or
indomethacin.

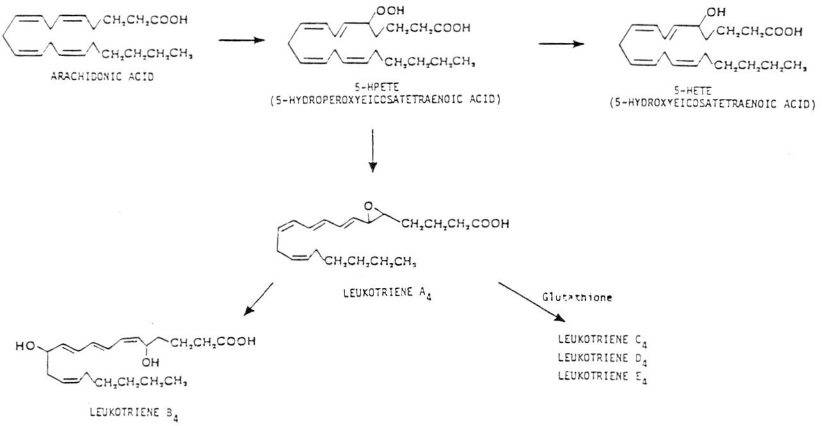

FIG 2.   5-lipoxygenase products of
arachidonic acid

The pathways leading to the leukotrienes are shown
in Figure 2. It can be seen that these involve the
formation of 5 HPETE (hydroperoxyeicosatetraenoic
acid) and epoxide intermediates (LTA₄) with the
subsequent conversion to the dihydroxy derivative
(leukotriene B₄) LTB₄ or to the glutathione
derivative LTC₄ and its metabolites.

In our work on the possible roles of leukotrienes
and related compounds on steroidogenesis in Leydig
cells, we have studied the effects of the available
inhibitors of arachidonic acid on LH-stimulated
steroidogenesis stimulated by LH, a LHRH (LH-
releasing hormone) agonist and dibutyryl cyclic AMP
(3,13). Our results indicate that leukotrienes but
not prostaglandins are involved. Furthermore [14]C-
arachidonic acid was metabolized to a number of
products some of which co-migrated with authentic 5-
HETE (hydroxyeicosatetraenoic acid), 12-HETE and
LTB₄ (3). The production of these metabolites was
potently inhibited by NDGA (nordihydro-guaiaretic
acid).

In our recent work which is described here we have
assessed the effect of a specific lipoxygenase

inhibitor RG5901 on steroidogenesis. We have also
examined in more detail the kinetics of the effects
of NDGA and indomethacin. We have also determined
the effects of the addition of various arachidonic
acid products on steroidogenesis. Finally we have
studied the regulation and formation of LTB_4 in
Leydig cells.

METHODS

Rat testis Leydig cells were purified on Percoll
density gradients and incubated at 32°C in DMEM in
10% CO_2; 90% air as described previously (1). The
cells were cultured at a concentration of 50,000
cells/200µl media. Assays for testosterone, (14),
cyclic AMP (4,11) and LTB_4 (8) were carried out as
described previously. Data were analysed by
Student's t-test.

RESULTS

We have examined the effects of RG5901 (a 5-
lipoxygenase inhibitor) (2) on Leydig cell
testosterone production, and found that this
compound inhibited both LH- and dibutyryl cyclic
AMP-stimulated steroidogenesis with an ED_{50} of
approximately 5µM (Fig. 3).

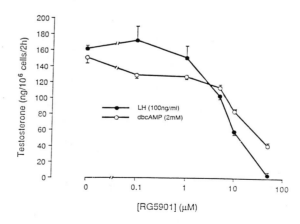

FIG 3. The effects of RG 5901 on
testosterone production stimulated by
LH (100ng/ml) or Dibutyryl cyclic AMP (2mM).

We also found that RG5901 decreased LH-stimulated
cyclic AMP production with a similar ED_{50}. These
results are the same as we previously found with

NDGA (3) and they indicate that leukotrienes are
involved at both pre- and post- cyclic AMP
production levels in the control of steroidogenesis.

In our earlier studies we demonstrated that
indomethacin had no effect on steroidogenesis
maximally stimulated by LH. However with a LHRH
agonist, which stimulates testosterone to a lower
level than LH there was an indomethacin-induced
dose-dependent increase in testosterone production
(13); this indicated that there may have been a mass
action effect in diverting the arachidonic acid from
the cyclooxygenase to the lipoxygenase pathway. In
our recent studies we have examined the effect of
indomethacin with sub-maximum stimulatory levels of
LH (Fig 4); it was found that at concentrations of
0.1pg to 0.1ng/ml LH there was a significant
stimulation of testosterone by 100 and 300µM
indomethacin.

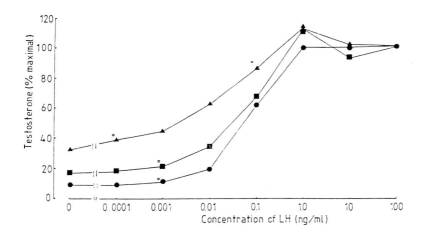

FIG 4. Effects of indomethacin on
LH-stimulated testosterone production.
Control (●), 100µM indomethacin (■),
300µM indomethacin (▲). All data are
means (n=3), all S.E.M<10%.

In our previous studies (3,13); we added the
inhibitors prior to the addition of LH etc. In
further studies we have examined the time required
for inhibition to take place by adding the
lipoxygenase inhibitors at various times before and

after the addition of LH (Fig 5). It is apparent
that there is a rapid decrease in the effectiveness
of the inhibitor if added after the LH; after 1 hour
of the 2 hour incubation with LH there was no
significant effect of NDGA. This indicates that the
lipoxygenase product(s) involved in steroidogenesis
are required in the early stages of hormonal
stimulation.

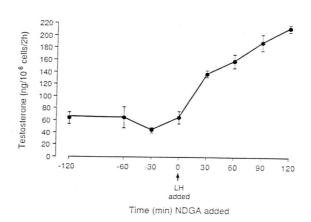

FIG 5. The effects of NDGA (10µM.) at
different times on LH stimulated
testosterone production. All data are means ±
S.E.M. (n=3)

We next attempted to stimulate testosterone by the
addition of known lipoxygenase products of
arachidonic acid metabolism. The compounds were
added 30 min after the addition of LH or dibutyryl
cyclic AMP since the above experiments indicated
that it is over this time period that the
lipoxygenase products are required.
5-HPETE was the most potent stimulant of
testosterone production in this system and was
capable of enhancing sub-maximal testosterone

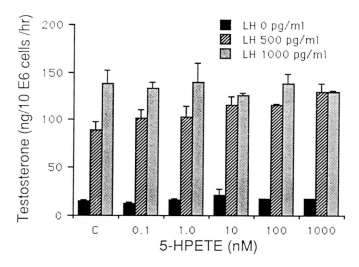

FIG 6.   Effects of 5-HPETE on
LH-stimulated testosterone production.
All data are means ± S.E.M. (n=3)

production to maximal levels (with 500pg of LH/ml)
(Fig 6).   At lower concentrations of LH, (<100
pg/ml) the effects of 5-HPETE were more variable and
at LH concentrations of <250pg/ml, 5-HPETE at
concentrations of 0.1-1000nM could not enhance
testosterone production to maximal levels.   Both
basal and maximally stimulated testosterone
production were unaffected by 5-HPETE at all
concentrations tested.   Similar results were
obtained with dibutyryl cyclic AMP, indicating that
5-HPETE exerts its effects after cyclic AMP
production (results not shown).   These results are
consistent with a role for 5-HPETE in hormone-
stimulated steroidogenesis.   Other arachidonic acid
metabolites tested (5-HETE, 15-HPETE, LTC₄) had no
effect at high LH concentrations (100ng/ml) and
inhibited testosterone production in the presence of
LH at 250-1000 pg/ml (results not shown)

Using the above incubation protocol, we studied the
effect of 5-HPETE on the inhibition of LH-stimulated
testosterone production by RG5901, NDGA and
mepacrine (a PLA₂ inhibitor).   These inhibitors were
added at appropriate concentrations (0-100μM) 30
minutes before the addition of LH, and the protocol
was followed as described above.   5-HPETE partially
antagonised the effects of RG5901 on LH- and
dibutyryl cyclic AMP-stimulated testosterone

production.   Similar results were found when NDGA
and mepacrine were used to inhibit testosterone
production.   Thus, 5-HPETE partially antagonizes the
effects of inhibitors of arachidonic acid release
and metabolism.

LTB_4 is one of the end products of arachidonic acid
metabolism and it can therefore be used to address
the question of whether or not the lipoxygenase
pathway is controlled by LH.   A specific
radioimmunoassay is also available for this
leukotriene (8).   Previously we showed that this
compound is synthesized and secreted by Leydig cells
(12).   Addition of the calcium ionophore A23187
increased LTB_4 production 6-fold within 10 min but
the effects of LH and hCG (human chorionic
gonadotropin) were variable.   Recently our attention
has focused on the contribution of other testis
cells that may synthesise LTB_4 and also whether or
not LH increases LTB_4 synthesis.

LTB_4 production has been determined in highly
purified Leydig cells and compared with impure
preparations.   The effects of various stimulants on
LTB_4 production in Leydig cells in vitro with and
without treatment in vivo with hCG has been
determined.

Testes from untreated rats were incubated with
collagenase to give a crude interstitial cell
preparation (Leydig cells 20%).   This was purified
on Percoll gradient (Leydig cells 85%) or the cells
were separated by elutriation and then further
purified on Percoll gradients (Leydig cells 97%).
Small increases in LTB_4 production following
incubation with LH or hCG were found in the purified
cells but not in the crude preparation.   When the
latter was mixed with either of the other two the
response to LH/hCG was lost.   Very high levels of
LTB_4 were produced in response to A23187 in the
crude preparation (approx 2500 pg/10^6 cell/3h)
compared to the purified cells (approx 400 pg/10^6
cells/3h).   However there was little difference
between the effect of A23187 on the two purified
preparations indicating that the 15% non-Leydig
cells in the Percoll purified cells did not
contribute to the LTB_4 production.   Extensive
metabolism of LTB_4 added to the crude preparation
took place indicating that the values obtained are
an underestimation of the actual production.
Determination of the macrophage content by an

immunocytochemical methods in the interstitial preparation showed that the crude cells contained $16 \pm 5\%$ macrophages compared with $0.02 \pm 0.01\%$ (means ± S.D. of 2 separate experiments) (G. Dirami & B.A. Cooke, unpublished results) in the elutriator-purified Percoll cells. It is thus possible that the macrophage content of the crude preparation explains the response to A23187.

In a further series of experiments with purified cells it was found that the response to LH/hCG was inconsistent, although A23187 always gave an increase. The effect of hCG in vivo on the subsequent LTB₄ production in vitro was therefore investigated. It was found that the levels of LTB₄ and response to A23187 in vitro in elutriator/Percoll purified cells increased with the time after administration of hCG; values they were low after 3 hours (158 ± 15 and 194 ± 29 pg/10^6 cells/2h respectively) but had not reached a maximum after 12 hours (424 ± 50 and 1096 ± 168 pg/10^6 cells/2h respectively). Little or no additional response to hCG added in vitro was obtained. HCG given in vivo increased PGF$_{2\alpha}$ levels in vitro and these had declined after 12h. Neither hCG nor A23187 had any effect in vitro on PGF$_{2\alpha}$ levels. Testosterone production in vitro showed a typical desensitization response after hCG in vivo.

We conclude that Leydig cells and other testis cell types form LTB₄. Although the response to LH/hCG in vitro is variable (possibly because of the short incubation times used), the Leydig cells isolated from hCG treated rats produced higher levels of LTB₄ which increased with the time after administration of hCG. No extra effect of hCG added in vitro was found but A23187 further increased LTB₄ levels. PGF2$_\alpha$ levels were also increased by hCG in vivo but they did not parallel LTB₄ and were not increased by A23187 or hCG in vitro.

These experiments demonstrate that the synthesis of LTB₄ can be stimulated by hCG (LH). However long periods are required (4-6h) so it is possible that this represents a trophic effect of hCG on the lipoxygenase enzymes rather than an acute stimulatory effect on phospholipase A₂. Also the kinetics of LTB₄ production indicate that this leukotriene is not involved in the control of steroidogenesis.

CONCLUSIONS

The inhibitor studies reported here and in earlier work (3) are consistent with a role for lipoxygenase products in steroidogenesis. Compounds which do not affect lipoxygenase activity (indomethacin, aspirin) either have no effect, or enhance testosterone production. The results obtained with RG5901, which does not inhibit cyclo-oxygenase activity (2) are also consistent with a role of a 5-lipoxygenase product in hormone stimulated steroidogenesis. 5-HPETE may be the metabolite involved in the stimulation of testosterone production by LH and dibutyryl cyclic AMP, since it enhances the effects of steroidogenically submaximal concentrations of both stimuli, but is without effect on basal and maximal testosterone production. It may be that 5-HPETE is not the sole limiting factor in steroidogenesis, since it will not enhance the effects of low LH concentrations (100-250 pg/ml) to maximal testosterone production. Furthermore, 5-HPETE cannot totally antagonise the effects of inhibitors known to decrease arachidonic acid metabolism to lipoxygenase products. It is not clear if this is due to only a limited amount of 5-HPETE entering the cells or in stability of 5-HPETE, or if the inhibitors used have other effects on Leydig cell function which preclude a complete reversal of inhibition by 5-HPETE. Similar results have been obtained by Hirai and co-workers (5) who demonstrated that only 5-HPETE enhanced submaximal steroidogenesis and that this metabolite was capable of antagonizing low concentrations of a lipoxygenase inhibitor. A more recent study has suggested that LTA_4 has inhibitory effects in adrenal cells (6).

Although rat Leydig cells produce LTB_4 (12), it is apparent that this production is not involved in steroidogenesis. Stimulation (in vivo) with hCG for 6-12 hours enhances LTB_4 production, particularly in response to ionophore A23187. It is not clear whether other cells (e.g. macrophages), which are known to respond to A23187 by producing LTB_4 (8) contribute to the production of LTB_4 by testicular cells. The stimulatory effect of hCG is not specific to the lipoxygenase system, since $PGF_{2\alpha}$ production by Leydig cells is also dramatically increased following in vivo hCG treatment. It remains to be determined whether these changes have any physiological counterpart.

ACKNOWLEDGEMENTS

We gratefully acknowledge the financial support of the M.R.C. for the work reported here. We also thank Mrs. L. Kurlak (Department of Biochemistry) and Drs. J. Jeremy and P. Dandona (Department of Chemical Pathology), of the Royal Free Hospital School of Medicine for assistance with the prostaglandin radioimmunoassays.

REFERENCES

1. Aldred, L.F. and Cooke, B.A. (1982): Int. J. Androl. 5: 191-195
2. Coutts, S., Khandwala, A., Van Inwegen, R., Chakraboty, U., Musser, J., Bruens, J., Jariwala, N., Dalley-Meade, V., Ingram, K., Pruss, T., Jones, H., Neiss, E. Weinryb, I (1985): In: Prostaglandins, Leukotrienes & Lipoxins (Ed: J.M. Bailey) Plenum pp 627-638
3. Dix, C.J., Habberfield, A.D., Sullivan, M.H.F. and Cooke, B.A. (1984): Biochem. J. 219: 529-537.
4. Harper, T.F. Brooker, G. (1975): Adv. Cycl. Nucl. Res. 1: 209-218
5. Hirai, A., Tahara, K., Tamura, Y., Saito, M., Terano, T. & Yoshida, S. (1985): Prostaglandins, 30: 749-767.
6. Jones, D.B., Marante, D., Williams, B.C. and Edwards, C.R.W. (1987): J. Endocrinol. 112: 253-258
7. Reich, R., Kohen, F., Naor, Z. and Tsafriri, A. (1983): Prostaglandins 26: 1011-1020
8. Salmon, J.A., Simmons, P.M. & Palmer, R.M.J. (1982): Prostaglandins 24: 225-235.
9. Samuelsson, B. (1982): Ang. Chemie. 21: (12) 902
10. Snyder, G.D., Capdevila, J., Chacos, N., Manna, S. and Falck, J.R. (1983): Proc. Natl. Acad. Sci. USA. 80: 3504-3507
11. Steiner, A.L., Parker, C.W. & Kipnis, P.M. (1972): J. Biol. Chem. 247: 1106-1113
12. Sullivan, M.H.F. and Cooke, B.A. (1985): Biochem. J. 230: 821-824
13. Sullivan, M.H.F. and Cooke, B.A. (1985): Biochem. J. 232: 55-59
14. Verjans, J.L., Cooke, B.A., de Jong, F.H., de Jong, C.M.M and van der Molen, H.J (1973): J. Steroid Biochem. 4: 665-676

Hormonal Control of Testicular Blood Flow Microcirculation and Vascular Permeability

A. Bergh[1], J.-E. Damber[2] and A. Widmark[3]

*Departments of [1]Anatomy Pathology, [3]Physiology and Urology & Andrology,
University of Umeå, S-901 87 Umeå, Sweden*

INTRODUCTION

The testicular interstitial space, particularly in the rat, is composed mainly of large lymphatic sinusoids that completely surround the tubules (8,25). Leydig cells secrete their products into this lymph and into the blood. Factors synthesized in the tubules are also secreted into this lymph, factors that locally modulate Leydig cells function (46,54). Testicular interstitial fluid (IF) thus serves as a medium for transport of factors between tubules, Leydig cells and blood (for review see 54). It is obvious that by modulating testicular blood flow and vascular permeability it is possible to influence both the secretion of hormones from the testis and the local milieu within the testis and in this way the paracrine control of testicular cells (54).

In this minireview, we try to summarize what is known about the hormonal regulation of testicular blood flow, microcirculation and vascular permeability . We focus our interest on recently published studies. Several excellent reviews covering both older and recent studies have been published by Setchell (47-49,52) and by Free (26).

Total Testicular Blood Flow

Several observations indicate that testicular blood flow could be controlled by hormones. Treatment of adult rats with human chorionic gonadotrophin (hCG) results in a delayed increase in blood flow occurring 16-24 h after treatment (15,50). This increase is probably preceded by a decrease in flow occurring 4-6 h after treatment (57,60). Similarly, treatment with LH results in a decreased blood flow at 6 h and increased flow 12 h after treatment (61). Treatment with a low dose LHRH administered intratesticularly (with no effect on endogenous LH) decreased blood flow within 2 h but treatment with a larger dose (increasing endogenous LH) increased testicular blood flow within 2 h (63). Treatment of hypophysectomized rats with a larger dose of LHRH increases blood flow within 2-4 h (18).

Hypophysectomy decreases testicular blood flow and this can be prevented by hCG substitution (13). Apparently, hormonal stimulation of the testis can induce time and possibly dose-dependent decreases and increases in testicular blood flow. It should be noted that these vascular effects occurred several hours after stimulation and most investigators have been unable to observe more acute effects (26,47), although Damber and Janson (14) observed a significant decrease in vascular resistance 20 min after LH stimulation.

The cellular origin and nature of the factors mediating these changes in blood flow are unknown. Leydig cell products are involved since hCG does not increase testicular blood flow in animals in which the Leydig cell population is depleted by EDS-treatment (22). Apparently the stimulation of Leydig cells results in secretion of factors which influence testicular blood vessels, but testosterone itself does not have any acute effects on blood flow (26). These factors could be of Leydig cell origin, but other testicular cells may also be involved. The testicular interstitium contains numerous macrophages which in general secrete vasoactive substances (56). Stimulation of Leydig cells with hCG induces morphological changes in testicular macrophages (3). It is thus possible that some of the vascular effects observed after Leydig cell stimulation could be mediated by testicular macrophages. Destruction of the seminiferous tubules by different means results in a decrese in blood flow that is parallel to the degree of destruction in the seminiferous tubules (51,59). EDS-treatment, which removes all Leydig cells, does not influence total testicular blood flow (22), suggesting that basal testicular blood flow could be maintained by tubular factors. Our observations that LHRH, a substance possibly secreted by Sertoli cells, influence blood flow (18,63) is also in line with this suggestion. Davidson et al. (23) report that FSH initially decreases and later increases testicular blood flow, but we were unable to influence testicular blood flow by PMSG treatment (pregnant mare serum gonadotrophin with documented FSH-like effect) in Leydig cell depleted rats (unpublished observation).

Decreases or increases in total organ blood flow are generally mediated by changes in the diameters of the precapillary resistance vessels. Thus it is likely that the hormone induced changes in testicular blood flow could be mediated by secretion of factors influencing the tonus in these blood vessels. Several substances with general effects on vascular tonus are produced and/or secreted locally in the testis. Arginine vasopressin (AVP), a potent vasoconstrictor is produced in the testis (37), and local injection of AVP in low doses acutely decreases testicular blood flow (unpublished observations). Oxytocin is produced by Leydig cells (44), but whether it is involved in the control of blood flow is not known. HCG treatment increases testicular prostaglandin synthesis within 4-8 h (31) and some prostaglandins decrease testicular blood flow (26). Mast cells are present under the testicular capsule (55) and serotonin decreases testicular blood flow (26). Sympathetic nerve stimulation of adrenaline/noradrenaline treatment decreases testicular blood flow (26,47). The ovary is innervated by several different types of peptidergic nerves containing different types of vasodilators such as VIP and substance P (42). Substance P is present in rat testicular arterioles (unpublished observations) but the role of nerves in the regulation of testicular blood flow remains to be investigated. Although the principal factors influencing testicular blood flow are probably substances affecting the tonus in precapillary vessels (and the testicular artery, see 26,47,48), their effect can sometimes be modulated by effects induced in the vasculature at other locations, i.e. increased venular permeability and leukocyte accumulation could decrease blood flow in spite of vasodilatation (see below).

In conclusion, it appears that gonadotrophins, LHRH, catecholamines, serotonin, testicular nerves and possibly also factors from the seminiferous tubules could influence total testicular blood flow. Which of these factors are really involved in the physiological control of testicular blood flow remains unknown.

Laser Doppler Flowmetry and Local Variations in Testicular Blood Flow

Testicular microcirculation can be studied using laser doppler flowmetry, a method permitting continuous registration. The laser probe is fixed just above the testicular surface and the total erythrocyte flux in fine calibre vessels in a tissue volume of approximtely 1 mm^3 is quantified (16,17). When studied in this way, testicular blood flow (in the anesthesized rat) shows large rhythmical variations with approximately 7-11 peaks per min. Bu studying the microcirculation in vivo with capillaroscopy simultaneously with laser doppler flowmetry, we found that the variations in laser signal were due to local variations in erythrocyte velocity (20). In a group of capillaries, supplied by the same arterioli, blood flow was synchronized and periods of high erythrocyte velocity alternated with periods of very slow or no flow. This type of microcirculation, called vasomotion, is probably a general phenomenon in most vascular beds. It may be involved in the formation of interstitial fluid. During periods with high flow there is filtration of plasma from the vasculature, but during stops the flow is reversed (27,34,35). Vasomotion is caused by spontaneous pacemaker activity in smooth muscle cells in the walls of arterioles and some observations suggest that this activity can be modulated or suppressed by humoral and neuronal factors, but the mechanisms controlling arteriolar vasomotion are largely unknown (27).

Interestingly, our observations suggest that the local blood flow pattern in the testis is influenced by hormones. HCG or LH treatment, inhibits vasomotion within 4 h (61,62), resulting in a continuous flow. Vasomotion then returns 12 h (for LH) or 24 h

(for hCG) after treatment. Similarly, treatment of hypophysectomized rats with an LHRH agonist inhibits vasomotion within 2 h
(21). The inhibition of vasomotion occurring within a week of hypophysectomy can be prevented by hCG substitution in a low dose
(65). Vasomotion also disappeared when the Leydig cells were removed from the testis by EDS treatment (22). Vasomotion is not
present in immature rats. It appears first in 24-day-old animals,
however hCG treatment may induce vasomotion in younger animals
(unpublished observations). These observations suggest that hormonal factors may induce developmental changes in the testicular
microvasculature inducing spontaneous vasomotion and that stimulation of the Leydig cells results in the secretion of factors
which directly or indirectly via some other testicular cell influences the precapillary blood vessels in the testis.

After hCG treatment there is an increase in the volume of interstitial fluid in the testis (see below). This increase is tempo-
rally related to the disappearance of vasomotion (62), and since
theoretically abolishing vasomotion could favor filtration of
plasma to the interstitium (34,35) we suggested that hormones by
modulating the local blood flow pattern in the testis could increase the transvascular filtration of substances (62). However,
as discussed below, the volume of interstitial fluid (IFV) in the
testis is controlled by several other factors. Thus inhibition of
vasomotion does not necessarily result in an increased IFV. That
changes in blood flow pattern could be one factor influencing the
volume and thus composition of testicular interstitial fluid is
demonstrated by the observation that it is still possible to increase the volume of IF by hCG treatment in rats in which the
hCG-induced increase in venular permeability is blocked (see below).

In conclusion, vasomotion is probably under hormonal control
in the adult rat testis, but the physiological significance of
testicular vasomotion remains to be established. The testis is
particularly suitable for studies of the general role of vasomotion since vasomotion in most other organs disappears after anaesthesia (27). Interestingly vasomotion is inhibited in testes
with experimental varicocele (43) and in experimental cryptorchidism (32) suggesting that alterations in blood flow pattern
could play a part in testicular pathophysiology.

Regulation of Vascular Permeability

The testicular microvessels show several peculiarities. The capillaries are unfenestrated which is unusual for an endocrine organ. Testicular blood vessels, like those in the brain, are imper-
meable to dyes that penetrate into the interstitium in other

organs. Therefore it was originally suggested that the blood testis barrier was located in the blood vessel walls (39). Testicular
endothelial cells have specialized transport mechanisms for amino
acids (49,52). The vascular permeability to albumin is of the
same magnitude as in dog muscle (41,52). These studies thus suggest
that the vascular permeability in the testis is rather low for being an endocrine organ. Other studies do, however, suggest a high
vascular permeability. The protein concentration in testicular
lymph is high and it contains macromolecules like immunoglobulins
(1), and at least in some species the lymph flow is very high (47,
49).

Testicular vascular permeability is probably under hormonal control. HCG treatment causes a marked increase in vascular permeability for albumin (41,52,55), as well as increases in the volume of
testicular interstitial fluid (50,53,54) and in testicular lymph
flow (50). These changes start at approximately 8 h and are maximal 16-30 h after hCG treatment (41,52,55).Similar increases in
the volume of testicular interstitial fluid are also observed after treatment with LH (61) and LHRH (see 54). Since the volume of
interstitial fluid is generally increased after hCG treatment it
appears that the hCG induced increase in vascular permeability is
not fully compensated for by the increase in lymph flow (see 41
for discussion). Since it is relatively easy to estimate the volume of IF in the testis, this is the method most used to quantitate
changes in vascular permeability (see 53). It should be noted, however, that the volume of this fluid is; apart from being dependent
on changes in vascular permeability; probably also influenced by
changes in filtration pressure, lymph flow and venous resistance;
the relative importance remains of the latter unknown.

The mechanisms mediating the hCG-induced increase in vascular
permeability are largely unknown. Interestingly, the hCG-induced
increase in IFV is preceded by an accumulation of polymorphonuclear leukocytes in the testicular blood vessels, particularly in
small venules. Simultaneously with the increase in IFV, leukocytes
can be observed in the interstitial space (2). This observation
suggests a marked increase in permeability also allowing cells to
migrate into the tissue. Using the colloidal carbon labelling
technique (12), we have shown that hCG treatment results in the
formation of large gaps (up to 1 μm in size) between endothelial
cells in postcapillary venules within 4 h (4), a type of vascular
response previously described only in inflammation or in pathological conditions (45,65). In vivo microscopy of the testicular
blood vessels after intravascular injection of dextran-150 shows
that this macromolecule leaks from the postcapillary venules (but
not from capillaries) at discrete sites (4), a type of vascular
leakage similar to that observed in vivo in other vascular beds
after administration of inflammation mediators (7,45). HCG treat
ment of the testis thus results in a situation with striking similarities to inflammation and the subsequent increase in IF could

perhaps be considered as an inflammatory exudate. The tissue oedema in inflammation is caused by two parallel, but independently
regulated, events (65): 1) dilatation of precapillary sphincters,
caused by secretion of vasodilators (principally prostaglandins)
resulting in increased hydrostatic pressure in capillaries and
postcapillary venules and 2) an increase in venular permeability,
caused by secretion of mediators that directly or indirectly result in the formation of interendothelial cell gaps (45,65). These
mediators are for instance histamine, with a direct effect on the
venular endothelium, or chemotactic factors like complement and
leukotrienes that cause gaps indirectly by attracting leukocytes.
In the testis, the accumulation of leukocytes appears to be of
major importance since it is not possible to induce endothelial
cell gaps by hCG treatment in leukopenic rats (64). The hCG-
induced effect on vasomotion is however not inhibited suggesting
that the hCG-induced changes in testicular venules are differently
regulated than are those in the arterioles (see above, 64). The
hCG induced increase in venular permeability can be blocked by
treatment with a β adrenergic agonist (5), possibly since β-
agonists prevent endothelial cell contraction and thus inhibit the
formation of gaps (45).

PMN-leukocytes could thus be involved in the control of testicular vascular permeability. The hormonally stimulated testis (LH
and LHRH treatment also result in intravascular leukocyte accumulation, 21,61) apparently secret a leukotactic factor, but the
nature and origin of this factor remains unknown. Interestingly,
the testis may secrete both interleukin-I (38), a substance causing leukocyte binding to the endothelium, and leukotriene B4 (11)
one of the most potent leucotactic factors yet known. We have recently observed that intratesticular injection of IL-1 β results
in a venular leakage similar to that seen after hCG treatment
(Bergh and Söder, unpublished), but whether LTB4 affects testicular
blood vessels has not yet been investigated. Theoretically, in-
flammation-mediators such as histamine, serotonin, or bradykinin
could be involved in mediating the venule leakage in the hCG stimulated testes, but current data suggest that this is not the case.
Histamine (28, unpublished observations) or serotonin (unpublished
observations) injections do not induce venular leakage in the testis, and substances antagonizing the effect of bradykinin do not
prevent the hCG-induced increase in vascular permeability (55).
Blocking testicular prostaglandin synthesis with indomethacin does
not prevent the hCG-induced increase in vascular permeability (55
58). In summary, it appears that a PMN-leukocyte dependent inflammation-like vascular reaction could be involved in the control of
vascular permeability in the testis. Our experiment with leukopenic rats, in which hCG could increase IF volume without causing
large endothelial cell gaps, may however suggest that other mechanism could also influence vascular permeability. On the other hand,
the increase in IFV could be caused by precapillary vasodilatation
(64). Hypothetically, by secreting leukotactic factors the

increase in permeability can be localized to the testis (no carbon leakage is observed in the pampiniform plexus after hCG treatment; unpublished observations).

<u>Physiological role of hCG/LH-induced changes in testicular micro-circulation - observations and speculations</u>

In the experiments described above large doses of hCG/LH/LHRH were used to induce changes in blood flow, vasomotion, permeability and lymph flow, doses that result in a maximal stimulation of testosterone synthesis. The lowest dose of hCG/LH affecting total blood flow has not been established. Testicular vasomotion is not inhibited by hCG doses lower than 25 i.u. (62). The lowest dose of hCG causing intravascular leukocyte accumulation and venular endothelial cell gaps is somewhere between 6.25 and 12.5 i.u. (ref. 2, and unpublished observations). No increase in IFV was noted until 32 h after treatment with 12.5 i.u. hCG (62), suggesting that the time-response curve for IFV, like that for plasma testosterone (33) is dependent on the hCG dose given. Perhaps inflammation-like changes in testicular microcirculation occur only during supra-physiological stimulation. Indeed focal tubule damage has been described after hCG and LHRH treatment in high doses (30,57). On the other hand, microcirculatory changes induced by low doses may have escaped our attention since, 1) IF volume is a crude way to esti-mate changes in filtration and permeability, 2) we do not know whether the laser doppler is able to detect discrete changes in blood flow pattern and the importance of the changes in vasomotion amplitude and frequency sometimes noted (unpublished observations) are also unknown and 3) a small increase in the number of open endothelial cell gaps, although difficult to detect, may neverthe-less be of physiological importance. Interestingly, recent studies suggest that the physiological control of macromolecular permeabi-lity in general takes place at interendothelial cell junctions in small postcapillary venules and not by static pores in the capil-lary endothelium as previously thought. By controlling the size of these interendothelial cell junctions permeability is regulated (9,10,29). What we observed after hCG treatment is perhaps an in-dication that macromolecular permeability, also in the testis, is controlled in a similar way.

One important experiment would be to elucidate the microvascu-lar effect of a physiological LH-peak. Mating of female rabbits results in an LH-peak that induces ovulation. This peak is follow-ed by intravascular and perifollicular leukocyte accumulation and oedema, and anti-inflammatory drugs prevent ovulation (24). Using the colloidal carbon-labelling technique we have observed that this LH-peak, within 4 h, results in endothelial cell gaps in ova-rian postcapillary venules of a similar nature to those in the testis after hCG treatment (Bergh and Cajander, unpublished ob-servations). An endogenous LH-peak, although much smaller than in females, can also be induced in male rats by mating (36). The

intravascular leukocyte concentration is doubled 4 h after mating
in male rats and, in such rats, we can observe some, but not many.
open interendothelial cell gaps in postcapillary venules (unpublished observations). A physiological stimulation may thus influence vascular permeability in the testis, although the response is
much more descrete than after large doses of hCG and the physiological relevance is therefore not known. It should also be noted
that there may be large species differences in testicular microcirculation. In anaesthethised male mice, vasomotion is not observed. LHRH or hCG treatment increase IFV and albumin permeability,
but result neither in leukocyte accumulation nor in the formation
of venular gaps (at least not large enough to allow passage of
carbon particles, 6). It is clear that further studies are needed
to elucidate the physiological relevance of gonadotrophin-induced
changes in testicular blood flow and microcirculation. In these
studies it is likely that new methods must be introduced, i.e.
methods that in contrast to the current ones allow detection both
of discrete and rapidly occurring changes in flow and permeability. As yet we have one example that disturbances in testicular
microcirculation could be of importance in testicular pathophysiology. HCG treatment results in an extreme increase in vascular
permeability in the unilateral abdominal testis in rats (ref. 19,
and unpublished observations) and in a major increase in intratesticular pressure (32). HCG is currently used in the treatment of
cryptorchid in boys and the clinical experience is that the cryptorchid testes in such boys is unusually firm the day after treatment (40). Hypothetically, this may indicate that pharmacological
hCG treatment could induce similar microvascular changes in humans
as in rats, and this should serve as a basis for further studies.

ACKNOWLEDGEMENTS

This work was supported by grants from the Swedish Medical Research Council (proj 5935 and 5053), the Maud and Birger Gustav-
son, the Lions, the Jeansson, and the Magn Bergvall Foundations.

Correspondence: Dr A Bergh, Department of Pathology, University of Umeå, S-901 87 Umeå, Sweden

REFERENCES

1. Beh, K.J., Watson, D.L., and Lascelles, A.K. (1974): Aust. J.
   Exp. Med. Biol., 52:81-86.
2. Bergh, A., Widmark, A., Damber, J.-E., and Cajander, S. (1986):
   Endocrinology, 119:580-590.
3. Bergh, A. (1987): Int. J. ANdrol., 10:765-772.
4. Bergh, A., Rooth, P., Widmark, A., and Damber, J.-E. (1987):
   J. Reprod. Fert. 79:135-143.
5. Bergh, A., and Damber, J.-E. (1987): J. Reprod. Fert., 80:623-
   627

6. Bergh, A., and Damber, J.-E.-E.(1988): Int. J. Androl. (in
    press).
7. Björk, J., Hedqvist, P., and Arfors, K.E. (1982): Inflammation,
    6:189-200.
8. Clark, R.V. (1976): Anat. Rec., 184:203-226.
9. Crone, C. (1986): Fed. Proc., 45:77-83.
10. Crone, C. (1987): Int. J. Microcirc.: Clin. and Exp., 6:101-
    122.
11. Cooke, B.;., Dix, C.J:, Habberfield, A.D., and Sullivan, M.H.F.
    (1984): Ann. N.Y. Acad. Sci., 438:269-282.
12. Cotran, R.S., and Majno, G. (1964): Amer. J. Path., 45:261-281.
13. Daehlin, L., Damber, J.-E., Selstram, G., and Bergman, B.
    (1985): Int. J. Andol., 8:58-68.
14. Damber, J.-E., and Janson, P.-O. (1978): Acta Endocrinol.
    (Coph.), 88:390-396.
15. Damber, J.-E., Selstam, G., and Wang, J.M. (1981): Biol. Re-
    prod. 25:555.
16. Damber, J.-E., Lindahl, O., Selstam, G., and Tenland, T.
    (1982): Acta Physiol. Scand., 115:209-215.
17. Damber, J.-E., Lindahl, O., Selstam, G., and Tenland, T.
    (1983): Acta Physiol. Scand. 118:117-123.
18. Damber, J.-E., Bergh, A., and Daehlin, L. (1984): Int. J.
    Androl. 7:236-243.
19. Damber, J.-E., Bergh, A:, and Daehlin, L. (1985): Endocrino-
    logy, 117:1906-1913.
20. Damber, J.-E., Bergh, A., Fagrell, B., Lindahl, O., and Rooth,
    P. (1986): Acta Physiol. Scand., 126:371-376.
21. Damber, J.-E., Bergh, A., and Widmark, A. (1987): Int. J. And-
    rol 10:785-791.
22. Damber, J.-E., Bergh, A., and Widmark, A. (1987): Biol. Re-
    prod., 37:1291-1296.
23. Davidson, O.W., Denis, J., and Gil, F. (1974): Fertil Steril,
    25:296 (abstract).
24. Espey, L.L. (1980): Biol. Reprod. 22:73-106.
25. Fawcett, D.W., Neaves, W.B., and Flores, M.N. (1973): Biol.
    Reprod. 9:500-532.
26. Free, M.J. (1977): In: The Testis. Vol. 4 PP 39-90. EDs.
    Johnsson AD & Gomez WR. Academic Press, New York.
27. Funk, W., and Intaglietta, M. (1983): Progr. Appl. Microcirc
    3:66-82.
28. Gabbiani, G., Badonnel, M.C., and Majno, G. (1970): Proc.
    Soc. Exp. Biol. Med. 135:447-452.
29. Grega, G. J., Adamski, S.W., and Dobbins, D.E. (1986): Fed.
    Proc. 45:96-100.
30. Habenicht, U.-F., Neuman, F., and El Etreby, M.-F. (1987):
    Andrologia 19:602-613.
31. Haour, F., Kouznetzova, B., Dray, F., and Saez, J.M. (1979):
    Life Sci 24:2151-2158.
32. Hjertkvist. M., Bergh, A., and Damber, J.-E. (1988): J. And-
    rology, in press.
33. Hodgson, Y.M, and de Kretser. D.M. (1982): Int. J. Androl.,

        5:81-91.
34. Intaglietta, M. (1981): Microvasc Res., 21:153-164.
35. Intaglietta, M., and Gross, J.F. (1982): Int. J. Microcirc: Clin and Exp 1:55-65.
36. Kamel, F., Wright, W.W., Mock, E.J., and Frankle, A.I. (1977): Endocrinology, 101:421-429.
37. Kasson, B.G., Adashi, E.Y., and Hsueh, A.J.W. (1986): Endocrine Rev. 7:156-168.
38. Khan, S.A., Söder, O., Syed, V., Gustafsson, K., Lindh, M., and Ritzén, E.M. (1987): Int. J. Androl., 10:495-503.
39. Kormano, M. (1967): Histochemie, 9:327-338.
40. Läckgren, G. (1983): Thesis, University of Uppsala, Sweden.
41. Maddocks, S., Sowerbutts, S.F., and Setchell, B.P. (1987): Int. J. Androl., 10:535-542.
42. McNeill, D.L., and Burden, H.W. (1987): Am. J. Anatomy, 179:269-276.
43. Nagler, H.M., Lizza, E.F. House, S.D., Tomachefsky, P., and Lipowsky, H.H. (1987): J. Andrology, 8:292-298.
44. Nicholson, H.D., Worley, R.T.S., Guldenaar, S.E.F., Pickering, B.T. (1987): J. Endocrinology, 112:311-316.
45. Persson, C.G.A., and Svensjö, E. (1985): In: The Pharmacology of Inflammation , edited by I.L Bonta, M.A. Bray and M.J. Parnham, pp. 61-82. Elsevier, Amsterdam.
46. Saez, J.M., Tabone, E., Perrard-Sapuri, M.H., and Rivarola, M.A. (1985): Medical. Biol., 63:225-236.
47. Setchell, B.P. (1970): In: The Testis, edited A.D. Johnson, W.R. Gomez, and N.L. vanDemark, vol. 1, pp. 101-239. Academic Press, New York.
48. Setchell, B.P. (1978): The Mammalian Testis. Paul Elek, London.
49. Setchell, B.P. (1986): Aust. J. Biol. Sci, 39:193-207.
50. Setchell, B.P., Sharpe, R.M. (1981): J. Endocr., 91:245-254.
51. Setchell. B.P. and Galil, K.A.A. (1983):Aust. J. biol. Sci, 36:285.
52. Setchell, B.P., Bustamante, J.-C., Niemi, M. (1984): In: Progress in Microcirculation Research II, edited by F.C. Courtice, D.G. Garlick, M.A. Perry, pp. 291-296. Committee in Postgraduate Medical Education, University of N.S.W., Sidney.
53. Sharpe, R.M., and Cooper, I. (1983): J. Reprod. Fert., 69: 125-135.
54. Sharpe, R.M. (1984): Biol. Reprod., 30:29-49.
55. Sowerbutts, S.F., Jarvis, L.G., and Setchell, B.P. (1986): Aust. J. Exp. Biol. Med. Sci 64:137-147.
56. Takemura, R., and Werb, Z. (1984): Am. J. Physiol., 246:C1-6.
57. van Vliet, J., Wensing, C.G.J., Rommerts, F.F.G., Rooij, D.G., Saxena, P.R., and Zijlstra, F.J. (1986): IV European Workshop on Molecular and Cellular Endocrinology of the Testis. Capril April 1986. Miniposter F 7.

58. Veiola, M., and Rajaniemi, H. (1985): Int. J. Androl., 8: 69-79.
59. Wang, J.M., Galil, K.A.A. and Setchell, B.P. (1983): J. Endocrinol., 98:35-46.
60. Wang, J.M., Gu C.H., Oian, Z.M., and Jing, G.W. (1984): J. Reprod. Fertil., 71:127-133.
61. Widmark, A. (1987): Thesis. Umeå University Medical Dissertations, New Series no 189, Umeå, Sweden.
62. Widmark, A., Damber, J.-E., and Bergh, A. (1986): J. Endocr. 109:419-425.
63. Widmark, A., Damber, J.-E., and Bergh, A. (1986): Int. J. Androl., 9:416-423.
64. Widmark, A. Bergh, A., Damber, J.-E., Smedjegård, G. (1987): Moll. Cell. Endocrinol. 53:25-31.
65. Widmark, A., Damber, J.-E., Bergh, A. (1987): J. Endocrinol., 115:489-495.
66. Williams, T.J. (1985): In: The Pharmacology of Inflammation, edited by I.L. Bonta, M.A. Bray, M.J. Parnham, pp. 49-59. Elsevier, Amsterdam.

Do Contractions by Peritubular Myoid Cells Influence Local Transport of Interstitial Fluid in the Testis?

I.B. Fritz

Banting and Best Department of Medical Research
University of Toronto, Toronto, Canada M5G 1L6

While considering the topic presented by Bergh (this volume), I was struck by the notion that tissue pressure between seminiferous tubules might play a role in influencing local fluid exchange among vascular, lymphatic and interstitial compartments in the testis. For purposes of developing this hypothesis, three assumptions have been made:

1) Fluid filtered through the vascular walls is returned to the circulation by venules and lymphatics, with inappreciable uptake by seminiferous tubules.
2) The colloid osmotic pressures are similar in vascular, lymphatic and interstitial fluids.
3) The walls of testicular blood vessels and those of lymphatic vessels are very permeable to the passage of proteins.

Since protein levels in testicular lymph are approximately two-thirds as high as those in plasma (15), the latter two assumptions appear to be reasonably safe ones. Nevertheless, changes in degrees of permeability could occur in response to various stimuli, even though the capillary walls in testis are relatively leaky. Testicular capillaries are classified as "Type A-1-α", which indicates the presence of a basement membrane with an incomplete covering of pericytes around the wall, and the absence of intercellular spaces between endothelial cells (15).

On the basis of these assumptions, it follows that when the volume of interstitial fluid is in a steady state, the amounts filtered through the arterial ends of capillaries must equal the volumes taken up by venules and lymphatic vessels. It may be inferred that a hydrostatic difference exists between the pressure in the arterial end of the capillary and the pressure in the surrounding interstitial area. It is this pressure difference which presumably provides the force responsible for filtration of vascular fluid through the capillary wall. The above inferences are based on comparisons with events known to take place in other tissues. I am not aware of direct measurements of pressures within different kinds of testicular capillaries (14,15). What then creates the pressure gradient which drives the vascular filtrate into venules and lymphatics? In the classical laws of fluid exchange across the interstitial space formulated by Starling, the differences between the low protein concentrations in interstitial fluid and the high protein concentrations in blood would result in osmotic movement of fluid into the venous ends of capillaries. This, however, cannot account for fluid uptake by testicular venules or lymphatics because protein levels are so high in testicular interstitial fluid that the colloid osmotic pressure difference would be insufficient.

A remaining force for consideration is the tissue pressure within the tunica albuginea, generated by containment of tissue fluids and the mass of tubules within a relatively taut capsule. If the tissue pressure were very low, approaching zero, the interstitium would act as a sink for filtered vascular fluid, continuing to do so until the tissue pressure rose sufficiently to limit filtration at the arterial end of the capillary, and to favor fluid uptake at the venule end and by lymphatics. It has been well appreciated, at least since the time of de Graaf, that if a small incision is made in the testicular capsule, tubules and fluid immediately begin to seep out of the opening. Although the tissue pressure is thereby readily demonstrated to be greater than zero, the precise values in different regions of the testis do not appear to have been determined, and I have been unable to find published values. The prediction can be tested experimentally that if tissue pressure in the testis were increased with a suitable cuff, the interstitial fluid volume should decrease, and lymphatic uptake should increase. Lymph flow from testes of pigs has been observed to increase three-fold, in fact, when the spermatic venous pressure was increased (15).

From these general considerations, it follows that an understanding of the nature and modulation of volumes of testicular interstitial fluid during gonadal maturation or after various hormonal changes requires the following types of information:
1) The precise pressures inside testicular blood vessels, especially in the arterial and venous ends of "circumferential" capillaries present in testes of adult mammals (9,14,15).
2) The testicular interstitial tissue pressures in defined regions under various sets of physiological conditions.

Vasomotion occurs in blood vessels of mature testes, but not in those of immature gonads (4). The oscillating changes in pressure presumably reflect altered rates of blood flow. The onset of vasomotion during testicular development may be associated with the changes in the anatomy of the testis vasculature which take place around puberty (9,14). In any case, local pressure changes within vessels manifesting vasomotion are likely to be associated with pulsatile changes in pressure at the arterial ends of capillaries, thereby increasing net filtration during pressure peaks. Interestingly, hCG injection results in abolition of vasomotion (2,4), suggesting the possibility of a sustained, unchanging pressure.

Administration of high levels of hCG elicits the accumulation of increased levels of interstitial fluid in the testis (12). Lower levels of hCG, capable of augmenting androgen synthesis, do not increase the volume of testicular interstitial fluid (1). These data imply that the increases in interstitial fluid volume in the testis after injection of large amounts of hCG are not caused by increased levels of androgens. It is suggested that hCG may elicit an increase in permeability of testis blood vessels, perhaps in association with inflammatory reactions observed to follow the administration of large amounts of hCG (1,12). Polymorphonuclear leucocytes, which tend to accumulate in testicular blood vessels in the presence of high levels of hCG, are reported to penetrate blood vessel walls and migrate into the interstitium in testes of adult rats following hCG injection (2). It may be inferred, then, that the increase in testis interstitial fluid volume after hCG administration is a complex phenomenon, resulting perhaps from elevation of pressure in the arterial ends of capillaries, an increase in permeability across the capillary wall, or from a combination of both. Rates of blood flow, however, are reported to remain constant (1,2), even though vasomotion ceases (4).

In addition, consideration must be given to possible changes in tissue pressure following hCG administration. It has long been known that tubules in organ culture undergo rhythmic contractions, and that the presence of androgens augments these contractions (8,10). It therefore seems plausible that increased androgen levels would result in enhanced contractions by seminiferous tubules, from which it follows that hCG administration in vivo should have the same effect. Tubule contractions are postulated to generate increases in testis tissue pressure at discrete sites, thereby favoring the uptake of interstitial fluid into lymphatics and venules at these sites. Administration of androgen to intact adult rats, however, did not increase the interstitial volume in testis (2,12). In contrast, administration of androgens to rats depleted of Leydig cells did prevent the fall in interstitial volume which otherwise occurred several days after Leydig cell destruction (11).

Combined observations suggest that the hCG-induced increase in interstitial volume, which is dependent upon the presence of intact Leydig cells, may be mediated by actions of hCG to stimulate the synthesis of products other than androgens. Is it not possible that one or more of these other Leydig cell secretions might act on peritubular myoid cells to inhibit contractions, or to alter the coordinate responses of seminiferous tubules to androgen? Several potential candidates (pro-opiomelanocorticoids, activin, interleukin suppressing factor, etc) have been shown at this Workshop to be secreted by Leydig cells, and to be under hCG regulation. These products apparently are not required for the maintenance of spermatogenesis in adult rats deprived of Leydig cells, since replacement with androgens alone is sufficient for nearly normal rates of spermatogenesis (13), and also for maintaining interstitial volumes in the testis (11). However, various products of Leydig cells other than androgens might still play an important role in regulating the initial development of seminiferous tubules, and in the differentiation of peritubular myoid cells. Speculatively, hCG administration may result in the formation of a Leydig cell product other than androgens which impairs the coordinate contractions by peritubular myoid cells, thereby abolishing the "milking actions" of changing tissue pressures.

Peritubular myoid cells and Sertoli cells interact cooperatively in several ways to generate and maintain the cytoarchitecture of the seminiferous tubule. For example, basement membrane formation is most likely dependent upon metabolic cooperativity and upon initial direct contact between the two cell types (16,17). In addition, peritubular cells have been shown to secrete factors which stimulate various Sertoli cell functions (for reviews, see refs 5-7). A new possible function of peritubular cells, postulated in this presentation, remains to be tested. Although it is well appreciated that peritubular myoid cells are contractile (3,10), the possible functions of these contractions in the testis have remained conjectural. On the basis of points presented, I suggest that a local increase in tissue pressure, cause by coordinate tubule contractions mediated by peritubular myoid cells, results in increased uptake of tissue fluid by venules and lymphatics.

The hypothesis predicts that the interplay between levels of vascular filtration (perhaps influenced by vasomotion), and the uptake of interstitial fluid (mediated by local changes in tissue pressure) determines the net volume of interstitial fluid in the testis. If contractions were impaired, or if the tissue pressure were decreased, the hypothesis predicts that levels of interstitial volume in the testis would increase, simply because the high protein concentrations in interstitial fluid would prevent a sufficient colloid osmotic difference to drive fluid into lymphatics of venules. Does the administration of large amounts of hCG impair coordinate tubular contractions, somehow blocking the "milking action" of peritubular myoid cells?

SUMMARY

    The hypothesis was developed that coordinate contractions by peritubular myoid cells in seminiferous tubules create pressure gradients in the interstitium necessary for fluid exchange. Local increases in tissue pressure were postulated to favor the transport of interstitial fluid into the venules and lymphatic channels of the testis. Changes in tissue pressure would appear to be required because colloid osmotic differences are insufficient to drive fluid from the protein-rich interstitium into the vascular and lymphatic vessels. A physiological role for peritubular myoid cell contractions is thereby envisaged, namely to generate a "milking action" which would modulate the uptake of testis interstitial fluid, driving fluid in the vicinity of the contracting seminiferous tubule into the venous ends of capillaries and into lymphatic vessels at these sites. A corollary of this hypothesis was developed with respect to the actions of androgens which increase contractions of peritubular myoid cells and seminiferous tubules. It was postulated that androgens are required for maintenance of normal testis interstitial volumes because androgens are necessary for coordinate tubule contractions. Finally, the speculation was offered that hCG administration may increase testis interstitial fluid volumes by interfering with tubule contractions, presumably mediated via a Leydig cell product other than androgens.

REFERENCES

1. Bergh, A., Widmark, A., Damber, J-E., and Cajander, S. (1986): Endocrinol. 119:586-590.
2. Bergh, A. (1988): Testicular Microcirculation. This volume.
3. Clermont, Y. (1958): Exp. Cell Res. 15:438-440.
4. Damber, J-E., Bergh, A., and Widmark, A. (1988): This volume.
5. Fritz, I.B. (1978): Biochem. Actions of Hormones V:249-281.
6. Fritz, I.B. (1984): Les Editions de L'Inserm 123:15-54.
7. Fritz, I.B., and Tung, P.S. (1986): In: Gametogenesis and the Early Embryo (J. G. Gall, ed). N.Y: Alan R. Liss, Inc., pp. 151-173.
8. Hovatta, O. (1972): Z. Zellforsch 131:299-308.
9. Kormano, M. (1967): Z. Anat. Entwicklungsgesichte 126:138-153.
10. Kormano, M., and Hovatta, O. (1972): Z. Anat. Entwicklungsgesichte 137:239-248.
11. Maddocks, S., and Sharpe, R.M. (1988): This volume.
12. Sharpe, R.M. (1984): Biol. Reprod. 30:29-49.
13. Sharpe, R.M., Fraser, H.M., Cooper, I., and Ratnasooriya, W.D. (1988): This volume.
14. Setchell, B.P. (1970): Testicular blood supply, lymphatic drainage and secretion of fluid. In: The Testis (A.D. Johnson, W.R. Gomes and N.L. Vandemark, eds). N.Y.:Academic Press Vol. I: 101-239.
15. Setchell, B.P. (1978): The Mammalian Testis. London: Paul Elek pp. 50-76.
16. Tung, P.S., and Fritz, I.B. (1980): Biol. Reprod. 23:207-217.
17. Tung, P.S., and Fritz, I.B. (1987): Develop. Biol. 120:139-153.

Role of Arachidonic Acid Metabolites in Mediating the HCG-Induced Increases in Interstitial Fluid Volume in Rats

D.R.E. Abayasekara[1], L.O. Kurlak[1], B.A. Cooke[1],
J.Y. Jeremy[2], P. Dandona[2] and R.M. Sharpe[3]

[1]Dept. of Biochemistry,
[2]Dept of Chemical Pathology, Royal Free Hospital School of Medicine,
Rowland Hill St., London NW3 2PF;
[3]MRC Reproductive Biology Unit, Edinburgh

Introduction

Previous studies have shown that administration of hCG leads to an increase in interstitial fluid volume (IFV) within the testes (9,7,2). It has been suggested that this is due to an increase in capillary permeability. Recent reports have demonstrated that the increased IFV is preceded by intra vascular accumulation of polymorphonuclear leucocytes (PMNs) and migration of PMNs into the interstitial spaces (2,16). These changes are similar to vascular events associated with acute inflammation. Arachidonic acid metabolites .ie. prostaglandins (PGs) and leukotrienes (LTs) are known to be associated with these events (15). Furthermore it has been previously shown that hCG treatment **in vivo** leads to an increased production of leukotriene B_4 (LTB$_4$), prostaglandin F_2 (PGF$_{2\alpha}$) and prostaglandin E_2 (PGE$_2$) by isolated, purified Leydig cells **in vitro** (3,1). We have therefore investigated changes in levels of PG's and LT's in IF following hCG treatment **in vivo**.

Materials and Methods

Adult male rats were injected (a) s.c. with hCG (100 IU) and/or (b) intra-testicularly with indomethacin (300 ug) or (c) i.p. with ethane dimethyl sulphonate (EDS: 7.5 mg/100g body weight). Rats were killed at various intervals post treatment by cervical dislocation following inhalation anaesthesia. Testes were removed and IF was collected overnight at 4°C (10). IF was loaded onto a C_{18} Sep-Pak Cartridge (Waters Associates) in 10% methanol and Arachidonic acid metabolites were eluted in 100% methanol (11). The eluted sample was then evaporated to dryness under vacuum. LTB_4 (6), $PGF_{2\alpha}$ and PGE_2 (4) in extracts were measured by specific RIAs. Testosterone was measured by RIA prior to extraction (14).

Results

All results are expressed as mean + s.d. (n=5). HCG treatment led to an increase in IFV which was maximal 4h after treatment (table 1). A similar pattern of response was observed for increases in levels of testosterone and $PGF_{2\alpha}$. LTB_4 levels were found to be minimal at the time that $PGF_{2\alpha}$ levels were maximal. In a different series of experiments no significant increase in IFV was detected with any dose of hCG when rats were killed 16h after treatment. Testosterone and $PGF_{2\alpha}$ levels in IF were significantly increased by doses of hCG > 3 IU. Conversely LTB_4 levels were found to be significantly decreased following treatment with doses of hCG > 1 IU (fig.1).

EDS treatment caused a significant reduction in IFV and testosterone levels for up to 14 days post treatment. In contrast LTB_4 levels were unchanged over this period (fig.2).

The cyclooxygenase inhibitor indomethacin when given together with hCG increased IFV at 2h when $PGF_{2\alpha}$ levels were apparently decreased. HCG on its own increased IFV at 4h and at this time $PGF_{2\alpha}$ levels were markedly increased (table 2). LTB_4 measurements so far have proved inconclusive.

Discussion

The increase in IFV following hCG treatment observed in this study confirms several previous reports (9,7,2,16,10). It is interesting that LTB_4 levels in IF were found to be decreased following

Time after administration of hCG (hrs)	IFV (µl)	Testosterone (ng/ml)	LTB$_4$ (ng/ml)	PGF$_{2\alpha}$ (ng/ml)
0	66.8±4.3	645±179	3.95±1.54	6.74±0.61
2	101.2±5.9	2824±808	1.87±0.42	15.75±1.40
4	124.4±13.3	3051±716	1.01±0.29	280.50±40.20
8	116.0±21.0	2419±569	1.29±0.60	182.50±48.90
24	131.8±11.0	2364±401	2.13±1.24	10.55±2.60
48	90.3±10.6	1423±237	1.73±1.06	5.49±0.73
72	91.3±10.6	2004±340	2.56±0.15	4.20±2.30

TABLE 1 Time course of the effect of hCG (100 I.U.) on interstitial fluid volume (IFV) and IF-testosterone, LTB$_4$ and prostaglandins

Time after treatment (hrs)	Interstitial fluid Levels with hCG treatment			Interstitial fluid levels with hCG + Indomethacin treatment		
	Fluid volume (µl)	Testosterone (ng/ml)	PGF$_{2\alpha}$ (ng/ml)	Fluid volume/testis (µl)	Testosterone (ng/ml)	PGF$_{2\alpha}$ (ng/ml)
0	85.8±18	328±177	4.8±1.3	82.7±19	362±258	5.8±1.8
2	70.8±12	4498±760	3.8±1.2	116.8±15	2945±598	1.1±0.75
4	153.0±30	2000±514	39.4±12.6	167.0±29	1580±587	20.4±6.5
8	167.4±20	2819±348	31.3±9.2	163.0±10	2064±336	31.3±5.9

TABLE 2 Time course of the effect of hCG (100 I.U.) and/or indomethacin (300 ug) on interstitial fluid volume (IFV) and IF-testosterone and prostaglandins

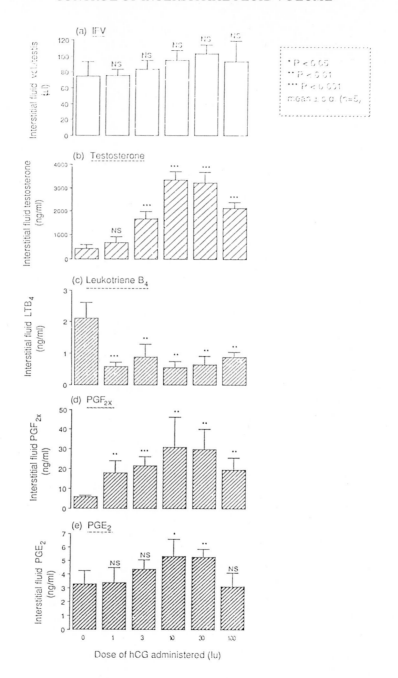

Figure 1 The effect of different doses of hCG (0-100 I.U.) on IFV, testosterone, LTB$_4$ and prostaglandins

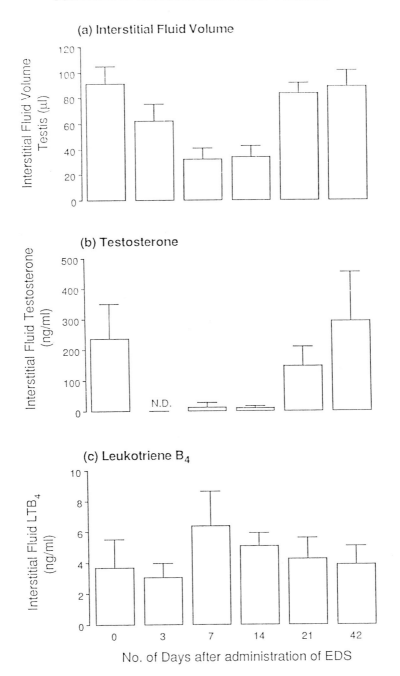

Figure 2 The time course of the effect of EDS (7.5 mg/100g body weight) on IFV, testosterone and LTB₄.

hCG treatment since it has been previously reported that Leydig cells **in vitro** produce significantly greater amounts of LTB_4 following hCG **in vivo** (1). No obvious explanation for this dichotomy is apparent at this time. The apparent lack of significant effect of different doses of hCG on IFV 16h post treatment may be explained by the variability within groups. EDS treament led to a significant decrease in IFV and testosterone levels in IF. This is in agreement with the suggestion that EDS treatment specifically destroys Leydig cells (5), and that Leydig cell products regulate the IFV (8). Since LTB_4 levels were unchanged following EDS treatment it is unlikely that LTB_4 is produced solely by Leydig cells within the testes and hence is unlikely to be the mediator of hCG-induced increases in IFV. Here we report for the first time dramatic increases in $PGF_{2\alpha}$ levels in IF following hCG treatment. The possibility that this change mediates the increases in IFV following hCG treatment was investigated using the cyclooxygenase inhibitor indomethacin. Indomethacin was found to have little or no effect on IFV in agreement with previous reports (12,13). However it is interesting to note that the inhibitory effect of indomethacin on prostaglandins was apparent only at the early time points. Previous studies (12,13) using indomethacin were conducted over much longer periods of time (14 and 24 hrs respectively) and although the present study confirms the conclusions of the aforementioned studies we have demonstrated that conclusions reached using inhibitors without measurement of the products need to be re-examined. From findings presented in this study we conclude that changes in levels of prostaglandins and leukotrienes do not appear to correlate with increases in IFV following hCG treatment **in vivo.**

Summary

Administration of hCG **in vivo** to rats has been shown to induce inflammatory like reactions in rat testes, the effect of hCG on potential mediators of these reactions - metabolites of arachidonic acid- have been measured in interstitial fluid (IF). HCG treatment significantly increased prostaglandin levels and decreased LTB_4 levels in IF. Ethane dimethyl sulphonate (EDS) treatment which specifically destroys Leydig cells significantly decreased interstitial fluid volume (IFV) without having any effect on LTB_4 levels. Indomethacin had little or no effect on IFV. These results suggest that arachidonic acid metabolites are not the primary mediators of the increases in IFV following hCG-treatment.

References

1) Abayasekara D.R.E., Kurlak L.O., Cooke B.A., Jeremy J.Y., Dandona P. and Sharpe R.M. (1987): J.Endocr.,(Suppl).115:Abst.No.33

2) Bergh A., Widmark A., Damber J.E. and Cajander S. (1986): Endocrinology.,119:586-590

3) Haour F., Kouznetzova B., Dray F. and Saez J.M. (1979): Life Sci.,24:2151-2158

4) Jeremy J.Y., Okonofua F.E., Thomas M., Wojdyla J., Smith W., Craft I.L and Dandona P. (1987): J.Clin.Endocrinol.Metab.,65:402-406

5) Molenaar R., de Rooij D.G., Rommerts F.F.G., Reuvers P.J. and Van der Molen H.J. (1985): Biol.Reprod.,33:1213-1218

6) Salmon J.A., Simmons P.M. and Palmer R.M.J. (1982): Prostaglandins., 24:225-235

7) Setchell B.P. & Sharpe R.M. (1981): J.Endocr.,91:245-254

8) Setchell B.P. and Rommerts F.F.G.(1985): Int.J.Androl.,8:436-440

9) Sharpe R.M.(1977):Biochem.Biophys.Res.Commun., 75:711-717

10) Sharpe R.M. and Cooper I.(1983): J.Reprod.Fert.,69:125-135

11) Shaw R.J., Cromwell O. and Kay A.B. (1984): Clin.Exp.Immunol.,56:716-722

12) Sowerbutts S.F., Jarvis L.G. and Setchell B.P.(1986): Aust.J.Exp.Biol.Med.,64: 137-147

13) Veijola M and Rajaniemi H (1985): Int.J.Androl.,8: 69-79

14) Verjans H.L., Cooke B.A., de Jong F.H.,
    de Jong C.M.M. and Van der Molen H.J. (1973):
    J.Steroid.Biochem.,4:665-676

15) Wedmore C.V. & Williams T.J. (1981):
    Nature.,289:646-650

16) Widmark A., Bergh A., Damber J.E. and
    Smedegard G. (1987): Mol.Cell.Endocrinol.,
    53:25-31

Regulatory of Interstitial Fluid Volume in the Rat Testis: A Role for the Seminiferous Tubules?

S. Maddocks and R.M. Sharpe

MRC Reproductive Biology Unit, Centre for Reproductive Biology, 37 Chalmers Street, Edinburgh EH3 9EW, Scotland, U.K.

INTRODUCTION

There is now considerable evidence that changes in vascular permeability and blood flow can alter interstitial fluid turnover in the testis (6,11), and that these parameters may be regulated from within the testis (6,11,16). Much of our current knowledge comes from studies using high doses of hCG or LH, the administration of which leads to a significant increase in vascular permeability and blood flow some 10-30 hours after injection (15,19,20). Because LH and hCG bind to receptors on the Leydig cell, and the observed responses are lost when the Leydig cells are destroyed with the toxin ethane dimethyl sulphonate (EDS;13), studies on paracrine control of the testicular vascular have focussed primarily on the interstitial region, and the Leydig cell as the likely source of any paracrine factors.

However, while the vascular network of the testis is confined to the interstitial region it is the seminiferous tubules that are the major user of most of the products transported into the testis, and it would therefore seem logical if the tubules, rather than the Leydig cells had an important controlling influence over the vasculature. There is already some evidence to this effect as testicular blood flow is correlated with the overall mass of seminiferous tubules (12).

As all blood-borne products must first pass into testicular interstitial fluid (IF) before they can gain access to the seminiferous tubules, it might be expected that the volume and rate of turnover of IF would also be under the control of the seminiferous tubules. This study assesses this possibility using a model system in which the Leydig cells of adult rats were destroyed with EDS, thus removing their possible influence on the vasculature, and the animals then supplemented with testosterone to assess the role of normal seminiferous tubule function.

MATERIALS AND METHODS

Animals

Adult male Sprague-Dawley rats (400-600 g) were maintained under standard conditions with food and water available ad libitum.

Treatments

Ethane dimethylsulphonate (EDS) was administered as a single intraperitoneal injection at a dose of 75 mg/kg bw in a solution of 1:3 DMSO:water (9).

Testosterone esters (Sustanon-250, Organon) were injected subcutaneously at a dose of 25 mg in 0.1 ml arachis oil every 3 days; a dose which has been shown previously to maintain spermatogenesis quantitatively in EDS-treated rats (18).

Protocol

Experiment 1
Seven groups of adult male rats (n=3 to 17) were injected with EDS. A control group (n=11) received DMSO vehicle. Three of the EDS-treated groups received testosterone replacement from the time of EDS administration. Groups of animals injected with EDS alone were killed at 3,6,12 and 21 days after EDS, and those receiving testosterone were killed at 6,12 and 21 days after EDS.

Experiment 2
In a second experiment, four groups of adult male rats (n=6) were used; one group of controls received no treatment, one group was injected with EDS on day 0, one group received testosterone by injection every 3 days beginning on day 0, and the fourth group were injected with EDS on day 0 and then given a single testosterone injection on day 6. All animals were killed on day 9.

In both experiments, animals were killed using carbon dioxide followed by cervical dislocation. Peripheral trunk blood was collected immediately and stored overnight at 4°C prior to centrifugation for serum collection. Both testes were removed and weighed, and interstitial fluid collected by drip-collection overnight at 4°C (16). Fluid from both testes was then pooled for each animal, the volume measured, and an aliquot diluted with medium 199 for subsequent hormone analysis as described previously (16,17). All samples were stored frozen at -20°C until assayed for testosterone and gonadotrophins.

Assays

Testosterone levels were measured in blood and interstitial fluid by radioimmunoassay as described previously (17). Serum levels of LH and FSH were measured by radioimmunoassay as described previously (3) using NIADDK kits.

RESULTS

Experiment 1

Figure 1 shows the interstitial fluid (IF) volumes recorded for animals in the first experiment. Following EDS administration only, testicular IF volume declined over time and was lowest at 12 days after treatment. Throughout this period, Leydig cells were absent from the testis. By 21 days however, Leydig cells have begun to regenerate, and IF volume had returned to control levels. In animals given EDS plus testosterone replacement from day 0, there was no reduction in IF volume, and levels remained at control values throughout the period of treatment.

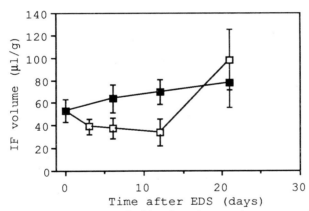

Fig. 1. Interstitial fluid volumes (Mean $\pm$ SD) in adult male rats treated with EDS (□) or EDS plus testosterone (■).

Testis weights showed a steady but significant (P< 0.05) decline after EDS treatment, which could be prevented with testosterone replacement (Table 1). Testosterone levels (Table 1) were similar to those obtained previously in EDS-treated rats given the same testosterone dose and in which spermatogenesis was maintained quantitatively (18).

Experiment 2

The results from this experiment are shown in Figure 2.

TABLE 1.   Testis weights, and serum and IF testosterone levels in rats treated with EDS plus/minus testosterone (T).

| Days after EDS | Testis weight (g) | | Testosterone (ng/ml) | | | |
| | | | Serum | | Interstitial fluid | |
	EDS	EDS+T	EDS	EDS+T	EDS	EDS+T
0	1.78+0.14 (11)		1.7+0.7 (11)		313+120* (11)	
3	1.59+0.13 (5)	n.d.	0.05 (5)	n.d.	2.5 (5)	n.d.
6	1.38+0.18 (5)	1.56+0.84 (8)	0.2+0.1 (5)	49+23 (8)	1.5 (5)	58+5 (6)
12	0.83+0.92 (3)	1.50+0.12 (6)	0.1 (3)	131+70 (6)	23+21 (3)	138+58 (6)
21	0.86+0.12 (6)	1.69+0.17 (17)	0.7+0.4 (6)	76+20 (17)	231+54* (6)	113+27 (17)

Values are Means+S.D. with the number of samples in brackets. n.d. : not determined. * : values are likely to be over-estimations of normal IF concentrations due to continued secretion of testosterone during collection of IF (see 6).

Following EDS treatment, IF volume declined as seen in the first experiment (see Fig. 1), and was significantly reduced by day 9 ($P < 0.01$). Furthermore, testosterone treatment from the time of EDS administration again maintained the IF volume at control levels. In animals given EDS on day 0, but in which testosterone replacement was not commenced until day 6, IF volume increased rapidly following testosterone injection to reach control levels within 3 days (day 9).

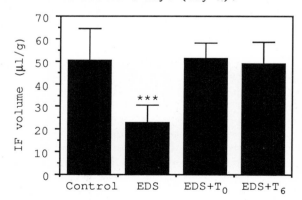

Fig. 2.   Testicular IF volumes in rats. Control: not treated, EDS: EDS on day 0, EDS+T_0: EDS on day 0 and testosterone every 3 days, EDS+T_6: EDS on day 0 and testosterone on day 6.

DISCUSSION

This study has demonstrated that androgens, but not Leydig cells, are required for maintenance of the interstitial fluid (IF) volume in the adult rat testis. How this is achieved remains to be determined, but the effect is probably mediated by the seminiferous tubules.

In the first experiment, treatment with EDS alone caused a significant reduction in IF volume up to 12 days after treatment (Fig. 1). Levels had returned to control values by 21 days in the absence of testosterone replacement. Leydig cells are destroyed within 3 days of EDS treatment and testosterone levels are undetectable at this time (1,4,5). That fluid volume did not reach minimum levels in this time, but took another 9 days to do so suggests that the Leydig cells are not involved in mediating this response. However, in the absence of androgen, the disruption of spermatogenesis and the decline in testis weight is much slower and is progressive between 6 and 21 days after EDS treatment (Table 1). This slow decrease parallels the decline in IF volume up to 12 days suggesting that it is the seminiferous tubules that are regulating IF volume. Beyond 9 days after EDS, Leydig cells begin to regenerate in the testis (4,5), and by 21 days are secreting large amounts of androgen; coincident with this change, the IF volume is returned to control levels. In the animals receiving testosterone from the time of EDS injection (Fig. 1), testicular IF volume was maintained at control levels throughout the period of study. With such treatment, Leydig cells do not repopulate the interstitium and spermatogenesis is not disrupted (1).

The second experiment was designed to test the response of the mechanism(s) involved to the presence of testosterone. By giving animals EDS alone for the first 6 days, testicular IF volume was allowed to reduce significantly in the absence of androgen, in parallel with testis weight (Fig. 2). Supplementation with testosterone at this time led to a dramatic increase in IF volume within the next 3 days, indicating the ability of the mechanisms involved in fluid regulation to respond rapidly to the presence of androgen. This time frame is now being examined in greater detail to further refine the time of the response. It is unlikely that there are any significant numbers of Leydig cells in the interstitial region at this time as no Leydig cells are present at 6 days after EDS treatment, and supplementation with this dose of testosterone is able to prevent Leydig cell regeneration completely over an extended period (1). It is therefore concluded that this data suggests further that the seminiferous tubules are mediating this response of testicular IF volume to testosterone.

The possibility that the seminiferous tubles are involved in an androgen-dependent regulation of the interstitial fluid volume is potentially significant for a number of reasons. As mentioned in the Introduction, testicular blood flow appears to be correlated with the mass of seminiferous tubules (12), although no physiological basis for this has been reported. Furthermore, there are few known specific actions of testosterone on the seminiferous tubules, despite the knowledge that testosterone is required for maintenance of spermatogenesis (2,10). Finally, recent evidence suggests that changes in blood flow and/or vascular permeability in the testis can affect the concentration of testosterone in teaticular IF and its distribution between IF and blood, and this is particularly evident in testes in which spermatogenesis has been disrupted experimentally (6,7,8).

Paracrine events in the testis remain an obviously important, but largely unknown, entity. In this study we have presented further evidence that such control extends to the vasculature of the testis.

ACKNOWLEDGEMENTS

The authors are grateful to the NIADDK for LH and FSH radioimmunoassay kits, to Dr. R.W. Kelly for synthesizing EDS, and to Denis Doogan, Jan Speed and Irene Cooper for skilled help. SM is a Sir Robert Menzies Memorial Scholar in Medicine.

REFERENCES

1. Bartlett, J.M.S., Kerr, J.B. and Sharpe, R.M. (1988): J. Androl., 9:31-40.
2. Cunningham, G.R. and Huckins, C. (1979): Endocrinology, 105:177-186.
3. Fraser, H.M. and Sandow, J. (1977): J. Endocr. 74:291-296.
4. Kerr, J.B., Donachie, K. and Rommerts, F.F.G. (1985): Cell Tissue Res., 242:145- 156.
5. Kerr, J.B., Bartlett, J.M.S., Donachie, K. and Sharpe, R.M. (1987): Cell Tissue Res., 249:367-377.
6. Maddocks, S. and Setchell, B.P. (1988): Ox. Rev. Reprod. Biol. 10:in press.
7. Maddocks, S., Zupp, J.L. and Setchell, B.P. (1987): Society for the Study of Fertility, Winter meeting, University of Reading, abstr. 13.
8. Maddocks, S., Zupp, J.L., Sowerbutts, S.F. and Setchell, B.P. (1987): Proc. Aust. Soc. Reprod. Biol. 19:85.
9. Molenaar, R., Rooij, D.G., Rommerts, F.F.G., Reuvers, P.J., and van der Molen, H.J. (1985): Biol. Reprod., 33:1213-1222.
10. Russell, L.D. and Clermont, Y. (1977): Anat. Rec., 187:347-366.

11. Setchell, B.P. (1986): Aust. J. Biol. Sci., 36:285-293.
12. Setchell, B.P. and Galil, K.A.A. (1983): Aust. J. Biol. Sci., 36:285-293.
13. Setchell, B.P. and Rommerts, F.F.G. (1985): Int. J. Androl., 8:436-440.
14. Setchell, B.P. and Sharpe, R.M. (1981): J. Endocr., 91:245-254.
15. Sharpe, R.M. (1979): J. Reprod. Fert., 55:365-371.
16. Sharpe, R.M. (1983). Qrt. J. Exp. Physiol., 68:265-287.
17. Sharpe, R.M. and Cooper, I. (1983): J. Reprod. Fert., 69:125-135.
18. Sharpe, R.M., Donachie, K. and Cooper, I. (1988): J. Endocr., 117:19-26.
19. Sowerbutts, S.F., Jarvis, L.G. and Setchell, B.P. (1986): Aust. J. Exp. Biol. Med. Sci., 64: 137-147.
20. Widmark, A., Damber, J.E. and Bergh, A. (1986): J. Endocr., 109:419-425.

Effect of Neurotransmitters and Lymphatic-Vascular Transfer of Prostaglandin $F_{2\alpha}$ on Ovarian Blood Flow and Hormone Secretion

R.B. Heap, A.J. Davis, I.R. Fleet, J.A. Goode, M.H. Hamon and A.P.F. Flint

*A.F.R.C. Institute of Animal Physiology and Genetics Research
Babraham, Cambridge CB2 AT*

INTRODUCTION

The local effect of the uterus on ovarian function in certain species is most clearly exemplified by the uterine luteolysin, prostaglandin $F_{2\alpha}$ ($PGF_{2\alpha}$; 11). Produced by the uterus, $PGF_{2\alpha}$ is transferred by a countercurrent mechanism from the uterine vein into the adjacent ovarian artery and thence to the ipsilateral ovary where it is believed to exert a destructive role in bringing about the demise of the corpus luteum (15). Evidence for the local vascular transfer of $PGF_{2\alpha}$ clarified the findings of earlier studies that revealed the importance of the uterus in the regulation of ovarian cyclicity, and provided an explanation of the original reports that hysterectomy in certain, though not all species, prolongs the life-span of the corpus luteum (4). One exception is to be found in the human female in which hysterectomy fails to extend the life-span of the corpus luteum or disrupt the duration of the menstrual cycle (4). Nonetheless the vascular disposition of ovarian vessels in the human female is characterised by a remarkably tortuous ovarian artery which is closely associated with the ovarian and utero-ovarian vein, a feature recorded by Blancardi (5,6) as early as 1687. This vascular arrangement is encountered in several mammalian species including those in which the local transfer of $PGF_{2\alpha}$ from the utero-ovarian vein to ovarian artery has been shown to play a major role in the regulation of ovarian function, as in sheep and pigs (9).

The lymphatic vessels form an important second tubular system in addition to the blood vessels. Present in all vertebrates except agnatha and cartilagenous fishes, the lymphatic vessels start as delicate lymph capillaries, which are closed at one end. They permit the trans- and inter-endothelial transfer of fluids and other substances from the tissue spaces to the lumen of the

vessel. Fluid passes into the lumen of lymph capillaries which
join to form complex networks opening into conducting vessels,
transport vessels and finally collecting ducts before terminating
in the lymphovenous connection of the thoracic duct (19). Lymph
capillaries have a greater permeability potential than blood
capillaries because the former have an incomplete or absent basal
membrane. The wall of lymphatic vessels is permeable to substances of small molecular weight to a limited degree leading to
a further concentration of the lymph when it travels a long dis-
tance from the peripheral region to the lymphovenous connection
of the thoracic duct.

Disposition of the lymphatic network in relation to ovarian vasculature

In 1966 Morris and Sass (18) showed that a profuse network of
lymphatics develops within the corpus luteum of the sheep during
the luteal phase of the oestrous cycle (approximately 16 days
duration) and in early pregnancy (approximately 148 days). These
lymphatics join in the subovarian plexus to form a variable
number of transport vessels (4 to 12) which drain from the ovary
and are joined by lymphatics from the proximal half of the oviduct. The lymphatics which drain the ovary are mainly associated
with the utero-ovarian vascular pedicle and, because the active
corpus luteum has a high lymph flow (14) these ducts are much
enlarged during the luteal phase and pregnancy.
Although earlier studies found little evidence for connections
between the lymphatics draining the ovary and those draining the
uterus itself, this subject has been re-examined (20). The
injection of small quantities (100 μl) of Evans Blue (0.5% in
0.9% NaCl) into the proximal half of a uterine horn revealed
lymphatics that drained towards the utero-ovarian pedicle where
they collected into at least two main vessels (Figure 1). Subsequent injection of Evans Blue into a corpus luteum of the adjacent ovary revealed an additional series of lymphatics which
frequently converged with, or ran in parallel to the uterine
lymphatic vessels. Connections between uterine and ovarian
lymphatics, visualised by dyes of different colour injected into
the ovary and uterus simultaneously, occurred almost exclusively
along the distal two-thirds of the pedicle before reaching the
lumbo-aortic node. There was a remarkably close apposition of
this network of lymphatic vessels with the ovarian artery (Figure
1). Anastomoses between lymphatics of ovarian and uterine origin
were observed in all animals studied but there was no evidence
for retrograde flow within uterine, ovarian or utero-ovarian
lymphatics (Figure 2). Whereas the lymphatic drainage in the
broad ligament was confined to one side, occasionally lymphatics
were observed that crossed to the opposite side and joined utero-
ovarian lymphatics that drained from the contralateral ovary and
uterus.

(a)

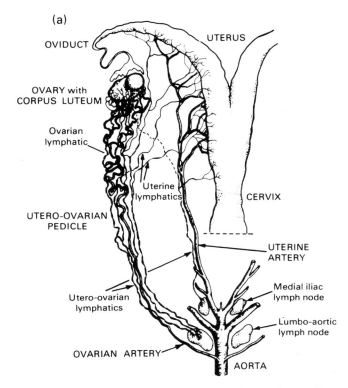

FIG. 1. Composite drawing showing the major pathways in sheep of lymphatic drainage from the ovary and uterus along the utero–ovarian pedicle to the lumbo-aortic node(s) and beside the uterine artery to the medial iliac lymph node(s). The interconnections between uterine and ovarian ducts to form the utero-ovarian lymphatic network are shown and also the connection (broken line) between an ovarian and uterine lymphatic parallel to the uterine artery. Valves in the lymphatic vessels are indicated as irregular narrowing of the black lines while the ovarian and uterine arterial supplies are shown as shaded ducts. The uterus is shown reflected about the broken line near the cervix to allow for clearer portrayal of the lymphatic and vascular pathways (20). Reproduced with permission of Journals of Reproduction and Fertility Ltd.

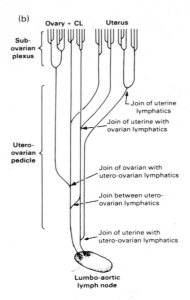

FIG. 2. Schematic diagram showing the anastomoses which have been observed between ovarian, uterine and utero-ovarian lymphatics along the utero-ovarian pedicle (20). Reproduced with permission of Journals of Reproduction and Fertility Ltd.

Lymph flow and composition

Afferent lymph was collected continuously from a utero-ovarian lymphatic located in the vascular pedicle. A lymphatic was cannulated surgically at mid-ventral laparotomy and the catheter exteriorised to enable collections to be made from conscious animals during early pregnancy. The results (Table 1) showed that lymph in the utero-ovarian network had a low number of leucocytes and a high concentration of protein being about 78-86% of plasma values, confirming earlier reports (18), and consistent with the highly permeable nature of the vessels of the corpus luteum (14). Similar results were also obtained in uterine lymph collected from a sheep between days 16 and 20 of pregnancy. Electrolytes in utero-ovarian lymph were similar to those in plasma with respect to K, but were consistently higher for Na and lower for Cl, though the Na/K ratio was not different. The most striking feature was the high concentration of progesterone in utero-ovarian lymph which, when corrected for lymph flow and a maximum of 12 draining lymphatics, accounted for less than 10% of

TABLE 1. The flow rate and composition of lymph recovered from a single lymphatic vessel in the utero–ovarian vascular pedicle adjacent to the ovary containing a corpus luteum in six pregnant sheep (between days 15 to 31 after mating) (20).

Variable	Lymph	Plasma (peripheral)	Difference
Flow (ml/h)	2.9±0.6	–	–
Leucocytes (per mm^3)	171±47	–	–
Na (mM)	149.5±1.4	138.8±2.3	P<0.001
K (mM)	4.26±0.13	4.11±0.19	N.S.
Na/K	35.5±1.2	34.7±1.6	N.S.
Cl (mM)	101.2±1.2	104.2±0.7	P<0.05
Protein (mg/ml)	74.9±3.1	87.0±3.4	P<0.05
Progesterone (nM)	1531±621	5.2±0.7	P<0.0001

the estimated daily production of ovarian progesterone. Uterine lymph, in contrast, contained a progesterone concentration similar to that in peripheral plasma. Regarding lymph flow and composition in utero–ovarian lymph, similar results were obtained in a goat except that flow rate was somewhat greater (20).

Sequential changes in the concentration of prostaglandins and steroids in uterine lymph of sheep have been determined during the oestrous cycle (1,2). The results showed that the concentrations of progesterone resembled those in peripheral plasma, though those of oestradiol-17β were inexplicably higher than those found in plasma at comparable stages of the oestrous cycle. Prostaglandin $F_{2\alpha}$ ($PGF_{2\alpha}$) showed episodic fluctuations in concentration, unlike prostaglandin E_2. The values of $PGF_{2\alpha}$ in uterine lymph increased to concentrations of about 4 ng/ml prior to the onset of luteal regression, and these levels were comparable to those obtained in uterine vein plasma at a similar time in the oestrous cycle (17). These findings, together with those already described concerning the close association of the utero–ovarian lymphatic network with the utero–ovarian vein and the ovarian artery, are consistent with the idea of a lymphatic–vascular exchange system whereby uterine $PGF_{2\alpha}$ is locally transferred to the adjacent corpus luteum to facilitate the process of luteal regression. Evidence for the lymphatic–vascular transfer of certain compounds was therefore examined.

Lymphatic–vascular transfer of $PGF_{2\alpha}$

Consideration of the disposition of the utero–ovarian lymphatic network in relation to the utero–ovarian vein and ovarian artery revealed the possibility that transfer may occur by concurrent and/or countercurrent routes, respectively. To test this

hypothesis experiments in sheep were carried out under pentobarbitone anaesthesia.

In a first series of experiments [^{3}H]PGF$_{2\alpha}$ was injected into
the uterine lumen of non–pregnant animals 7–15 days after
oestrus. Labelled PGF$_{2\alpha}$ was recovered in uterine lymph at an
increasing rate after a lag of about 20 minutes. Radioactivity
remained high for at least 60 min whereas that in uterine vein
plasma reached peak values within 20 min of the injection and
then declined. Both PGF$_{2\alpha}$ and 13,14–dihydro–15–keto prostaglandin F$_{2\alpha}$ were recovered from uterine lymph and utero–ovarian
vein plasma (10). The results of these experiments show that
uterine PGF$_{2\alpha}$ is readily transferred into uterine lymph and that
its concentration remains high, probably on account of the low
flow rate. These findings indicate that a concentration gradient
would exist between uterine lymph and ovarian artery plasma in
respect of PGF$_{2\alpha}$ particularly during the latter part of the
oestrous cycle when uterine secretion of PGF$_{2\alpha}$ is increased. The
lack of such a marked gradient between uterine lymph and the
utero–ovarian vein at this time has been noted above.

In a second series of experiments [^{3}H]PGF$_{2\alpha}$ was infused at a
constant rate either into a uterine lymphatic or a uterine vein
to compare its quantitative transfer into the ovarian vasculature. Details of the surgical preparation are shown in Figure 3.
The transfer was quantified in blood samples taken downstream
from a catheter in the utero–ovarian vein (lymphatic to utero-
ovarian vein transfer) and upstream from an ovarian vein in the
sub–ovarian plexus within 2 cm of the ovarian hilus (lymphatic to
ovarian vein transfer). Samples were taken from the ovarian vein
rather than ovarian artery to avoid disturbance of ovarian
haemodynamics and to enable measurements of ovarian tissue
concentrations of labelled PGF$_{2\alpha}$ at the end of the experiment.

[^{3}H]PGF$_{2\alpha}$ was infused into a uterine lymphatic at a constant
rate and produced a maximum concentration of radioactivity which
was 5.6– and 1.7–fold higher in the adjacent utero–ovarian and
ovarian vein, respectively, than in carotid artery plasma. Chromatography of plasma extracts showed that [^{3}H]PGF$_{2\alpha}$ accounted for
61.3, 60.6 and 30.8% of the total activity in ovarian vein,
uterine vein and carotid artery plasma. Estimations of the
amount of infusate transferred from a lymphatic into ovarian vein
blood gave a value (0.4%) similar to that for transfer from a
uterine vein (0.3%), the latter figure being similar to that
reported by Land et al., 1976 (12) but lower than that of
McCracken et al., 1981 (17). From Figure 4 it can be seen that
transfer from a uterine lymphatic into the adjacent utero–ovarian
vein precedes that which occurs into ovarian vasculature and that
in both instances there is a relatively slow transfer during the
first 15 minutes of the infusion followed by a more rapid process. This aspect will be considered in more detail in the next
section.

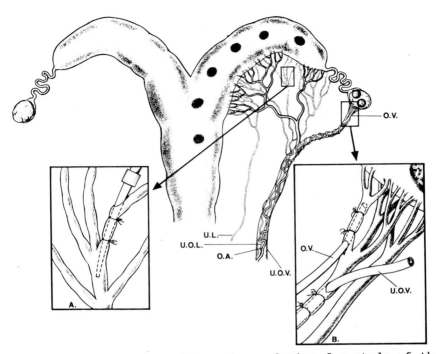

FIG. 3. Diagram to show sites of cannulation for study of the transfer of [³H]prostaglandin $F_{2\alpha}$ from a uterine lymphatic into the adjacent ovarian vasculature. Evans Blue was injected into the myometrial layer at 6 different sites along the length of the uterine horn (shaded). A tapered catheter was inserted into a uterine lymphatic vessel (A), or into a uterine vein in a similar region. Blood samples were taken from a catheter placed into an ovarian vein (O.V.) in a retrograde direction (B), and from a second catheter placed in the same ovarian vein and inserted 8–10 cm to lie downstream in the utero–ovarian vein (U.O.V.). U.L., uterine lymphatic; U.O.L., utero–ovarian afferent lymphatic; O.A., ovarian artery; U.O.V., utero–ovarian vein (10). Reproduced with permission of Journals of Reproduction and Fertility Ltd.

Further evidence for the local transfer of $PGF_{2\alpha}$ from a uterine lymphatic into the adjacent ovarian vasculature was provided by the presence of significantly higher concentrations of ³H-labelled compounds in the ovary and corpus luteum adjacent to the site of intra–lymphatic infusion compared with those in the opposite organs. The concentrations in the adjacent ovary and corpus luteum were significantly greater when an intra–lymphatic rather than intra–uterine vein infusion was adopted (Figure 5). Furthermore, ³H-labelled compounds were concentrated in the uterine portion of the oviduct rather than in the middle

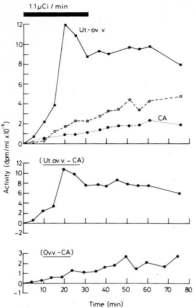

FIG. 4. Rate of occurrence of ^{3}H-labelled
compound in the adjacent utero-ovarian
vein and ovarian vein after infusion of
[3H]PGF$_{2\alpha}$ (1.1 μCi/min) into a uterine
afferent lymphatic (black bar) in Sheep
H351, 15 days after oestrus. Top; concentration of radioactivity in the adjacent
utero-ovarian (solid line) and ovarian
vein (dashed line) and carotid arterial
plasma (dotted line): middle; veno-
arterial difference across the adjacent
uterine horn and ovary (utero-ovarian
vein - carotid artery): lower; veno-
arterial difference across the adjacent
ovary (ovarian vein - carotid artery)
(10). Reproduced with permission of
Journals of Reproduction and Fertility
Ltd.

or proximal regions after an intra-lymphatic infusion, but not
after an intra-uterine vein infusion (Figure 6). This is
consistent with the proposal that there is an additional pathway
for PGF$_{2\alpha}$ transport involving oviducal vessels (3). According to
this suggestion, labelled PGF$_{2\alpha}$ infused into a uterine lymphatic
would diffuse into adjacent arterial branches supplying initially
the distal and middle segments of the oviduct.

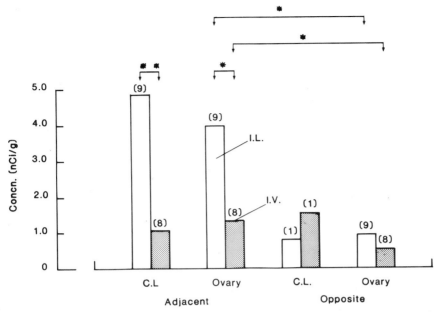

FIG. 5. Transfer of [^{3}H]prostaglandin F$_{2\alpha}$ from a uterine lymphatic vessel (I.L.) or from a uterine vein (I.V.) into the adjacent and opposite ovary or corpus luteum (C.L.) in sheep 8–15 days after ovulation (10). *, P < 0.05; **, P < 0.01.

Mechanisms of transfer

As indicated above, transfer from a lymphatic vessel into the adjacent ovarian vasculature may be achieved by countercurrent (lymphatic to ovarian artery) or concurrent (lymphatic to utero-ovarian vein) diffusion. The kinetics of transfer indicate that the occurrence of radioactivity in utero–ovarian vein blood precedes that in the ovarian vein by about 10 min and exceeds it in concentration by 2- to 3-fold (Figure 4). However, uptake by ovarian tissues may have obscured the rate of transfer in the initial stages so that the question of whether there is a two-stage (lymphatic → utero–ovarian vein → ovarian artery) or one-stage transfer (lymphatic → ovarian artery) cannot be answered conclusively from these data. Evidence from several studies implies that diffusion down a concentration gradient plays an important part in the transfer process, though proof of the nature of this pathway is lacking. Countercurrent transfer from the utero–ovarian vein to the ovarian artery has been reported not only for PGF$_{2\alpha}$ but also for xenon and krypton, and between

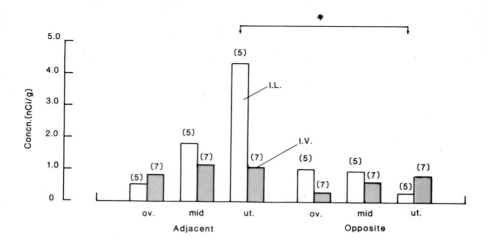

FIG. 6. Transfer of [³H]prostaglandin F$_{2\alpha}$ from a uterine lymphatic vessel (I.L.) or from a uterine vein (I.V.) into the oviduct (ut., uterine segment; mid., middle segment; ov., ovarian segment) in sheep 8–15 days after ovulation (10). * P < 0.05.

the ovarian or uterine vein and the ovarian artery for progesterone. In the male a similar transfer between the spermatic vein and artery has been reported for heat, xenon, krypton, testosterone and tritiated water. Moreover, steroid transfer in the ovarian vascular pedicle is related to lipid solubility, less polar steroids being transferred more rapidly than their hydroxylated counterparts (16).

Whereas the transfer of gas through the walls of the vascular pedicle occurs very readily, steroid hormones and small peptides such as relaxin and oxytocin take several minutes. With PGF$_{2\alpha}$ there is an initial delay of about 15 min (Figure 4) and in male rhesus monkeys testosterone was transferred only when the endogenous concentration reached high values (16).

To investigate the pathways of transfer, we have infused [³H]PGF$_{2\alpha}$, [¹⁴C]mannitol and [³⁶Cl]Na simultaneously into a uterine lymphatic and determined their appearance in uteroovarian vein blood and ovarian vein blood. In an experiment carried out at day 15 of the oestrous cycle the concentration of

[^{3}H]PGF$_{2\alpha}$ in utero–ovarian vein plasma reached a maximum at 70 min, and [^{14}C]mannitol and [^{36}Cl]Na at 45 min after the start of a constant infusion (which lasted 58 min) (Figure 7). The results of several experiments carried out in the second half of the luteal phase show that the rate of transfer of these three compounds follows the sequence [^{36}Cl]Na > [^{14}C]mannitol > [^{3}H]PGF$_{2\alpha}$. A similar sequence of transfer was observed between the uterine lymphatic and the ovarian vein in the subovarian plexus, though accurate values were difficult to obtain unless indomethacin (170 μg/min into the dorsal aorta at the origin of the ovarian arteries) was infused simultaneously. This dose level increased the amount of labelled compounds transferred into the ovarian vasculature.

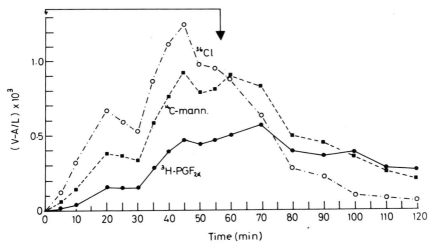

FIG. 7. Transfer of [^{35}Cl]Na, [^{14}C]mannitol and [^{3}H]prostaglandin F$_{2\alpha}$ from a uterine lymphatic (infused at a constant rate, 4.1 ml/h) into the adjacent utero–ovarian vein of a non–pregnant anaesthetised sheep at day 15 of the oestrous cycle. The arrows denote the duration of the infusion and the amount transferred is expressed as the utero–ovarian vein concentration minus arterial concentration divided by the estimated concentration in the uterine lymphatic.

The results show that three radiolabelled compounds of different molecular weight (NaCl, 58; mannitol, 182; PGF$_{2\alpha}$, 354) and hydrophobicity were transferred from an afferent lymphatic vessel into adjacent blood vessels. The fact that they are transferred at different rates shows that transfer is not achieved by local interconnecting channels, and that these afferent conducting lymphatics are differentially permeable to small molecules.

Transfer of small molecules across lymphatics with their open and closed endothelial junctions is not unexpected, but transfer

across an adjacent vein or artery wall is more difficult to
envisage. Passive diffusion down a concentration gradient via
interstitial fluid is the most probable interpretation for the
transfer of mannitol (an extra-cellular marker) whereas diffusion
across cell membranes would occur with Cl and possibly $PGF_{2\alpha}$.
The results also show that transfer occurs between lymphatic and
blood vessels whether the direction of flow in the two vessels is
concurrent or countercurrent. Transfer is presumably facilitated
by the difference in flow rate of at least 100-fold between a
lymphatic and its adjacent blood vessel, together with the large
surface area of the tortuous lymphatic in close proximity to the
ovarian artery and utero-ovarian vein. The question to be considered next is whether such transfer has an effect on ovarian
function.

Ovarian response to lymphatic-vascular transfer

Earlier studies demonstrated that cloprostenol, a synthetic
analogue of $PGF_{2\alpha}$, will cause the rapid release of oxytocin from
the ovary of sheep containing a corpus luteum (7). The question
we have to consider is whether intra-lymphatic $PGF_{2\alpha}$ is capable
of affecting the release of ovarian oxytocin.

Close-arterial infusion of $PGF_{2\alpha}$ into the dorsal aorta through
a femoral artery catheter placed close to the origin of the
ovarian artery stimulated the rapid release of ovarian oxytocin.
$PGF_{2\alpha}$ was infused at a constant rate of 17 and 170 ng/min (estimated concentration, in the ovarian artery 23 and 230 pg/ml) for
5 min. Furthermore, infusion of $PGF_{2\alpha}$ into a uterine lymphatic
(28 ng/min) was found to stimulate the release of oxytocin from
the adjacent ovary (Figure 8). Peak concentrations of oxytocin
in the ovarian vein were reached by 50 min after the start of
infusion and they remained high for a further 10 min after the
infusion was stopped. The results show that the transfer of
$PGF_{2\alpha}$ from a uterine lymphatic into ovarian vasculature facili-
tates the release of ovarian oxytocin from the corpus luteum.
Increased concentrations of $PGF_{2\alpha}$ occur episodically in uterine
lymph after day 10 of the oestrous cycle in sheep (1,2), so that
the close association of lymphatics and ovarian vasculature may
have an important functional role in luteal regression. The
enhanced pulsatile release of ovarian oxytocin from day 12
onwards is believed to increase the pulsatile secretion of luteal
$PGF_{2\alpha}$ which, by means of a positive feedback mechanism (8) drives
luteolysis to its completion.

Intra-lymphatic $PGF_{2\alpha}$ infusions have been found to cause the
simultaneous release of oxytocin from the opposite ovary containing a corpus luteum implying that the effects are not confined to the adjacent ovary and its vascular pedicle. Colour
lymphography has revealed that certain uterine lymphatics

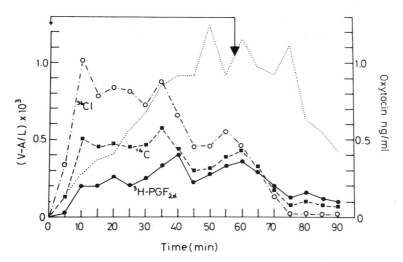

FIG. 8. Transfer of [^{36}Cl]Na, [^{14}C]mannitol and [^{3}H]prostaglandin F$_{2\alpha}$ from a uterine lymphatic (infused at a constant rate, 4.1 ml/h) into the adjacent utero-ovarian vein of a non-pregnant anaesthetised sheep at day 14 of the oestrous cycle. The arrows denote the duration of the infusion and the amount transferred is expressed as the utero-ovarian vein concentration minus arterial concentration divided by the estimated concentration in the uterine lymphatic. Concentration of oxytocin in ovarian vein plasma is shown by the dotted line.

traverse the broad ligament to reach the uterine vasculature on the opposite side. However, the disposition of these lymphatics relative to the contralateral vascular pedicle and the slow rate of lymph flow which would be expected to give a delayed response from the contralateral ovary suggest that alternative mechanisms should be sought to elucidate the functional interactions between uterine lymphatics and ovarian vasculature in respect of PGF$_{2\alpha}$-induced oxytocin release.

Results of experiments in which neurotransmitters were infused into the dorsal aorta via a femoral artery catheter placed close to the origin of the ovarian arteries showed that both noradrenaline and acetylcholine elicited a rapid release of ovarian oxytocin. Dose response curves gave a near maximum response in terms of oxytocin concentration in ovarian vein plasma at 7×10^{-8} and 1.1×10^{-5} mol/min for noradrenaline and acetylcholine, respectively (Table 2). Both neurotransmitters produced a marked vasoconstriction at these doses when ovarian blood flow was monitored by an ultrasonic flow probe located around the ovarian artery (Transonics Systems, Inc., New York; Table 2). Ovarian vasoconstriction was related to the expected hypertensive effect of noradrenaline, but with acetylcholine it resulted from a marked fall in blood pressure which, when blocked by atropine, revealed

TABLE 2. Effect of neurotransmitters on ovarian oxytocin release
and ovarian blood flow in anaesthetised sheep 8 to 10 days after
ovulation.*

Treatment	Oxytocin		Ovarian blood flow	
	Ovarian vein conc. before treatment (pg/ml)	Maximum fold increase after treatment	Blood flow before treatment (ml/min)	% change after treatment
Noradrenaline (7×10^{-8} mol/min)	203 ± 51	24.7 ± 6.0 (4)	14.3 ± 3.8	-21.9 ± 0.3 (5)
Acetylcholine (1.1×10^{-5} mol/min)	219 ± 68	61.2 ± 20.3 (3)	21.6 ± 6.1	-38.4 ± 5.6 (6)

*Animals were superovulated and had an average number of corpora
lutea of 4.6 ± 0.3.   When corpora lutea were present on both
ovaries the mean of the two values was used. After infusion of
neurotransmitter into the dorsal aorta close to the origin of the
ovarian arteries, ovarian vein blood samples were taken at 2.5,
5.0, 10 and 15 minutes. Ovarian blood flow was monitored by an
ultrasonics flow probe placed around an ovarian artery to provide
continuous flow recordings.

the expected cholinergic vasodilatation. It should be noted that
the neurotransmitter concentration reaching the ovary was reduced
by nearly three orders of magnitude (measured by a dye dilution
method) compared with that infused into the dorsal aorta.   In
addition acetylcholine is rapidly metabolised in blood such that
luteal cells would be exposed to very low concentrations.   The
results show that the sheep corpus luteum is sensitive to noradrenaline and acetylcholine both in terms of its vascular
response and oxytocin release. Our findings differ from those of
recent studies on cultured bovine granulosa cells in that whereas
catecholamines stimulated oxytocin secretion in vitro, acetylcholine was without effect (13). This may mean that acetylcholine brings about its effect in vivo by an indirect mechanism
and work is in progress to investigate the role of neural pathways in the bilateral release of ovarian oxytocin in response to
a unilateral intra-lymphatic infusion of $PGF_{2\alpha}$.

References

1. Abdel Rahim, S.E.A., Bland, K.P., and Poyser, N.L. (1983): Prostaglandins Leuk. and Med., 10:157–161.
2. Abdel Rahim, S.E.A., Bland, K.P., and Poyser, N.L. (1984): Prostaglandins Leuk. and Med., 14:403–410.
3. Alwachi, S.N., Bland, K.P., and Poyser, N.L. (1981): J. Reprod. Fert., 61:197–200.
4. Anderson, L.L. (1973): In: Handbook of Physiology, Section 7 Endocrinology, vol. II, part 2, edited by R.O. Greep and E.B. Astwood, pp. 69–86. American Physiological Society, Washington D.C.
5. Bendz, A. (1982): Prostaglandins, 13:355–362.
6. Blandcardi, S. (1687): Anatomia Reformata. Joannemten Hoorn, Amstelodami.
7. Flint, A.P.F., and Sheldrick, E.L. (1982): Nature, Lond. 297:587–588.
8. Flint, A.P.F., and Sheldrick, E.L. (1986): J. Reprod. Fert. 76:831–839.
9. Ginther, O. (1976): Vet Scope (Kalamazoo), 20:1–17.
10. Heap, R.B., Fleet, I.R., and Hamon, M. (1985): J. Reprod. Fert. 74:645–656.
11. Horton, E.W., and Poyser, N.L. (1976): Physiol. Rev., 56:595–651.
12. Land, R.B., Baird, D.T., and Scaramuzzi, R.J. (1976): J. Reprod. Fert., 47:209–214.
13. Luck, M.R., and Jungclas, B. (1987): J. Endocr. 114:423–430.
14. Lindner, H.R., Sass, M.B., and Morris, B. (1964): J. Endocr. 30:361–376.
15. McCracken, J.A., Carlson, J.C., Glew, M.F., Goding, J.R., Baird, D.T., Green, K., and Samuelsson, B. (1972): Nature New Biol., 238:129–134.
16. McCracken, J.A., Schramm, W., and Einer-Jensen, N. (1984): Steroids, 43:293–303.
17. McCracken, J.A., Schramm, W., Barcikowski, B., and Wilson, L. Jnr. (1981): Acta Vet. scand., Suppl. 77:71–88.
18. Morris, B., and Sass, M.B. (1966): Proc. Roy. Soc. B. 164:577–591.
19. Schummer, A., Wilkens, H., Vollmerhaus, B., and Habermehl, K.H. (1981): In: The Circulatory System, the Skin, and the Cutaneous Organs of the Domestic Mammals, pp. 292–308. Verlag Paul Parry, Berlin.
20. Staples, L.D., Fleet, I.R., and Heap, R.B. (1982): J. Reprod. Fert., 64:409–420.

The Fate of Fetal Leydig Cells in the Developing Rat Testis

J.B. Kerr

Department of Anatomy, Monash University,
Victoria, 3168, Melbourne, Australia

A characteristic feature of the developing mammalian testis is the appearance of the two generations of Leydig cells, i.e. the fetal and adult Leydig cells which exhibit distinct morphological and functional properties (1,4,8,15). The relative abundance of these Leydig cells during the life history of the testis suggests a biphasic pattern of development (Fig. 1). Fetal Leydig cells are thought to decline in number during the perinatal period, followed later by the postnatal maturation of the adult-type Leydig cells.

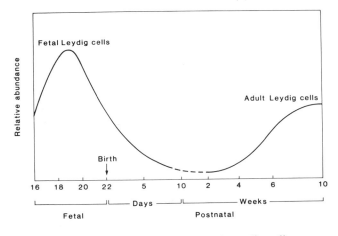

Fig.1 Biphasic appearance of Leydig cells

Various suggestions have been proposed to account for the disappearance of the fetal Leydig cells: 1) cell degeneration or 2) regression or dedifferentiation back to interstitial fibroblast type cells. However due to the uncertain identity of interstitial cells in the early postnatal testis, no unequivocal evidence favoring either theory has been available. Previous quantitative studies of fetal Leydig cells of the rat testis (12,16) have suggested that few if any fetal Leydig cells remain within the testis by the second week of postnatal life. Other studies (13,19) have shown no perinatal decline in fetal Leydig cells although they were not observed in the adult rat testis. The aim of this study was to trace the developmental history of fetal Leydig cells using light and electronmicroscopy together with a quantitative assessment of their numbers per testis from day 17 of fetal life to 100 days after birth.

Sprague-Dawley rats were time-mated and a minimum of 6 male fetuses were obtained at daily intervals from day 17 to 22 of gestation. After birth, 6-10 males were obtained at daily intervals from day 1 to 10 of life and thereafter similar numbers were selected on days 14, 21, 28, 35, 56 and 100. Testes were collected, fixed by immersion or perfusion with buffered glutaraldehyde (9), weighed and after cutting into slices or blocks, the tissues were processed for electronmicroscopy. One micron sections were stained with toluidene blue and the number of fetal Leydig cells per testis was estimated using morphometric procedures (9). Fetal Leydig cells and adult-type Leydig cells were identified by light and electronmicroscopy as described below. Numerical density (Nv) of fetal Leydig cells was calculated using the equation $Nv = Na \div D + T\text{-}2h$ (2) using methods previously described (10,11). Na = number of visible nuclei within a defined reference area (a), D = mean diameter of the nucleus, T = section thickness and h = the height of the smallest visible cap of the nucleus. Reference areas were scored at random over all sections examined (total 444) and the number of recognisable fetal Leydig cell nuclei was recorded regardless of the proportion of intertubular vs. tubular tissue observed within the reference areas (total = 15,000). Over 35,000 such cells were manually counted in $1\mu m$ sections using a x40 oil-immersion objective lens. D was calculated from measurements of 10,000 nuclei from all age groups. The number of fetal Leydig cells per testis was calculated by multiplying Nv by the weight (equal to volume) of the same testes from which the Nv data were obtained.

Fetal Leydig Cells

On day 17 of gestation, fetal Leydig cells were recognised using three criteria 1) ovoid nucleus at times containing a nucleolus 2) a thin rim of cytoplasm 3) variable degrees of basophilia (Fig. 2). From day 18 to 22, fetal Leydig cells were intensely basophilic and now contained numerous lipid inclusions (Figs. 3 & 4). In the postnatal testis, fetal Leydig cells retained their basophilia, showed numerous cytoplasmic lipid inclusions and were often aggregated into clusters partly bordered by attenuated endothelial cytoplasm (Figs. 5,6,7). From 5 weeks until 100 days postnatally their morphology remained essentially unchanged being arranged into distinct cell clusters (Figs. 8,9).

Adult Leydig cells

The interstitial tissue of the postnatal testis contained numerous fusiform-shaped cells (Fig. 5) a proportion of which developed into the adult Leydig cells. From 3 to 4 weeks postnatally, the precursor mesenchymal cells showed increasing hypertrophy and began to exhibit the morphological features of immature Leydig cells (Fig. 7). These cells occurred singly or in loose clusters and exhibited circular or elliptical nuclei and characteristically contained few lipid inclusions (Figs. 7,10). With further maturation of the testis, the immature Leydig cells transformed into typically adult-type Leydig cells (Fig. 11) showing highly pleomorphic shapes and very few, if any, cytoplasmic lipid droplets.

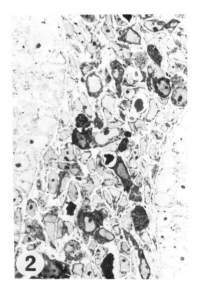

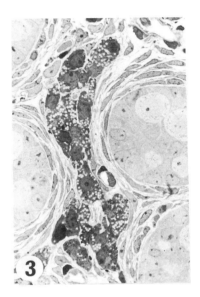

Fig. 2   17-day fetal testis   Fig. 3   22-day fetal testis

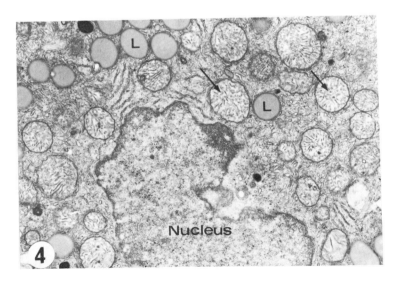

Fig. 4   Fetal Leydig cell showing lipid inclusions (L)
and tubular mitochondrial cristae (arrows)

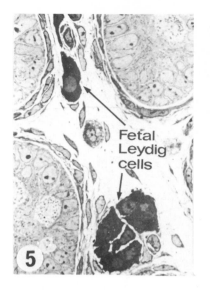
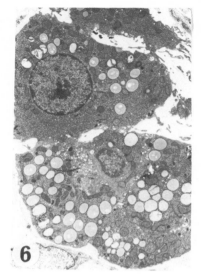

Fig. 5   5-day postnatal testis   Fig. 6   5-day fetal Leydig cells

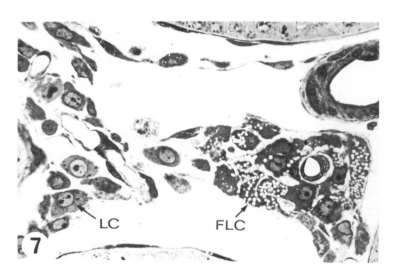

Fig. 7   4 week postnatal testis showing fetal Leydig cells (FLC)
              and immature forms (LC) of adult Leydig cells

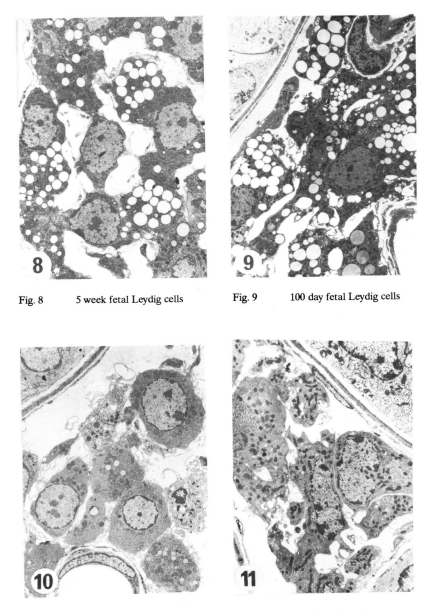

Fig. 8   5 week fetal Leydig cells

Fig. 9   100 day fetal Leydig cells

Fig. 10   4 week immature Leydig cells

Fig. 11   Adult Leydig cells

Quantitative Studies

Testis weight on day 17 of fetal life was 0.271 ± 0.006 mg (mean ± s.d.) increasing to 2.13 ± 0.05 mg by day 22 of gestation (Fig. 12). With postnatal maturation, testis weight increased rapidly up to 1567 ± 40 mg on day 100 after birth. Nv of fetal Leydig cells ($\text{X}10^2$/cubic mm of testis) achieved a maximum value of 1078 ± 76 (mean ± s.d.) on day 18 of fetal life and declined by day 100 postnatally to 0.35 ± 0.11 $\text{X}10^2$ cells/cubic mm (Fig. 13). On day 17 of gestation the testis contained approximately 25 ± 2 $\text{X}10^3$ (mean ± s.e.m.) fetal Leydig cells on day 17 of gestation and increased to 90 ± 9 X 10^3 cells on day 21. Thereafter, up to 2 weeks after birth, fetal Leydig cell numbers per testis remained unchanged. From 21 to 100 days after birth the numbers of fetal Leydig cells showed variation, ranging from 45 ± 10 to 60 ± 19 X 10^3 cells per testis (Fig. 14).

The persistence of fetal Leydig cells

The results show that fetal Leydig cells do not decline in numbers or disappear from the perinatal rat testis. The presence of fetal Leydig cells throughout the postnatal development of the testis and in the fully mature testis raises some doubts about previous suggestions that the fetal Leydig cells degenerate soon after birth. One of the difficulties encountered in following the developmental fate of fetal Leydig cells is due to their decreasing, relative abundance within the developing testis in which a simple inspection of tissue sections gives the subjective impression of a rapid disappearance of the fetal Leydig cells. Initially of high concentration within the fetal testis, the fetal Leydig cells become widely scattered in the intertubular tissue as the volume of the testis expands after birth, but when their Nv values are multiplied by testis volume, considerable numbers of fetal Leydig cells persist within the postnatal testis.

However the present data may not necessarily represent the pattern of fetal Leydig cell development in other species, an example of which is the human testis, where numerous studies have proposed a marked attrition of fetal Leydig cells in the late fetal or early neonatal testis (3,5,6,14,18). Morphological analysis of human fetal testes have suggested pyknotic changes to the fetal Leydig cells leaving few recognisable Leydig cells within the testes during the early postnatal period (see reviews 4,15). Until appropriate tissue becomes available the fate of fetal Leydig cells in the human testis remains to be fully understood. For species which have a relatively rapid period of postnatal sexual maturation such as the mouse, guinea pig, hamster and rabbit the previously held notion of degeneration of fetal Leydig cells may require modification in view of the present results for the rat. What is the physiological function of two generations of Leydig cells which appear to represent two distinct and unrelated classes of cells? In fetal life the fetal Leydig cells are steroidogenically very active (8) and the androgens produced ensure sexual differentiation of the hypothalamus, pituitary and genitalia. The pubertal elevation of steroidogenesis in rats is characterized by increased ratios of C19/C21 steroids and activation of C17-20 lyase, 5α-reductase and 17β-HSD enzymes leading to an increase in testicular endogenous testosterone in late puberty (7,17). The qualitative change in steroid secretion of fetal vs. adult Leydig cells is perhaps a reflection of the androgen supplies necessary for maintenance of spermatogenesis.

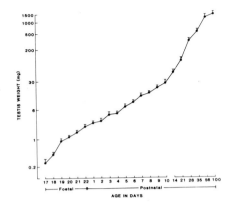

Fig. 12   Log testis weight vs. increasing age

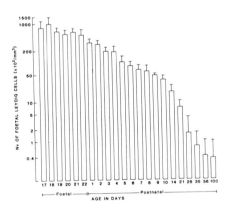

Fig. 13   Log numerical density of fetal Leydig cells vs. age

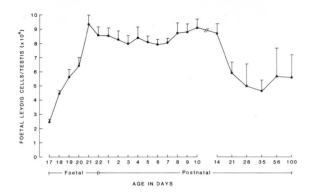

Fig. 14   Fetal Leydig cell no. per testis vs. age

In conclusion this study has demonstrated the persistence of fetal Leydig cells within the postnatal rat testis and their continuity in the testes of adult rats does not support earlier proposals of significant or complete Leydig cell degeneration soon after birth. The data obtained in the rat may be applicable to other laboratory species although the life history of fetal Leydig cells in the human testis remains to be clarified.

Acknowledgement

Supported by the N.H. & M.R.C. of Australia.

REFERENCES

1.   Christensen, A.K. (1975): In: *Handbook of Physiology, vol. 5*, edited by D.W. Hamilton and R.O. Greep, pp. 57-94. American Physiological Society, Washington, D.C.

2.   Floderus, S. (1944): *Acta Pathol. Microbiol. Scand. (Suppl.)*, 53: 1-276.

3.   Gondos, B., and Golbus, M.S. (1976): *Andrologia* 8: Suppl 1, 116.

4.   Gondos, B. (1977): In: *The Testis, vol. 4*, edited by A.D. Johnson and W.R. Gomes, pp. 1-37. Academic Press, New York.

5.   Hayashi, H., and Harrison, R. (1971): *Fertil. Steril.*, 22: 351-355.

6.   Holstein, A.F., Wartenberg, H., and Vossmeyer, J. (1971): *Z. Anat. Entwickl-Gesch.*, 135: 43-66.

7. Huhtaniemi, I., Nozu, K., Warren, D.W., Dufau, M.L. and Catt, K.J. (1982): *Endocrinology*, 111: 1711-1720.

8. Huhtaniemi, I., Warren, D.W. and Catt, K.J. (1984): *Ann. New York Acad. Sci.*, 438: 283-303.

9. Kerr, J.B., and Knell, C.M. (1988): *Development*, 103: in press.

10. Kerr, J.B., Bartlett, J.M.S., Donachie, K., and Sharpe, R.M. (1987): *Cell Tiss. Res.*, 249: 367-377.

11. Kerr, J.B., and Sharpe, R.M. (1985): *Endocrinology*, 116: 2592-2604.

12. Lording, D.W., and de Kretser, D.M. (1972): *J. Reprod. Fert.* 29: 261-269.

13. Mendis-Handagama, C., Risbridger, G.P., and de Kretser, D.M. (1987): *Int. J. Androl.*, 10: 525-534.

14. Pelliniemi, L., and Niemi, M. (1969): *Z. Zellforsch.* 99: 507-522.

15. Prince, F.P. (1984): *Anat. Rec.* 209: 165-176.

16. Roosen-Runge, E.C., and Anderson, D. (1959): *Acta Anat.*, 37: 125-137.

17. Tapanainen, J., Kuopio, T., Pelliniemi, L.J., and Huhtamiemi, I. (1984): *Biol. Reprod.* 31: 1027-1035.

18. Vilar, O. (1970): In: *The Human Testis*, edited by E. Rosenberg and C. Paulsen, pp. 95-111. Plenum Press, New York.

19. Zirkin, B.R., and Ewing, L.L. (1987): *Anat. Rec.*, 219: 157-163.

Leydig Cell Cytotoxicity of Putative Male Antifertility Compounds Related to Ethane-1, 2-Dimethanesulphonate

G. Edwards, B.W. Fox[1], H. Jackson and I.D. Morris

Reproductive Research Group, Physiological Sciences,
University of Manchester, Manchester M13 9PT and
[1]Paterson Laboratories, Christie Hospital and Holt Radium Institute,
Manchester M20 9BX

INTRODUCTION

The testis is a very complex organ, not only does it contain many cell types but the anatomical and paracrine relationships that exist to enable the testis to function as an integrated tissue are of a highly regulated and specific nature. The complexity of the testis is a great obstacle to experimental analysis in vivo as well as to the interpretation of experiments using isolated cells. The classical endocrine techniques of surgical removal of a defined part of the system are not possible but sophisticated techniques have been developed. One of the most popular approaches is to manipulate the function of a testicular compartment or cell by exploiting the reproductive toxicity of drugs or chemicals thus providing a convenient means by which to alter selectively testicular cell populations. However, these compounds are rarely selective to the testis and although many authors ignore the non testicular effects they should always be an important consideration when interpreting the results. The seminiferous tubule is probably the most sensitive compartment to pharmacological manipulation. The development of the spermatogenic epithelium can be partially or completely inhibited if rats are treated with busulfan in utero (5). Damage to the Sertoli cell population can also be achieved by neonatal treatment with cytoarabinoside (12) or when adult by tolnidamine (14). In the adult rat the germ cell population can be reversibly depleted by busulfan (11) or permanently depleted by use of other anticancer drugs such as adriamycin (15). The Leydig cell is apparently not affected by these treatments, any changes in Leydig cell activity, which are usually small, have been attributed to paracrine influences arising from the severely damaged tubule.

Recently the invincibility of the Leydig cell has been overcome by the discovery of the Leydig cell cytotoxin ethane-1,2,-dimethane sulphonate (EDS) which has opened many new avenues of research. EDS can be used to produce a Leydig cell-depleted or enriched testis (8, 10, 16). The antigonadal activity of EDS was first reported by one of us in 1965, (9) during the investigation of the reproductive effects of the alkane sulphonate drugs. It soon became clear that the antifertility effects of EDS were related to the withdrawal of androgen rather than a direct effect upon the spermatogenic epithelium (6, 7). The first microscopical examination (2) and subsequent more extensive studies (8, 10) showed that EDS caused the destruction of the Leydig cell, the debris from which was subsequently phagocytosed by macrophages so that by 4 days after injection the interstitium was devoid of Leydig cells. Precursor cells appear unaffected as the Leydig cells regenerate and testicular functions are restored several weeks later. One of the most convincing demonstrations of the Leydig cell cytotoxicity of EDS is given in Fig 1 and 2. The interstitium, which is normally difficult to visualise, is readily seen after retrograde pressure atrophy of the seminiferous epithelium induced by a high dose of the antifertility compound alpha chlorohydrin (Fig 1). It is very clear that EDS destroys the interstitium: at 7 days after EDS injection to the aspermatogenic rat only the barest architecture of the testis remains (Fig 2).

The mechanism by which EDS kills Leydig cells is not understood. Busulfan, a close homologue of EDS, is a reactive biological alkylating agent and has actions upon both the spermatogenic epithelium and the bone marrow but not upon the Leydig cell (11). It is not clear why EDS should selectively destroy the non proliferating Leydig cell yet spare the proliferating populations in the bone marrow and spermatogenic epithelium. To try and identify the components of the EDS molecule responsible for Leydig cell cytotoxicity we have investigated a variety of compounds which are structurally related to EDS.

MATERIALS AND METHODS

Adult male rats were treated with the compounds described in Table 1. Rats were killed 7 days after treatment except in the case of Compound 4 when the toxicity of this compound necessitated killing the rats 2 days after injection. Serum and testis testosterone and testicular ^{125}I-hCG binding to LH receptors were determined as described elsewhere (10).

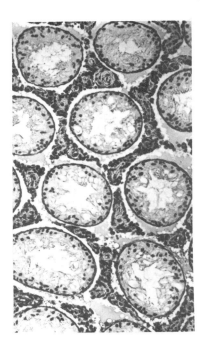
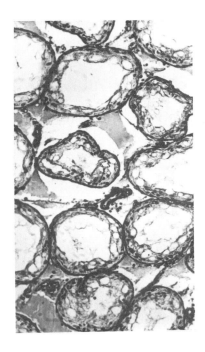

Fig 1. Interstitial tissue
and spermatogenic tubules 7
days after injection vehicle.

Fig 2. The interstitial spaces
are devoid of Leydig cells 7
days after treatment with EDS.

RESULTS

Compounds **1, 2 and 3**   EDS (Compound 2) decreased all Leydig
cell parameters when compared to DMSO injection vehicle Compound
1. The potential metabolite (Compound 3) of EDS had no effect.

Compounds **4, 5 and 8**   Substitution of a hydrogen by a methyl
group on one of the carbon atoms bearing the methane sulphonate
group, Compound 8, caused loss of activity. Substitution of a
hydrogen on both carbon atoms bearing the methane sulphonate
group, Compound 4, produced falls in serum and testicular
testosterone. This compound did not change the testicular
^{125}I-hCG binding capacity and was severely toxic to the rats
so it is probable that the changes represent non-specific
toxicity. . Extension of the carbon chain between the alkylating
methane sulphonate groups in Compound 5 also caused loss of
specific, i.e. no change in testicular ^{125}I-hCG binding,
^{15}I-hCG and the appearance of non specific activity, i.e.
systemic toxicity and falls in serum and testicular testosterone. Busulfan is another member of this series which has
antispermatogenic activity at doses which cause haematological

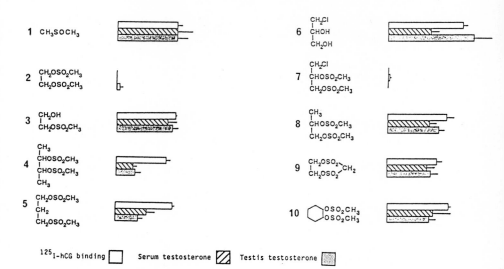

1 CH_3SOCH_3

2 $CH_2OSO_2CH_3$
   $CH_2OSO_2CH_3$

3 CH_2OH
   $CH_2OSO_2CH_3$

4 CH_3
   $CHOSO_2CH_3$
   $CHOSO_2CH_3$
   CH_3

5 $CH_2OSO_2CH_3$
   CH_2
   $CH_2OSO_2CH_3$

6 CH_2Cl
   $CHOH$
   CH_2OH

7 CH_2Cl
   $CHOSO_2CH_3$
   $CH_2OSO_2CH_3$

8 CH_3
   $CHOSO_2CH_3$
   $CH_2OSO_2CH_3$

9 CH_2OSO_2
   CH_2OSO_2 CH_2

10 OSO_2CH_3
   OSO_2CH_3

^{125}I-hCG binding ☐   Serum testosterone ▨   Testis testosterone ▦

Table 1: The in vivo effects of EDS and various related compounds.
Dose: [1], 2 ml/kg; [2], [4], [5], [6], [7], [8], 0.46 mmol/kg;
[3], [10], 0.34 mmol/kg; [9], 0.23 mmol/kg. Doses of [3], [9] and
[10] limited by systemic toxicity.

damage but Leydig cell activity remains unaffected (11). Consequently this compound was not re-examined.

Compounds **6, 7 and 8**   Substitution of a hydrogen by a chlorine in the methyl group of Compound 8 resulted in the reappearance of Leydig cell toxicity in Compound 7.   The cytotoxicity is probably not due to a simple halogen substitution in the molecule, unrelated to the alkane sulphonate groups as the potential metabolite, Compound 6, was not active.

Compound **9**   Cyclic SOSO is a potent antitumor drug whose activity related to alkylation after metabolism. Opening of the ring could yield a compound with an EDS type structure. Cyclic SOSO was severely toxic to the rats yet no effect upon the Leydig cells was found.

Compound **10**   The bifunctional alkylating groups are held in a rigid conformational position in this derivative.   No Leydig cell effects were seen at doses which were toxic to the rats.

DISCUSSION

These experiments have demonstrated that structural changes in the EDS molecule cause the total loss of Leydig cell toxicity with the appearance of general systemic toxicity. Introduction of a chloro methyl group ($-CH_2Cl$) into the EDS molecule produces a compound with both Leydig cell toxicity and dramatic antispermatogenic activity. However the specificity of this drug was not as great as that of EDS because systemic toxicity was also increased.

The experiments give few clues to the mechanism of action of EDS, the conversion to an active metabolite is unlikely as a potential metabolite was inactive. The antitumor effects of this series of methane sulphonates is generally attributed to alkylation, so that the action of EDS on Leydig cells may have a similar explanation (1). EDS will alkylate proteins both in vivo and in vitro (4, 13) however, this reaction is not tissue specific. The reactivity of EDS is low, in aqueous solution at 37°C the degradation is slow ($T_{\frac{1}{2}}=12$ days) and after injection of EDS into the rat 70-80% is excreted unchanged into the urine. Approximately 20% appears as methane sulphonic acid which could indicate that a significant degree of alkylation has taken place (3). However the pattern of metabolism in the mouse is exactly the same as in the rat yet EDS is not toxic to murine Leydig cells.   Alkylation of DNA is probably the most important biological reaction which leads to cell death, while alkylation of protein may not be lethal. The ability to cause interstrand DNA cross links by the dimethanesulphonic acid esters has been examined in Yoshida lymphosarcoma cells (1).   It was demonstrated that cross linking is directly associated with cytotoxicity.   EDS was not cytotoxic and did not form DNA interstrand cross links.

These present studies have confirmed the unusual and specific cytotoxicity of EDS in the rat Leydig cell.   The mechanism by which this is brought about remains a mystery.   The specificity of this drug must rely upon some unique target within the Leydig cell.   In order to affect this target EDS may require activation within this cell, if so this also would require a Leydig cell specific mechanism.   It is clear that the elucidation of the mechanism of action of EDS will contribute towards our understanding of the biology of the Leydig cell as well as cytotoxic drugs in general.

This work was supported by the Wellcome Trust.

REFERENCES

1.   Bedford, P. and Fox, B.W. (1983): Biochem. Pharmac. 32: 2297-2301.

2.   Dixon, J., Lendon, R., Jackson, N.C. and Jackson, H.J. (1983):   Presented to the Society for the Study of Fertility, Manchester. Abstract 55.

3.   Edwards, K., Craig A.W. and Jackson, H. (1969): Biochem. Pharmac. 18: 1693-1700.

4.   Edwards, K., Jackson, H. and Jones, A.R. (1970): Biochem. Pharmac. 19: 1793-1789.

5.   Hemsworth, B.N. and Jackson, H. (1962): Nature, 195: 816-817.

6.   Jackson, C.M. and Jackson H.J. (1984): J. Reprod Fertil. 71: 393-401.

7.   Jackson, C.M. and Morris, I.D. (1977): Andrologia 9:   29-35.

8.   Jackson, N.C., Jackson, H., Shanks, J.H., Dixon, J.S. and Lendon, R.G. (1986):   J. Reprod. Fertil. 76: 1-10.

9.   Jackson, H. (1965): In: Agents affecting fertility.   Edited by C.R. Austin and J.S. Perry, p.62-75.   Churchill, London.

10. Morris, I.D., Phillips, D.M., and Bardin, C.W. (1986): Endocrinology, 118: 709-719.

11. Morris, I.D., Bardin, C.W., Musto, N.A., Than, R.A. and

Gursalus, G.L. (1987): Int. J. Androl. 10: 681-700.

12. Orth, J.M., Gunsalus, G.L. and Lamperti, A.A. (1988): Endocrinology, 122: 787-794.

13. Rommerts, F.F.G., Teerds, K.J. and Hoogerbrugge, J.W. (1988): Molec. Cell. Endoc. 55: 87-94.

14. Spitz, I.M., Gunsalus, G.L., Mather, J.P. Than, R. and Bardin, C.W. (1985): J. Androl., 6: 171-178.

15. Ward, J.A. and Morris, I.D. (1988): Repro. Toxicol. (in press).

16. Zaidi, A., Lendon, R.G., Dixon, J.S. and Morris, I.D. (1988): J. Reprod. Fertil., 82: 281-392.

The Role of Reactive Oxygen Species in the Aetiology of Male Infertility

R.J. Aitken

MRC Reproductive Biology Unit, Centre for Reproductive Biology,
37 Chalmers Street, Edinburgh EH3 9EW, U.K.

Approximately 1 in 6 couples will have cause to visit a specialist infertility clinic during their reproductive life span (12). Within this population the most frequently encountered, defined condition is defective sperm function, which alone accounts for about 25% of all cases (12). In addition, studies employing bioassays of sperm-oocyte fusion indicate that in about one third of couples exhibiting idiopathic infertility defects of sperm function can be detected, even though the semen profile is normal (4). In the light of such information it seems probable that a male factor predominates in at least 40% of all infertile couples.

Despite the widespread occurrence of male infertility there are few, if any, effective treatments to correct this condition. This situation is a direct reflection of our poor state of knowledge concerning both the fundamental cell biology of the human spermatozoon and the precise nature of the lesions present in the spermatozoa of infertile patients.

Our understanding in this area has recently been increased by studies indicating that a large proportion of men exhibiting defective sperm function, produce spermatozoa which cannot develop a capacity for oocyte fusion in response to the calcium signal generated by the calcium ionophore A23187 (5,6). These results have helped to define the lesions present in defective spermatozoa in that they point to a breakdown in the membrane fusion process downstream from calcium influx. In order to pursue this lead we have been investigating the way in which calcium acts upon the human spermatozoon to induce the cascade of events leading to the acrosome reaction and sperm-oocyte fusion. In the studies reviewed in this chapter we have used the sensitive, chemiluminescent reagent, luminol (5-amino-2,3-dihydro-1, 4-phthalazinedione) to investigate the influence of calcium on the generation of reactive oxygen species by these cells and examined the way in which this activity contributes to the aetiology of male infertility.

In their resting state, normal functional human spermatozoa produce very low levels of reactive oxygen, chiefly superoxide anion (2,7). However, following the addition of divalent calcium ionophores, such as A23187 or ionomycin, a sudden burst

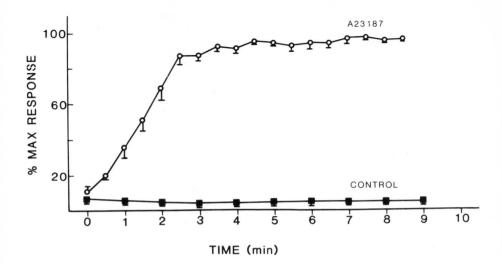

Fig. 1 Generation of reactive oxygen species by human
spermatozoa following addition of the divalent cation ionophore
A23187. The spermatozoa were prepared by repeated
centrifugation (3) in medium BWW (8).

of activity is observed (Fig. 1), via mechanisms dependent upon
the presence of mM levels of extracellular calcium (Fig. 2).
This activity is exhibited by cells which have been prepared by
the conventional centrifugation technique, recovered from 7.5%
albumin columns, isolated by the 'swim-up' procedure or
fractionated on discontinuous Percoll gradients, indicating
that none of the minor cellular contaminants present in human
semen (chiefly leucocytes and squamous epithelial cells) could
have been a major contributor to the levels of reactive oxygen
recorded.

Several features of this reactive oxygen species generating
system suggest regulation by protein kinase C. Hence,
treatment with activators of this kinase, including phorbol 12-
myristate, 13-acetate (Fig. 3) and 1-oleoyl, 2-acetyl glycerol
result in a profound stimulation of activity. The specificity
of this response is indicated by the fact that related
compounds which do not activate protein kinase C, such as 4-
phorbol 12,13-didecanoate or 1,2-dioleoyl glycerol, exhibit a
corresponding inability to influence reactive oxygen species
production.

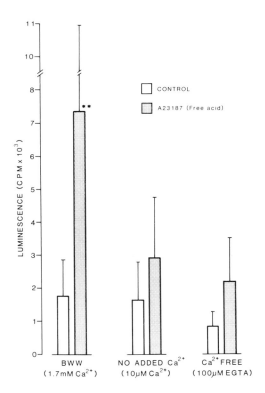

Fig. 2. The generation of reactive oxygen species by human spermatozoa in the presence of A23187 and 1.7 mM external calcium. ** = P < 0.01 Wilcoxon paired rank sum test on 7 independent experiments. If calcium is omitted from the medium a significant response to A23187 is not obtained (2).

The generation of reactive oxygen depends upon the presence of glucose in the external medium. If the glucose is removed or replaced with an equivalent concentration (5.56 mM) of 2-deoxyglucose (Fig. 4) both the resting level of reactive oxygen species production and the response to A23187 are considerably reduced, despite the fact that both pyruvate and lactate are present in the medium and the motility of the spermatozoa is unimpaired. Studies employing ^{14}C-labelled glucose tracers indicate that the degree of reactive oxygen species generation by human spermatozoa is highly correlated (r=0.89) with both the proportion of glucose flux through the pentose phosphate pathway and the activity of the key enzyme in this pathway,

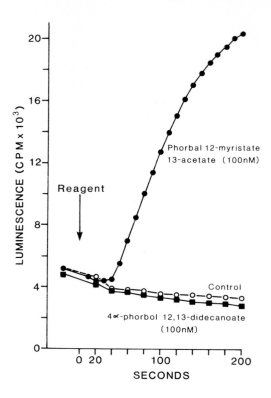

Fig. 3. Generation of reactive oxygen species by human spermatozoa in response to stimulation of protein kinase C by phorbol 12-myristate, 13-acetate. Phorbol esters which do not influence protein kinase C, such as the 4 α-phorbol 12,13-didecanoate, do not accelerate the production of reactive oxygen species (RJ Aitken, unpublished observations).

glucose-6-phosphate dehydrogenase (r=0.82) (RJ Aitken and WC Ford, unpublished observations).

Since one of the major functions of the pentose phosphate pathway is to generate NADPH, the influence of this pyridine nucleotide on the generation of reactive oxygen species by human spermatozoa was investigated (10). Neither NADH or NADPH influenced the generation of reactive oxygen species by intact human spermatozoa. However, in broken-cell preparations (Fig. 5) 100,000g particulate fractions and isolated plasma membrane vesicles, both of these compounds were effective in stimulating

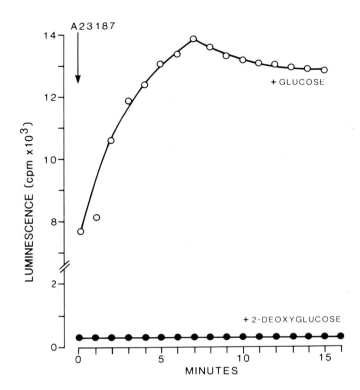

Fig. 4. Influence of 5.56mM glucose or 2-deoxyglucose on the generation of reactive oxygen species by human spermatozoa (R.J. Aitken - unpublished observations).

an immediate burst of activity. Permeabilization of the cells with triton-X also enabled the spermatozoa to exhibit a rapid burst of activity in the presence of NADPH or NADH. Calculation of the respective Km values, revealed that NADPH was the preferred substrate, yielding a Km value of 3.8 μM compared with 11 μM for NADH. Non-specific electron donors such as ascorbate were not effective in stimulating the production of reactive oxygen species at doses up to 10 mM. Furthermore, a mitochondrial origin for this activity can be excluded because the inhibitors oligomycin (0.033mM) antimycin (0.01mM) and rotenone (0.01mM) failed to influence the responses of intact cells to A23187 or of permeabilized cells to NADH /NADPH.

Scavengers of either singlet oxygen (histidine HC1,

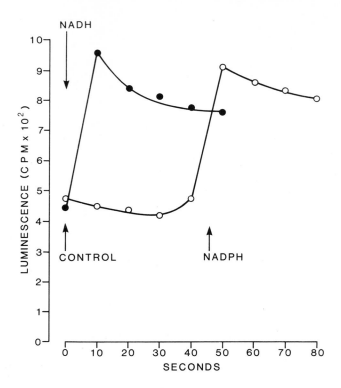

Fig. 5. Influence of NADH and NADPH on the generation of
reactive oxygen species by washed preparations of human
spermatozoa which had been disrupted in a ground glass Dounce
homogenizer in 0.34M sucrose and 1mM NaHCO$_3$ on ice (R.J.
Aitken, unpublished observations).

diazobicyclo octane, bilirubin, dimethyl-furan) or the hydroxyl
radical (ethanol, mannitol, Na benzoate, histidine HCl) did not
suppress the capacity of triton-permeabilized cells to generate
reactive oxygen in response to NADH or NADPH; diazobicyclo
octane and bilirubin even stimulated this activity. Similarly
in intact cells, none of these scavengers had a significant
inhibitory effect on the generation of reactive oxygen in
response to A23187. In contrast, cytochrome C was a powerful
scavenger of the responses of intact cells to A23187 or of
triton-permeabilized cells to NADH and NADPH (2), suggesting
that the primary product of this oxygen radical generating
system is superoxide anion (7).

The biological significance of this superoxide generating system has yet to be elucidated. It may be pertinant that NADPH oxidase activity has also been detected in other types of non-phagocytic cell including adipocytes and thymocytes, (14,15) and that the hydrogen peroxide formed by this system is thought to act as a second messenger, mediating the action of such hormones as insulin, oxytocin and nerve growth factor. It is possible that the reactive oxygen species generated by the human spermatozoon serve a similar role in mediating the action of signals, derived from the female reproductive tract or ovum, which control those calcium-dependent, membrane fusion, events associated with the acrosome reaction and fertilization of the oocyte.

The clinical significance of this superoxide generating system, in terms of male infertility, was indicated by recent studies in which the capacity of human spermatozoa to exhibit sperm-oocyte fusion in response to A23187 was correlated with their ability to produce reactive oxygen species (2). Samples exhibiting a normal capacity for oocyte fusion (> 26% of oocytes penetrated) (6) were characterized by a low level of reactive oxygen species production when the cells were in a resting state, and a small, 2-3 fold, rise on exposure to A23187. In contrast, specimens exhibiting a poor capacity for oocyte fusion (11-25% oocyte penetration), and particularly those in which < 10% of oocytes were penetrated following treatment with A23187, were extremely active in the generation of reactive oxygen species yielding mean values which were 40x higher than the levels recorded for normal functional cells (Fig. 6).

Fig. 7 presents data for a cohort of 61 patients exhibiting oligozoospermia in which this relationship between the excessive generation of reactive oxygen species and impaired sperm function can be clearly seen. Approximately 50% (33/61) of these patients exhibited penetration rates of less than 10% following exposure to A23187. The mean production of reactive oxygen species by such defective cells was 10x higher than in patients exhibiting 10-25% penetration and 70x higher than in samples scoring within the normal fertile range of 26-100% (R.J. Aitken, unpublished observations).

Failure to respond to a calcium influx by undergoing sperm-oocyte fusion is a specific defect which has been observed in all classes of infertile men examined to date, including those with varicoceles, oligozoospermia or unexplained infertility (4,5,6). These findings indicate that the presence of this particular defect is frequently associated with the excessive activity of a novel superoxide generating system, probably located in the sperm plasma membrane. This activity may be directly responsible for the loss of membrane function through the peroxidation of unsaturated fatty acids (13) or the denaturation of proteins in the sperm plasma membrane (11).

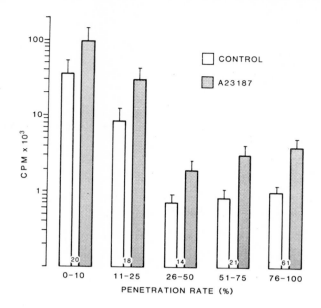

Fig. 6   Clinical significance of the superoxide generating system.   Graph showing the inverse relationship between the capacity of human spermatozoa to generate reactive oxygen species and sperm-oocyte fusion (2).

Alternatively, the hyperactive generation of reactive oxygen species may be a consequence of a primary defect in the organization of the plasma membrane, such that the control mechanisms regulating this activity are no longer effective. Elucidating the relationship between superoxide generation and sperm pathology will be of clinical value, since if the loss of sperm function is a direct consequence of oxidative damage to the plasma membrane, rational therapeutic options will be presented for the correction of human sperm function, including the use of antioxidants (9,11,12,16).   In vitro studies have already demonstrated the potential of vitamin E in this respect (1).

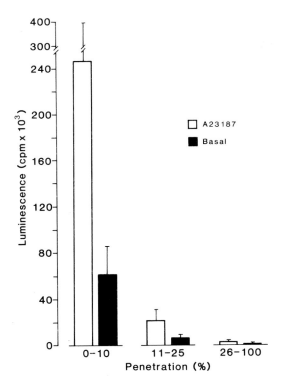

Fig. 7 Generation of reactive oxygen species by oligozoospermic samples before and after addition of the divalent cation ionophore, A23187 (R.J. Aitken, unpublished observations).

REFERENCES

1. Aitken, R.J. (1987): Human Reproduction. 3: 89-95.

2. Aitken, R.J. and Clarkson, J.S. (1987): J. Reprod. Fert., 81: 459-469.

3. Aitken, R.J., Best, F.S.M., Richardson, D.W., Djahanbakhch, O. and Lees, M.M. (1982): Fertil. Steril., 38: 68-76.

4. Aitken, R.J., Best, F.S.M., Richardson, D.W., Djahanbakhch, O., Mortimer, D., Templeton, A.A. and Lees, M.M. (1982): Fertil. Steril., 38: 212-221.

5. Aitken, R.J., Clarkson, J.S., Huang, G-F. and Irvine, D.S. (1987): In: Recent Advances in Spermatology, edited by H. Mohri, pp 75-90. Japanese Scientific Societies Press, Tokyo.

6. Aitken, R.J., Ross, A., Hargreave, T., Richardson, D. and Best, F. (1984): J. Androl., 5: 321-329.

7. Alvarez, J.G., Touchstone, J.C., Blasco, L. and Storey, B.T. (1987): J. Androl., 8: 338-348.

8. Biggers, J.D., Whitten, W.K. and Whittingham, D.G. (1971): In: Methods in Mammalian Embryology, edited by J.C. Daniel Jr., pp. 86-116. Freeman, San Francisco.

9. Burton, G.W., Cheeseman, K.H., Doba, T., Ingold, K.U. and Slater, T.F. (1983): In: Biology of Vitamin E. Ciba Foundation Symposium 101, edited by R. Porter and J. Whelan, pp. 4-18. Ciba Foundation, London.

10. Gabig, T.G. and Babior, B.M. (1979): J. Biol. Chem. 254: 9070-9074.

11. Halliwell, B. and Gutteridge, J.M.C. (1986): Free Radicals in Biology and Medicine. Universities Press, Belfast.

12. Hull, M.G.R. (1986): In: Human Embryo Research: Yes or No, edited by G. Bock and M. O'Connor, pp. 24-35. Ciba Foundation, London.

13. Jones, R., Mann, T. and Sherins, R. (1979): Fertil. Steril. 31: 531-537.

14. Mukherjee, S.P. and Mukherjee, C. (1982): Biochem. Pharmacol. 31: 3163-3172.

15. Mukherjee, S.P. and Mukherjee C. (1982): Arch. Biochem. Biophys. 214: 221-222.

16. Pursel, V.G. (1979): Biol. Reprod. 21: 319-324.

Identification of Spermatids with "Aprotruded Tails" in Human Semen by Monoclonal Antibodies and Electron Microscopy

A. Jassim and H. Festenstein

*Department of Immunology, London Hospital Medical College,
Turner Street, London E1 2AD, UK*

Transmission electron microscopy (TEM) has been widely used in the study of morphological abnormalities of germ cells in both testis and semen. Different types of abnormal spermatids have been described in the testis of infertile patients (6). Also, in semen samples from fertile (7) and infertile men (3,10,11,15), a wide spectrum of defective sperm has been observed.

In this study we have used immunological techniques as a new approach for the identification and quantitation of certain abnormal spermatids in semen samples of some oligospermic donors. The abnormality involved the failure of the tails to protrude as free flagella; instead they coiled up inside. The advantages of this approach over TEM are discussed together with the importance of these spermatids as a model in the study of sperm tail morphogenesis and oligospermia.

MATERIALS AND METHODS

Semen Samples

The semen samples were obtained from medical students who were previously shown to produce low sperm counts (oligospermic) and high numbers of nucleated cells other than sperm (NCOS) (8).

Preparation Of Dried NCOS

Following their separation on ficoll/triosil (8), the NCOS were counted and their numbers adjusted to 8×10^5/ml. 100 µl of each cell suspension was dispensed onto slides and left to dry at room temperature. The slides were sometimes stored frozen at $-20°C$ before use.

Freezing And Thawing Of Sperm

Following washing, the sperm were pelleted and snap frozen in liquid nitrogen. The samples were then thawed in a $37°C$ water bath. The freezing and thawing was repeated 5 times.

Indirect Immunofluorescence (IIF) Test

The details of IIF testing of both cell suspensions and dried NCOS have been described elsewhere (9).

Monoclonal Antibodies (MoAbs)

GDA-J/F3 MoAb was previously produced in this laboratory (9). This antibody was used as undiluted supernatant. The anti-alpha- (Code N°.356) and beta-tubulin (Code N°.357) MoAbs were purchased from Amersham (England). They were ascites fluid and were diluted 1:100 with phosphate buffered saline before use.

Transmission Electron Microscopy (TEM) of NCOS

The details of this technique have been published elsewhere (8).

RESULTS

Reaction Of GDA-J/F3 MoAb With Dried NCOS

In dried samples the GDA-J/F3 MoAb produced circular immunofluorescence around the periphery of 10-20% NCOS (Fig.1). In addition, the antibody stained the principal piece of mature sperm tail.

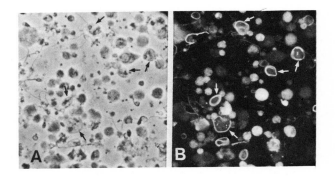

FIG.1. Indirect immunofluorescence test of dried NCOS with GDA-J/F3 MoAb. The antibody stains the tails which are encircled inside the spermatids (arrows). (A) Phase contrast. (B) Fluorescence microscopy. (x440).

Reaction Of Anti-Alpha- And Beta-Tubulin MoAbs With Dried NCOS

The anti-alpha- and beta-tubulin MoAbs showed similar reactivity with NCOS. Both antibodies reacted with the whole tail of mature sperm (principal and middle piece) and circular immunofluorescence was seen on the periphery of the spermatids (Fig.2). In addition, diffuse staining was observed with other types of cells (Fig.2).

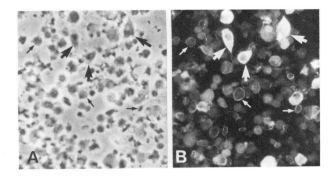

FIG.2. Indirect immunofluorescence test of dried NCOS
with anti-beta-tubulin MoAb. The antibody stains the
tails of the abnormal spermatids (thin arrows) as well
as other types of cells (thick arrows). (A) Phase contrast.

Reaction of GDA-J/F3, Alpha- And Beta-Tubulin MoAbs With Frozen-Thawed Sperm

Following the disruption of spermatozoal cell membranes by repeated
freezing and thawing, GDA-J/F3 MoAb stained only the principal piece
of all sperm (Fig.3 A,B). The anti-alpha- and beta-tubulin MoAbs, on
the other hand, reacted with the whole tails of all sperm, ie. the
immunofluorescence was seen on both the middle and principal piece
(Fig.3 C,D).

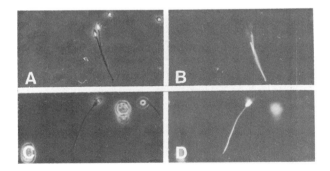

FIG.3. Indirect immunofluorescence test of frozen-thawed
sperm with GDA-J/F3 (A,B) and anti-beta-tubulin MoAb
(C,D). GDA-J/F3 stains the principal piece while anti-
beta-tubulin MoAb reacts with both middle and principal
pieces. (A,C) Phase contrast. (B,D) Fluorescence
microscopy. (x440).

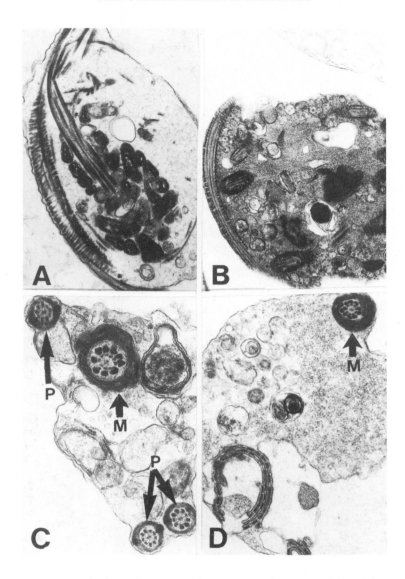

FIG.4. Transmission electron microscopy of spermatids with aprotruded tails.   The tails which are sectioned longitudinally are seen
coiled up beneath the cytoplasmic membrane (A & B).   In (C & D)
the tails were sectioned transversely at the middle (M) or principal
piece (P). A (x17000). B (x13000). C (x22000). D (x17000).

Ultrastructural Characterisation Of The Abnormal Spermatids

The TEM of NCOS revealed the presence of mainly germ cells at various stages of differentiation (data not shown). Among these were a group of spermatids with abnormal tails. These tails were seen spanning the periphery of the spermatids just beneath their cytoplasmic membranes. In some spermatids, the tails were simultaneously sectioned in the middle and principal piece (Fig. 4C). The ultrastructures of the aprotruded tails were sometimes defective.

DISCUSSION

Normally during spermiogenesis, the distal centriole migrates to the caudal part of the spermatid to give rise to the tail. The tail will then continue its development and elongate by pushing the cytoplasmic membrane outwards to form a free flagellum (2). In this study however we describe abnormal spermatids in which the tails failed to protrude as free flagella; instead they coiled up inside. These were called "aprotruded tails". Although this abnormality has been previously described as "coiled tail" by using TEM (4,12,13), the term "aprotrusion" was introduced to emphasise the significance of the flagellar protrusion as an essential step in the tail morphogenesis. As discussed later, the study of the causes and mechanism of aprotrusion could enlighten our knowledge about the process of protrusion itself.

The use of immunological techniques for the first time has greatly helped in the identification and quantitation of the abnormal spermatids. TEM is labour-intensive and requires special equipment and trained personnel. Furthermore, quantitation of these abnormal spermatids by TEM is not possible as the tails should always be sectioned before such spermatids can be identified. By using the GDA-J/F3 MoAb which recognises an intracellular antigen inside the principal piece (9) the aprotruded tails were seen spanning the periphery of the spermatids. This was further supported by using MoAbs against the alpha- and beta-tubulins which constitute the structural proteins of the axonemal microtubules. Although GDA-J/F3 and anti-alpha- and beta-tubulin MoAbs react with sperm tails, the three antibodies recognise different antigens. GDA-J/F3 has a limited tissue distribution (9) while alpha- and beta-tubulin are widely distributed in tissues forming the cytoskeletal microtubules (14). Furthermore GDA-J/F3 MoAb reacts only with the principal piece of the tail while the other antibodies react with both the principal and middle pieces.

The intracellular localisation of the aprotruded tails shown by the immunological approach was confirmed by TEM which showed the spermatids with their abnormal tails encircled just beneath their cytoplasmic membranes.

The cause of the tail aprotrusion could be due to the absence of one or more of the known tail ultrastructures (5) or alternatively to a molecular or anatomical defect. The first possibility could be ruled out since all the known tail ultrastructures were detected by TEM. The second possibility argues that although present, the flagellar ultrastructural components could be defective. There is evidence that disulphide bonding gives some stiffness to the tail to enable its movement (1). Whether the aprotrusion is due to a defect in the disulphide bonding or in other processes can only be established by biochemical analysis of the abnormal tails. The last possibility to explain the aprotrusion argues that if the distal centriole fails to migrate caudally, the tail would develop anteriorly in the direction of tissues where there is no chance for its protrusion. This can be investigated by examining testicular biopsies from patients having this abnormality.

The study of the causes of aprotrusion might enable us to understand better the sperm tail development and probably help in the identification of some factor(s) that could contribute in the pathogenesis of certain types of oligospermia. It is possible that these abnormal spermatids, by their large size, could physically interfere with the proper development and maturation of other normal germ cells resulting in their premature shedding from the testis. This could happen if the attachment sites to Sertoli cells are already occupied by the abnormal spermatids.

ACKNOWLEDGEMENT

We are indebted to Prof JP Blandy (Dept. of Urology), Drs. RTD Oliver (Dept. of Oncology) and A Biro (Dept. of Immunology) for their continuous help and advice. We are also grateful to A Gray (Morbid Anatomy) for his technical assistance with the TEM. The financial support of the RAC and Leverhulme Trust is greatly appreciated. Finally we thank Denny Williams for preparation of the manuscript.

REFERENCES

1. Bellve, A.R., and O'Brien, D.A. (1983): In: Mechanism and Control of Animal Fertilization, edited by J.F. Hartmann, pp.55-137.
2. DeKrester, D.M. (1969): Z. Zellforsch., 98:477-505.
3. Eliasson, R., Mossberg, B., Camner, P., and Afzelius, B.A. (1977): New Engl. J. Med., 297:1-6.
4. Escalier, D., and Georges, D. (1984): Biol. Cell., 50:37-52.
5. Fawcett, D.W. (1975): Dev. Biol., 44:394-436.
6. Holstein, A.F., and Schirren, C. (1979): In: The Spermatozoon, Maturation, Motility, Surface Properties and Comparative Aspects, edited by D.W. Fawcett and J.M. Bedford, pp. 341-353. Urban & Schwarzenberg, Baltimore-Munich.
7. Hunter, D.G., and Kretzer, F.L. (1986): Arch. Androl., 16:1-12.
8. Jassim, A., and Festenstein, H. (1987): J. Reprod. Immunol., 11:77-89.
9. Jassim, A., and Festenstein, H. (1987): J. Reprod. Immunol., 12:173-189.
10. McClure, R.D., Brawer, J., and Robaire, B. (1983): Fertil. Steril., 40:395-399.
11. Moryan, A., Guay, A.T., Kurtz, S., and Nowak, P.J. (1985): Fertil. Steril., 44:539-542.
12. Nistal, M., Paniagua, R., and Herruzo, A. (1977): Virchows Arch. B. Cell Path., 26:111-118.
13. Schieferstein, G., and Wolburg, H. (1986): Andrologia, 18:341-352.
14. Schliwa, M. (1986): The Cytoskeleton: An Introductory Survey: Cell Biology Monographs 13. Springer-Verlag, Wein/New York.
15. Serres, C., Feneux, D., and Jouannet, P. (1986): Cell Motil. Cytoskeleton, 6:68-76.

The Finnish Sauna Does Not Disturb Testicular Function

O. Hovatta, L. Bäck, S. Kaukoranta-Tolvanen
and I. Huhtaniemi*

*Infertility Clinic of The Finnish Population
and Family Welfare Federation "Väestöliitto", SF-00100 Helsinki,
and Department of Physiology*, University of Turku, SF-20520 Turku, Finland*

It has been suspected that the Finnish sauna bath, as a form of heat exposure, can disturb sperm production. Nevertheless, bathing in the sauna has been very popular in Finland for hundreds of years. Nearly everyone from infancy to old age goes to the sauna at least once a week.

Male infertility in Finland is not more frequent than reported elsewhere (7). Procope (6) studied the effect of excessive sauna bathing (eight times in two weeks) on sperm production of 12 men. He observed a slight transient decrease in sperm counts two months after the sauna period. However, the counts remained within the normal range. There were no changes in sperm morphology. Sperm motility was not examined. Brown-Woodman et al. (1) studied 5 men after a single sauna exposure (20 min) and observed electron microscopical changes in sperm morphology. Hormonal effects of the sauna bath have been studied by Leppäluoto et al. (5). Very intensive bathing (1 hour twice a day for 7 days, at 80 °C) caused a rise in serum prolactin levels, but testosterone, FSH and LH levels were unchanged.

We have now studied the effects of the Finnish sauna on semen parameters, scrotal temperature, salivary testosterone and serum testosterone, prolactin, LH and FSH levels.

SUBJECTS AND METHODS

Ten healthy men, aged 22-25 yrs, volunteered for the study. In the first part, semen, collected by masturbation, and serum samples were taken at the same time of day (10.00 - 12.00 h) one week before and immediately after one intensive sauna bath in well-controlled conditions. The men bathed for 30 min in a temperature of 73-85 °C, absolute moisture of 52-64 g/kg and relative moisture of 15-18 %. The scrotal temperature was measured by thermography (Varicoscreen, Medicon, Belgium) before the sauna, during the bath at 20 min, and 15 min after the sauna. Two-ml samples of mixed saliva for testosterone measurements was collected immediately before the sauna, at 10 min intervals during bathing, and 10 minutes after. Testosterone levels were measured by a sensitive radioimmunoassay as described by us previously (3). The serum hormone levels were measured by radioimmunoassays using commercial kits.

In the second part of the study, half of the men took their normal sauna bath once a week according to the traditional Finnish custom and served as controls. The other half bathed excessively, eight times in two weeks. Semen samples were taken before, immediately after and three months after the bathing period.

RESULTS

A slight but significant increase was observed in scrotal temperature (from 31.9 to 33.6 °C) during the sauna (Table 1). The temperature was still elevated 15 minutes after the bath.

Table 1. Effect of one intensive sauna bath (30 min at 73-85 °C) on scrotal temperature (°C) in 10 healthy young men (mean ± SD).

Before sauna	31.9 ± 0.9
During sauna (at 20 min)	33.6 ± 0.8 *
After sauna (15 min)	33.2 ± 0.3 *

* $p < 0.01$ vs. before the sauna, paired Student's t test.

There were no changes in any parameters of the semen analyses taken before and after one intensive sauna bath (Table 2). All the men were normospermic.

Table 2. Effect of one intensive sauna bath on semen parameters. Other details are as in Table 1.

	Sperm count (million/ml)	Motility (%)	Morphology (% normal sperms)
1 week before sauna	73 ± 86	62 ± 7	77 ± 8
immediately after sauna	78 ± 82	62 ± 5	77 ± 9

Serum testosterone, LH and FSH levels were unchanged (Table 3), and within reference ranges. However, a slight but significant elevation was observed in prolactin after the bath.

Table 3. Effect of one intensive sauna bath on serum testosterone, LH, FSH and prolactin levels. Other details are as in Table 1.

	Testosterone (nmol/l)	LH (U/l)	FSH (U/l)	Prolactin (mU/l)
1 week before sauna	15.4 ± 3.6	4.1 ± 1.0	3.0 ± 2.1	198 ±137
immediately after sauna	17.7 ± 6.3	3.7 ± 1.4	3.0 ± 2.1	276 ± 177[*]

*, $p < 0.05$

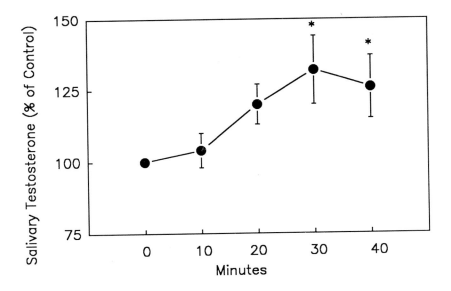

Figure 1. Salivary testosterone immediately before (0), at 10, 20 and 30 min during the sauna, and 10 min after (40 min) in 10 healthy young men. The values (mean ± SEM) are expressed as percents of the 0-value (260 ± 25 pmol/l). *, $p < 0.05$ vs. the 0-level.

Salivary testosterone levels increased significantly during the sauna, from 260 ± 25 to 334 ± 33 pmol/l (mean ± SEM), an increase of 32 % of the control level (Fig. 1). Ten min after the sauna it was still higher than the level immediately before bathing.

In the second part of the study, the semen samples were analyzed before and immediately after two weeks of intensive sauna bathing. A third semen analysis was carried out 3 months after the sauna period. There were no significant changes in any semen parameters between any of the groups analyzed (Table 4).

Table 4. Effect of excessive sauna bathing (8 times in 2 weeks) on semen of 5 healthy young men (group S, mean ± SD). The control data are from another group of 5 men (group C) who exercised moderate sauna bathing (once a week) at the same time.

		Sperm count (million/ml)	Motility (%)	Morphology (% normal sperms)
Before the sauna period	S	100 ± 119	62 ± 7	77 ± 9
	C	46 ± 21	61 ± 8	77 ± 7
Immediately after the sauna period	S	89 ± 83	52 ± 18	70 ± 13
	C	59 ± 20	54 ± 5	76 ± 6
3 months after the sauna period	S	154 ± 174	50 ± 4	69 ± 3
	C	87 ± 47	43 ± 20	71 ± 5

DISCUSSION

We were unable to detect any disadvantageous effects of the Finnish sauna on semen quality, even during excessive bathing. The morphological changes in spermatozoa after a single sauna bath observed by Brown-Woodman et al. (1) on electron microscopy remain to be confirmed. Our data are therefore in agreement with the previous study of Procope (6) in which the semen was collected from condoms. Since we examined fresh semen samples produced by masturbation, also the sperm motility could be studied, and was found to be unaffected by the sauna.

The heat exposure in traditional Finnish sauna is short and moderate, and the increase of scrotal temperature of less than two degrees is unlikely to have any effects. In cases of varicocele higher temperatures are seen

(4). A hot bath probably increases the scrotal temperature more efficiently than the sauna. Since sauna bathing is in Finland a custom adopted in childhood, it is an intriguing question whether testicular physiology is able to adapt to the frequent increases, though small, in scrotal temperature. Evidence for such adaptation or conditioning, though still without scientific proof, is the fact that most of the reports on the harmful effects of the sauna are from outside Finland. The Finnish studies, and even folklore, do not indicate any harmful effects of sauna bathing on male fertility.

The increase in salivary testosterone levels and hence indirectly that of the serum free testosterone during the sauna is a new finding. We also confirmed the previous finding of an increase in prolactin during the sauna bath (5). The prolactin rise is probably a stress response. Since prolactin has effects on Leydig cell function (3), the concomitant prolactin and testosterone increases can also be related. On the other hand, the rise in testosterone may also be the result of increased testicular blood flow or increased steroidogenesis, caused by the elevated scrotal temperature.

REFERENCES

1. Brown-Woodman, P.D.C., Post, E.J., Gass, G.C., and White, I. (1984) Arch. Androl. 12:4-15.
2. Huhtaniemi, I. (1983) Clin. Endocr. Metab. 12:117-132.
3. Huhtaniemi, I., Dunkel, L., and Perheentupa, J. (1986) Pediat. Res. 20:1324-1327.
4. Kormano. M., Kahanpää. K., Swinhufvud, U., and Tähti, E. (1970) Fertil. Steril. 21:558-563.
5. Leppäluoto, J., Huttunen, P., Hirvonen, J., Väänänen, A., Tuomonen, M., and Vuori, J. (1986) Acta Physiol. Scand. 128: 467-470.
6. Procope, B.J. (1965) Int. J. Fertil. 10: 333-339.
7. Rantala, M.L. (1988) Acta Obstet. Gyn. Scand., in press.

Contraception for Men Using Continuous Administration of LHRH Agonist and Androgen

C.W. Bardin, A. Moo-Young, C.C. Chang, C. Monder,
J. Bertolini and R. Thau

The Population Council, 1230 York Avenue, New York, NY 10021 USA

There are numerous studies suggesting that LHRH analogs are antigonadotropic, and that these peptides may be useful contraceptives in men (2,5,10). When administered alone, LHRH agonists and antagonists suppress LH and FSH; such treatment will provide acceptable contraception in men provided androgen supplementation is available. A review of previous studies in primates suggests that continuous rather than intermittent administration of both the LHRH analog and the androgen will be required to provide the best chance of suppressing spermatogenesis (4,11,12). In order to achieve this goal, the Population Council decided to design an implant system that would deliver an LHRH analog and an androgen continuously for one year.

SELECTION OF AN LHRH ANALOG

Both LHRH agonist and antagonist will suppress LH and FSH, but their mechanisms of action are entirely different. Administration of an agonist at first elevates LH and FSH in accordance with its ability to mimic the action of native LHRH, but subsequently reduces the level of these gonadotropins due to down regulation of gonadotrophs in the pituitary (3). The advantages of agonists are that they are highly potent and relatively soluble in physiological fluids; their disadvantage is that three to four weeks of treatment are required before LH and FSH levels are suppressed. By contrast, currently available antagonists have the advantage of suppressing LH and FSH secretion quite rapidly since they act by blocking the action of the native peptide at the LHRH receptor (7,8); their disadvantages, at least at present, are that they are relatively less potent than agonists and are less soluble in physiological fluids. In view of these considerations, we chose to develop an implant for an LHRH agonist. Based on previous studies, we elected to test [(imBzl) DHis^6-Pro^9-EA]-LHRH and [DTrp^6-Pro^9-EA]-LHRH.

SELECTION OF A MATERIAL TO BE USED IN THE COMPOSITION OF THE IMPLANT FOR PEPTIDE DELIVERY

There is considerable experience with the continuous adminis-tration of steroids from implants composed of Silastic rubber (6,9). This material, as it is usually manufactured, would not be suitable for delivering charged molecules such as peptides. Several delivery systems were therefore selected according to their ability to release peptides based upon the principles of molecular sieving. The cross-linking of these materials can be varied to release peptides at a constant rate depending on their size and the dose desired. Several models of implants containing LHRH-13 were tested and shown to suppress gonadotropin and testos-terone secretion in male rats and dogs. Methods for mechanized manufacture of these implants are currently under investigation.

SELECTION OF AN ANDROGEN

Since the major function of androgen replacement during treat-ment with LHRH analogs is to maintain anabolic and sexual activi-ties, it would be desirable to administer testosterone. However, since the daily production rate of this steroid in men is 5 to 7 mg, it could be impossible to produce an implant that would deliver this amount of testosterone over a one-year period. If such an implant is to be developed, then androgen replacement with a smaller mass of steroid per day must be achieved. Consequently, androgens with greater potency than testosterone were sought and tested in a variety of bioassays. From over ten compounds, 7α-methyl 19-nortestosterone acetate (7MNTA) was selected for further study.

Androgen receptor binding was first examined in mouse kidney. Following single injections of testosterone or 7MNTA, nuclear androgen receptors were comparable one hour later. However, after five hours, androgen receptor concentrations in renal nuclei remained at 50% of maximal in 7MNTA-treated animals whereas in testosterone-treated mice, receptor levels declined to control levels. These studies suggested that 7MNTA was retained by andro-gen receptors for a longer period of time than testosterone.

Studies of biological activity indicated that a single injec-tion of 7MNTA produced a 7- to 8-fold greater response in ornithine decarboxylase activity in the mouse kidney than did tes-tosterone. When implants of both androgens were prepared and administered to female mice, 7MNTA was 10-fold more potent than testosterone using induction of ornithine decarboxylase as an end point. Steroid-delivering implants were then prepared and administered to castrated male rabbits to determine their ability to maintain the male reproductive tract. Testosterone, at a dose of 250 μg/day, was required to maintain prostate and seminal vesicle weights in the normal range over a two-month period of time. By contrast, only 20 μg of 7MNTA were required to maintain these organs. Similar results were obtained from replacement therapy experiments in castrated male rates. The potency of 7MNTA was also 10 times that of testosterone in this species.

A study in intact male monkeys was next performed to determine whether 7MNTA would maintain sexual activity. Animals were first treated with minipumps containing an LHRH agonist. This caused a reduction of serum testosterone levels to <1.0 ng/ml after 1.5 months, and after 2 months the animals stopped ejaculating. Treatment was then continued with the agonist for an additional 6 months. During this time the animals were unable to produce a semen sample. Androgen treatment was then initiated by way of subdermal implants. The ability to ejaculate was re-established during 6 months of treatment. Following discontinuance of androgen and analog treatment, the animals returned to normal.

METABOLISM OF 7α METHYL-19-NORTESTOSTERONE ACETATE

In view of the greater potency of 7MNTA, it was desirable to study its metabolism in liver and in organs of the male reproductive tract. [^{3}H]-7MNTA was prepared and incubated with tissue homogenates, microsomes, or cytosol. [^{3}H]-Testosterone and [^{3}H] 19-nortestosterone (19NT) were used as reference preparations.

In liver microsomes, testosterone was completely metabolized after a 15-minute incubation period. By contrast, only 10 and 60% of 7MNTA and 19NT, respectively, were metabolized over the same period. Studies on the metabolism of these steroids in liver cytosol yielded qualitatively similar results. We concluded that rat liver metabolized 7MNTA much more slowly than testosterone or its 19-nor derivative (1).

The metabolism of testosterone, 19NT, and 7MNTA in prostate and epididymal homogenates from mature rats was next examined. The dominant metabolites of testosterone and 19NT, respectively, were 5α-dihydrotestosterone and 5α-dihydro-19NT in prostate and 5α-diols in epididymis. Interestingly, no 5α-reduced products were detected following incubation of prostate and epididymis with 7MNTA.

Metabolites from all of the tissues studied were fractionated using a variety of chromatographic procedures and then identified by mass spectral analysis. From the patterns of steroids found, we conclude that the 7MNTA does not undergo 5α-reduction even in organs that contain very large amounts of 5α-reductase. This androgen is metabolized by 5β-reduction, oxidation to the dione, and hydroxylation at the 16α-position (1).

SUMMARY

Development of a double implant system for use as a contraceptive in men has been initiated. One implant will deliver an LHRH analog to suppress LH and FSH. The other implant will deliver a testosterone analog for the maintenance of anabolic and sexual activities.

REFERENCES

1. Agarwal, A.K. and Monder, C. (1988): Endocrinology (submitted).
2. Bardin, C.W. (1983): Internatl. Sym. Res. Reg. Human Fert., Stockholm, Sweden, 835-840.
3. Conn, P.M., Hsueh, A.J.W., and Crowley, W.F. Jr. (1984): Fed. Proc., 43: 2351-2361.
4. Heber, D. and Swerdloff, R.S. (1981): Endocrinology, 108: 2019-2021.
5. Hsueh, A.J. W. and Jones, P.B.C. (1981): Endocr. Rev., 2: 437-461.
6. Nash, H.A., Robertson, D.N., Moo Young, A.J., and Atkinson, L.E. (1978): Contraception, 18: 367-393.
7. Rivier, C., Rivier, J., and Vale, W. (1980): Science, 210: 93-94.
8. Rivier, C., Rivier, J., and Vale, W. (1981): Endocrinology, 108: 1998-2000.
9. Robertson, D.N., Sivin, I., Nash, H., Braun, I., and Dinh, J. (1983): Contraception, 27: 483-495.
10. Sandow, J., Engelbart, K., and Rechenberg, W. von (1985): Med. Biol., 63: 192-200.
11. Swerdloff, R.S., Steiner, B.S., and Bhasin, S. (1985): Med. Biol., 63: 218-224.
12. Weinbauer, G.F. and Nieschlag, E. (1985): Med. Biol., 63: 210-217.

Male Contraception Based on Androgen/Gestagen Combinations

U.A. Knuth and E. Nieshlag

*Mac Planck Clinical Research Unit for Reproductive Medicine and
Institute of Reproductive Medicine
Westfälische-Wilhelms Universität
Steinfurter Str. 107, D4400 Münster, Federal Republic of Germany*

Spermatogenesis is predominantly regulated by pituitary gonadotropins. LH influences gamete production via stimulation of Leydig cells, resulting in high intratesticular testosterone concentrations, while FSH exerts its effects on Sertoli cells. Theoretically azoospermia can be achieved by suppression of gonadotropins, whereby, however, a severe decrease in androgen production would also occur. Since testosterone is required for normal male sexual function, maintenance of secondary sex characteristics, bone and protein metabolism as well as for gender identity, androgens must be an integral part of any male contraceptive method acting via suppression of gonadotropins.

HORMONES USED FOR MALE FERTILITY CONTROL

Testosterone Esters

Since testosterone by itself suppresses gonadotropins, testosterone esters seem to be the ideal substances for male fertility control. Although the general validity of this concept was demonstrated over the last 3 decades (3, 13, 10, 12) homogeneous azoospermia in all participating men could not be achieved.

Combination of antigonadotropic substances with testosterone esters

The effectiveness, however, was increased when testosterone esters were combined with other antigonadotropic substances such as gestagens. Multicenter trials were sponsored by WHO and the Population Council (for reference see 15, 18). Among different combinations tested testosterone oenanthate and depot medroxyprogesterone acetate were used most frequently. Instead of gestagens other antigonadotropic substances such as danazol, cyproterone acetate and GnRH analogs have been tested (for detailed review see 5). But again azoospermia, the final goal of all these investigations, could not be induced reproducibly in all participants.

There is accumulating data in men and non human primates that testosterone alone without LH may allow spermatogenesis to continue at a certain level, if testosterone concentrations within the testes are above a critical level (8, 9). This could mean that testosterone supplementation with presently available esters is detrimental to the goal of 100 % azoospermia. Available testosterone preparations cause considerable fluctuations in serum levels with high levels after injection. These peaks may be sufficient to guarantee a certain proportion of receptor occupancy with maintenance or recovery of spermatogenesis.

As a consequence of these considerations a search for an androgenic substance with longer half-life, slow release characteristics and strong antigonadotropic activity was started.

19-NORTESTOSTERONE FOR MALE FERTILITY CONTROL

During this exploration 19-nortestosterone-esters were identified as potential candidates. Among them 19-nortestosterone-hexyloxyphenylpropionate (Anadur) showed the best pharmakokinetic properties with a half-life of 21 days (2). This drug had been on the market for more then 20 years without reports of serious side effects and could be used for clinical trials without lengthy toxicological testing.

Monotherapy with Anadur

In a pilot study with 5 volunteers azoospermia was achieved in all of them after 12 weeks of injection (16). A follow-up study with a higher number of participants (n=12), a more elaborate design and a longer time of treatment showed that Anadur as a single entity and at longer injection intervals proved to be at least as effective as gestagen/testosterone enanthate combinations (5).

Semen analysis.

Azoospermia occurred in 2 volunteers as early as 9 weeks after the first injection of Anadur with a rising frequency throughout the treatment period. Twenty-one days after the last injection, 27 weeks after the start of the treatment and theoretically the time point at which a maximal impact of treatment could be expected, 6 volunteers presented with azoospermia; further 2 showed only single sperm in the sediment of the ejaculate and 2 had sperm counts below 5 mill/ml. Only 2 out of 12 men treated with Anadur revealed sperm counts in the normal range above 20 mill/ml with unimpaired motility, representing a failure rate of 17%. One of them, however, had been azoospermic after 9 and 12 weeks of treatment with a recovery of sperm counts thereafter.

Side effects.

Complaints about impaired somatic functions or reduction of general well-being were not reported by any of the volunteers. Administration of Anadur did not affect liver enzymes, creatinine, uric acid, serum electrolytes or serum lipids. Hemoglobin, erythrocytes, hematocrit and MCV, however, were significantly elevated following 13 weeks of treatment when compared to pretreatment values, although they did not leave the range considered normal by our standard values.

Combination of Anadur with DMPA

To test whether the promising results of Anadur mono-therapy could be improved, the substance was combined with DMPA in a consequent study.

Volunteers were treated for 7 weeks with weekly i.m. injections of 200 mg Anadur followed by 3-weekly injections of Anadur through week 15. DMPA (250 mg i.m.) was administered at the start of treatment and during weeks 6 and 12.

Serum hormone concentrations.
Measured at 3-week-intervals prior to the next injection 19NT serum levels reached their peak during week 6, while MPA concentrations in serum were highest during week 12. The steroid administration suppressed serum FSH to undetectable levels in all participants within 3 weeks, although 3 men showed detectable values 4 weeks after the last injection. LH serum levels remained below the detection limit until week 12 of follow-up. The decrease in LH caused a steep decline in serum testosterone, although, in general, libido was not impaired.

Semen analysis.
Concentration. Compared to the last pretreatment analysis sperm concentrations were already reduced significantly after 3 weeks of treatment. Azoospermia was achieved in individual volunteers within 9 weeks of treatment. The maximum effect on sperm concentrations was seen 8 weeks after the last injection, when 5 men showed azoospermia and 5 volunteers revealed only single sperm in the sediments of their ejaculates. The remaining two participants showed sperm concentrations of 2.1 and 3.0 x 10^6/ml, respectively. In one of them this number decreased further to single sperm in the sediment during follow-up week 12 and 16.

After 43 weeks of follow-up sperm concentrations of 2 men (4.5 and 11.5 mill/ml) were still below the pretreatment range. One of them had reached normal sperm concentrations of 38.9 x 10^6/ml when tested 75 weeks after the end of treatment. The remaining man had a sperm concentration of 14.8 x 10^6/ml during week 86 of follow-up. But the interval between the previous ejaculation and the time of investigation was only 12 hrs, so that a normalization of sperm production can be assumed.

Motility and morphology. Percentage of normally shaped sperm as well as the proportion of motile sperm was impaired by the treatment. Within 3 weeks a significant drop of motile sperm was observed in all participants (71.6% ± 2.8% vs. 57.1% ± 5.3%; p = 0.004). The percentage of normally shaped sperm decreased too during this interval (63.0% ± 1.9% vs. 54.1% ± 3.9%; p = 0.03). For both parameters lowest values were seen during week 12 in the remaining sperm, although no reasonable parametric statistics could be computed due to the high number of azoospermic ejaculates during the time course of treatment and follow-up.

Motion analysis. According to computerized image analysis the drop in motile sperm was corroborated by a significant decrease of other motion parameters such as mean sperm velocity (35.4 um/s ± 1.8 um/s vs. 25.7 um/s ± 1.7 um/s; p < 0.001), linearity (60.6% ± 2.3% vs. 47.4% ± 2.0%; p < 0.001), beat frequency (8.1 hz ± 0.2 hz vs. 6.5 hz ± 0.4 hz; p = 0.001) and lateral head displacement (3.4 um ± 0.2 um vs. 2.41 um ± 0.2 um; p = 0.003) within the first 3 weeks.

Fertility Regulation in the Male

Volunteers	n=54	n=42	n=15	n=18	n=17	n=12
>5 mill/ml	15%	7%	14%	94%	11%	0%
<5 mill/ml	50%	45%	33%		24%	33%
Azoospermia	35%	48%	53%		65%	67%
Androgen	TE	TE	TE	TU	19NT	19NT
Dose (mg)	200	200	250	120	200	200
Interval	/7d	/30d	/30d	/1d	/21d	/21d
Suppl.	none	Danazol	DMPA	Buserelin	none	DMPA

FIG.1: Comparison of success rates in representative experimental trials for male fertility regulation using different approaches to suppress gonadotropins. "Androgen" indicates substance used to maintain virility: TE=testosterone enanthate, TU=testosterone undecanoate, 19NT = 19-nortestosterone-hexyloxyphenylpropionate. "Interval" describes the frequency of androgen administration per multiple of days. "Suppl." lists the antigonadotropic substance given in addition. Based on (3, 5, 6, 10, 13, 15, 16).

DISCUSSION

Results from our studies using Anadur as an androgen replacement compare favorably to similar trials with testosterone esters (FIG). This suggests that pharmacokinetic properties of the androgen substituiton are of critical importance to achieve the goal of 100% azoospermia in all participants. At present this is the only generally accepted criterion to ensure complete infertility in men. The presence of only a few sperm may be sufficient to induce pregnancy. Pregnancies have occurred in partners of men testing DMPA and testosterone at levels below 10 and even below 1 mill sperm per ml (1). Therefore, the question prevails whether severe oligozoospermia combined with impaired morphology and decreased motility will be sufficient for male fertility regulation.

ACKNOWLEDGEMENTS

Anadur[R] was a gift from Pharmaleo GmbH, Ratingen, FRG. MPA was kindly measured by Dr. S. Cekan, Reproductive Endocrinology Research Unit, Karolinska Sjukhuset, Stockholm, Sweden. Semen analyses and hormone determinations were performed by Ms. C. Krüsemann, Ms. I. Upmann and Ms. M. Möller. Secretarial help was provided by Ms. S. Baha and Ms. B. Dinkhoff.

REFERENCES

1. Barfield, A., J. Melo, E. Coutinho, F. Alvarez-Sanchez, A. Faundes, V. Brache, P. Leon, J. Frick, G. Bartsch, W.-H. Weidke, P. Brenner, D. Mishell Jr, G. Bernstein, A. Ortiz (1979): Contraception 20:121-127

2. Belkien, L., Schürmeyer, T., Hano, R., Gunnarsson, P.O. and Nieschlag, E. (1985): J. Steroid. Biochem. 22:623-629.

3. Heller, C.G., Nelson, W.O. and Hall, I.C. (1950): Fertil. Steril., 1: 415-422.

4. Knuth, U.A., Behre, H., Belkien, L., Bents, H. and Nieschlag, E. (1985): Fertil. Steril. 44:814-821.

5. Knuth, U.A. and Nieschlag, E. (1987): Bailliers's Clin. Endocrinol. Metab., 1:113-130.

6. Leonard, J.M. and Paulsen, C.A. (1978): In: Hormonal Control of Male Fertility by J.D. Patanelli, pp 223-238. Department of Health, Education and Welfare, National Institutes of Health, Bethesda.

7. Michel, E., Bents, H., Akhtar, FB, Hönigl, W., Knuth, U.A., Sandow, J. and Nieschlag, E. (1985): Clin. Endocrinol., 23:663-675.

8. Marshall, G.R., Wickings, E.J., Lüdecke, D.K. and Nieschlag, E. (1983): J. Clin. Endocrinol. Metab., 57:152-159.

9. Marshall, G.R., Wickings, E.J. and Nieschlag, E. (1984): Endocrinology, 114: 2228-2233.

10. Mauss, J., Börsch, G., Richter, E. and Bormacher, K. (1974): Andrologia 10:149-153.

11. Paulsen, C.A., Leonhard, J.M., Burgess, E.C. and Ospina, L.F. (1978): In: Hormonal Control of Male Fertility by J.D. Patanelli, pp 17-35. Department of Health, Education and Welfare, National Institutes of Health, Bethesda.

12. Patanelli, D.J., editor (1978): Hormonal Control of Male Fertility. Department of Health, Education and Welfare, National Institutes of Health, Bethesda.

13. Reddy,P.R.K. and Rao, J.M. (1972): Contraception 5:295-301.

14. Sanchez, F.A., Brache, V., Leon, P. and Faundres, A. (1979): Int. J. Androl., 2:136-149.

15. Schearer, S.B. (1978): Int. J. Androl. 1 (Suppl 2): 680-711.

16. Schürmeyer, T., Knuth, U.A., Belkien, L. and Nieschlag, E. (1984): Lancet I, 417-420.

17. Schürmeyer, T., Knuth, U.A., Freischem, C.W. and Nieschlag, E. (1984): J. Clin. Endocrinol. Metab., 59:19-28.

18. World Health Organization (1972-83): Special Programme of Research Development and Research Training in Human Reproduction. Annual Reports, WHO, Geneva.

Suppression of Sperm Function in Steroid Male Contraception

F.C.W. Wu and R.J. Aitken

MRC Reproductive Biology Unit, Centre for Reproductive Biology,
37 Chalmers Street, Edinburgh EH3 9EW, Scotland, United Kingdom

INTRODUCTION

Sex steroids, via negative feedback inhibition of gonadotrophins, are known to suppress spermatogenesis in normal adult men (1,2,3). However, this has not to date been vigorously pursued as a potential hormonal method for reversible male contraception because only 50-70% of subjects become azoospermic while the rest continues to be oligozoospermic even after treatment with the most effective steroid regimes. Pregnancies have been reported in partners of men being treated with DMPA and TE when sperm counts were below 10 million/ml with half of the pregnancies occurring in those with sperm counts below 1 million/ml (4). This is in contrast to another report where only 7 unplanned pregnancies occurred in almost 300 volunteers using various steroid suppressive regimes over a period of 6 years (5). Significantly, none of the pregnancies occurred when sperm densities were below 5 million/ml. Thus the fertility in those men who continue to produce small numbers of sperm during steroid suppression remains uncertain.

The availability of in vitro tests of sperm fertilization potential (6) has provided a reliable method of assessing the fertility of oligospermic men (7) which can also be applied to examine the effectiveness of potential regimes. The aim of this study was to assess the in vitro fertilizing capacity of residual sperm from men rendered oligospermic by a combination of depot medroxyprogesterone acetate (DMPA) and testosterone oenanthate (TE) by means of an interspecific hamster oocyte penetration (HOP) assay.

SUBJECTS AND METHODS

Ten healthy normal fertile male volunteers, mean age (33.1±4.8 SD years), with normal sperm density (>20 million/ml), motility (>40%), morphology (>40%normal) and hamster oocyte penetration rates (>15%) received 3 intramuscular injections of 200 mg of DMPA (Upjohn) and 250 mg of TE (Schering) at 4-weekly intervals. In addition, 2 placebo (saline) injections were administered in a single-

incorporated into the assay by increasing oocyte numbers to compensate for any deficiencies in the density of motile spermatozoa. To further standardise the HOP assay for oligozoospermic samples, results were corrected to a constant motile sperm concentration of 5 million/ml using formulae based on the Poisson model (11). Thus our data demonstrate the presence of defective function in residual spermatozoa independent of the reduction in sperm numbers in steroid-induced oligozoospermia.

Although other aspects of sperm function such as movement characteristics and zona interaction were not examined, the HOP test revealed that one of the critical steps during fertilization, sperm-oocyte fusion was absent or severely curtailed during or following DMPA and TE treatment. The accuracy of the HOP assay, combined with sperm motility, in predicting fertility in oligozoospermic infertile men followed up for 4 years was about 80% accurate (15). The significantly lower sperm densities encountered in the present study combined with the repeatedly negative oocyte penetration in an assay with improved sensitivity would lend support to the contention that the state of steroid-induced oligospermia may constitute a sufficiently safe target for male contraception. Further studies are required to confirm the clinical efficacy of this and other sex steroid contraceptive regimes.

The mechanism whereby endocrine suppression of the pituitary-testicular axis can produce defects in sperm maturation and function is not known. Intratesticular deficiency of testosterone, as a result of gonadotrphin suppression, may impair Sertoli cell function (16) or prevent normal condensation of sperm heads (17) thus leading to defective sperm maturation and failure in the subsequent expression of sperm function. The findings in subject 1 also suggest that high T concentrations as a result of booster injections may have had certain protective effects which hastened the return of normal sperm function. This may be similar to the protective effect of testosterone observed during GnRH agonist suppression of spermatogenesis (18). MPA, in addition to gonadotrophin suppression, may also have exert direct effects on the Sertoli cells, the epidiymus and spermatozoa (19, 20).

All subjects attained normal sperm counts although the recovery process took 12 months in 1 subject due to circumstances unconnected with the study. Oocyte penetration normalised in 9 subjects by 8 months after treatment. The remaining subject, though normal before treatment, first showed low egg penetration during placebo treatment which did not return to the normal range at 9 months after treatment.

treatment months. In these 22 samples, the mean sperm density was 4.59±1.78 million/ml (<1-35.0); total and motile sperm counts were 12.9±5.5 (1.0-117.5) and 3.2±1.2 (0-26.3) million respectively. Of the 27 oligospermic samples with sperm densities <5 million/ml during treatment and recovery, 20 showed absent oocyte penetration, 5 yielded less than 0.6 million/ml of motile sperm which was the minimal concentration required for the oocyte penetration assay, 1 was not tested due to non-availability of hamster oocytes and 1 with sperm density of 2 million/ml (Subject 1 post-treatment month 2) showed 52% oocyte penetration. Mean sperm motilities of 26.8±14.4 (0-65) and 35.1±8.5 (2-56)% in the third treatment and the first post-treatment month respectively were significantly (P<0.05) lower than pre-treatment values of 53.3±2.7 and 53.2±3.1% (Figure 1).

During recovery, total sperm count, sperm density and the concentration of motile spermatozoa returned to within the pretreatment range in the 6th post treatment month. By the 4th post treatment month, mean HOP rates were not significantly different from pretreatment levels (Figure 1). However, in subject 1, who received additional testosterone injections during treatment, normal HOP capacity was re-established as early as 1 month after treatment.

Mean plasma T and MPA concentrations increased significantly (P<0.001) on Day 2 after each injection of TE and DMPA (Figure 2). T declined to the lower limit of the normal range (9.2±1.1, 8.9±1.4 and 11.2±3.3 nmol/l for first, second and third treatment month respectively) by day 28 (immediately before the next injection). Both LH and FSH were suppressed to the limit of detection by day 7 following the first treatment. LH increased significantly on day 28 from the nadir of the first and second month (P<0.01 & 0.05 respectively) but FSH rose significantly on day 28 only after the first injection. Plasma MPA was still detectable in 3 men at the end of the 6th post treatment month but the mean concentration (0.52±0.10 nmol/l) was not significantly different from pretreatment (below detection limit of assay 0.34 nmol/l). T, LH and FSH returned to pretreatment concentrations at the 5th or 6th post treatment month.

The only significant side effect encountered was a decline in sexual function in 1 subject which was immmediately alleviated by booster TE injections in the second and third months.

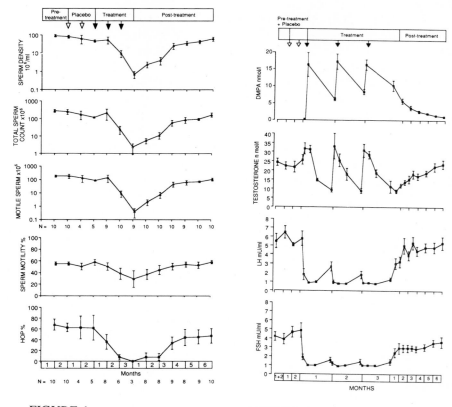

FIGURE 1
The effects of IM DMPA 200mg and TE 250mg (▼) monthly for 3 months on mean±sem sperm density, total and motile sperm counts, sperm motility and hamster oocyte penetration (HOP) rate in 10 normal men. Five received placebo (▽) for 2months.

FIGURE 2
Changes in MPA, testosterone, LH and FSH before, during and after IM DMPA 200mg and TE 250 mg (▼) at monthly intervals for 3 months in 10 normal men. Five received placebo (▽) for 2 months.

DISCUSSION

These results show, for the first time, the effective suppression of in vitro fertilizing potential in men with oligozoospermia induced by short-term treatment with DMPA and TE. Over 95% of non-azoospermic ejaculates with sperm densities of less than 5 million/ml failed to exhibit any capacity for fertilization. To be certain that this decline in fertilizing potential indicated a genuine disruption of sperm function rather than an effect secondary to the reduction in sperm numbers, a sufficient concentration of gametes (10) were incorporated into the assay by increasing oocyte numbers to compensate for any deficiencies in the density of motile spermatozoa. To further standardise the HOP assay for oligozoospermic samples, results were corrected to a constant motile sperm concentration of 5 million/ml using formulae based on the Poisson model (11). Thus our data demonstrate the presence of defective function in residual spermatozoa independent of the reduction in sperm numbers in steroid-induced oligozoospermia.

Although other aspects of sperm function such as movement characteristics and zona interaction were not examined, the HOP test revealed that one of the critical steps during fertilization, sperm-oocyte fusion was absent or severely curtailed during or following DMPA and TE treatment. The accuracy of the HOP assay, combined with sperm motility, in predicting fertility in oligozoospermic infertile men followed up for 4 years was about 80% accurate (15). The significantly lower sperm densities encountered in the present study combined with the repeatedly negative oocyte penetration in an assay with improved sensitivity would lend support to the contention that the state of steroid-induced oligospermia may constitute a sufficiently safe target for male contraception. Further studies are required to confirm the clinical efficacy of this and other sex steroid contraceptive regimes.

The mechanism whereby endocrine suppression of the pituitary-testicular axis can produce defects in sperm maturation and function is not known. Intratesticular deficiency of testosterone, as a result of gonadotrphin suppression, may impair Sertoli cell function (16) or prevent normal condensation of sperm heads (17) thus leading to defective sperm maturation and failure in the subsequent expression of sperm function. The findings in subject 1 also suggest that high T concentrations as a result of booster injections may have had certain protective effects which hastened the return of normal sperm function. This may be similar to the protective effect of testosterone observed during GnRH agonist suppression of spermatogenesis (18). MPA, in addition to gonadotrophin suppression, may also have exert direct effects on the Sertoli cells, the epidiymus and spermatozoa (19, 20).

All subjects attained normal sperm counts although the recovery process took 12 months in 1 subject due to circumstances unconnected with the study. Oocyte penetration normalised in 9 subjects by 8 months after treatment. The remaining subject, though normal before treatment, first showed low egg penetration during placebo treatment which did not return to the normal range at 9 months after treatment.

This work was supported by the World Health Organisation Special Programme of Research, Development, and Research Training in Human Reproduction.

REFERENCES

1. Shearer SB, Alvarez-Sanchez F, Anselmo J, Brenner P, Coutinho E, Latheon-Faundes A, Frick J, Heinild B, Johansson EDB. International Journal of Andrology 1978; Suppl2: 680-711.
2. Paulsen CA, Leonard JM, Burgess EC, Ospima LF. In: Hormonal Control of Male Fertility. pp 17-35. Ed. D.J. Patanelli. Department of Health Education and Welfare. National Institutes of Health 1978; Bethesda.
3. Leonard, J.M. and Paulsen, C.A. (1978). In Patanelli, D.J. (ed). Hormonal control of Male Fertility. pp. 223-238. Bethesda. Department of Health Education and Welfare, National Institutes of Health
4. Barfield A, Melo J, Coutinho E, Alvarez-Sanchez F, Faundes A, Brache V, Leon P, Frick J, Bartsch G, Weiske W, Brenner P, Mishell D, Bernstein G, Oritz A. Contraception 1979; 20: 121-127
5. Paulsen CA, Bremmer WJ, Leonard JM. In: Advances in Fertility Research pp 157-170. Ed. D.R. Mishell Jr. Raven Press 1982; New York.
6. Yanagimachi R. Gamete Research 1984; 10: 187-232.
7. Aitken RJ. International Journal of Andrology 1985; 8: 348-356.
8. Belsey MA, Eliasson R, Gallegos AJ, Moghissi KS, Paulsen CA, Prasad MRN. Press Concern 1980; Singapore.
9. Aitken RJ, Ross A, Hargreave T, Richardson D, Best F. Journal of Andrology 1984; 6: 180-193.
10. Aitken RJ, Elton RA. Journal of Reproduction and Fertility 1986; 78: 733-739.
11. Aitken RJ, Elton RA. Journal of Reproduction and Fertility 1986; 77: 670-674.
12. Hunter WM, Bennie JG. Journal of Endocrinology 1979; 80: 59-68.
13. Corker CS, Davidson DW. Journal of Steroid Biochemistry 1978; 9: 373-374.
14. Shrimanker K, Saxena BN, Fotherby K. Journal of Steroid Biochemistry 1978; 9: 359-363.
15. Aitken RJ. International Journal of Andrology 1985; 8: 348-356.
16. Cunningham GR, Huckins C. Endocrinology 1979;105: 177-189
17. Huang HFS, Nieschlag E. Journal of Reproduction and Fertility 1984; 70: 31-38.
18. Michel E, Bents H, Bint Akhtar F, Honigl W, Knuth UA, Sandow J, Nieschlag E. Clinical Endocrinology 1985; 23: 663-675.
19. Worgal T, Baker HWG, Murray FT, Jefferson LS, Bardin CW. Journal of Andrology 1979; 2: 408-418.
20. Lobl J, Musto NA, Gunsalus GL, Bardin CW. Biology of Reproduction 1983; 29: 697-712.

The Potential Uses and Misuses of Compounds Affecting Spermatogenesis

P. M.D. Foster

ICI Central Toxicology Laboratory,
Alderley Park, Macclesfield,
Cheshire, SK 10 4TJ

A large number of non-drug compounds (ie where human exposure is unintentional) are now recognised to affect adversely the male reproductive system of experimental animals. This phenomenon has been accompanied by a growing awareness of Industry, Regulatory Authorities and Trade Unions of the potential of workplace exposure to materials to impinge upon human reproduction.

In such a complex, co-ordinated system as that controlling male reproduction, it is possible to envisage a large number of potential target sites where the action of a xenobiotic will eventually lead to an impairment in reproduction. These could range from effects on the hypothalamic-pituitary-testicular axis, for example on the Central Nervous System (eg the cannabinoids), the pituitary (synthetic oestrogens), spermatogenesis (dinitrobenzene), epididymal maturation (methyl chloride) to fertilization and paternally mediated developmental toxicity (cyclophosphamide), although the latter has not been conclusively proven.

Consideration should also be given to indirect mechanisms by which foreign compounds may produce testicular toxicity, for example by action on the testicular vasculature (Cadmium), through nutritional deficiences (Vitamin A, 29; Zinc, 20) or on other organs, such as the liver (CCl4), involved in steroid metabolism and clearance. Of all the compounds studied, the vast majority appear to be producing their effects by disturbing spermatogenesis directly. This may be via an effect on the germ cells ie spermatogonia (busulphan, 18), or spermatocytes (for example by glycol ether solvents, 9), or spermatids (ethyl methane sulphonate, 17) or through effects directed at the Sertoli (eg phthalate esters, 10, dinitrobenzene, 1, hexanedione, 3) and Leydig cells (EDS, 25, acetaldehyde, 30), or perhaps myoepithelial peritubular cells.

Having demonstrated toxicity, it is important to realise the processes involved in producing the toxic end point, if such a compound is going to prove useful as a tool, then toxicity should occur at the target organ at the same, or preferably a lower dose, than toxicity to other organ systems. In order to produce toxicity at the target it is important to remember that the compound must be absorbed, distributed, probably metabolised and achieve a critical concentration at the target site, before cellular toxicity will ensue.

We have developed and used a rationale (Fig 1) to attempt to address and understand why any particular compound should adversely affect spermatogenesis. This involves a careful morphological characterization of the lesion, coupled with a metabolism and pharmacokinetics package to determine tissue concentration and metabolite profile, leading on to more detailed in vitro investigations of mode of action and finally, a component involved in detecting functional reproductive deficits.

Figure 1.

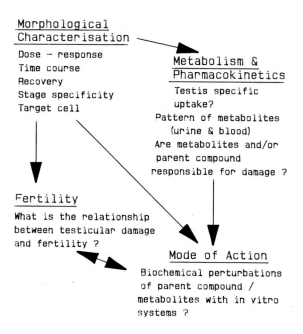

Rationale for the investigation of
Testicular Toxicants

Morphological
Characterisation

Dose - response
Time course
Recovery
Stage specificity
Target cell

Metabolism &
Pharmacokinetics

Testis specific
uptake?
Pattern of metabolites
(urine & blood)
Are metabolites and/or
parent compound
responsible for damage ?

Fertility

What is the relationship
between testicular damage
and fertility ?

Mode of Action

Biochemical perturbations
of parent compound /
metabolites with in vitro
systems ?

There may be a number of reasons why it may be important to understand the mechanism of action of a testicular toxicant (Fig 2). These would range from an ability to improve the assessment of reproductive hazard and from this a more accurate estimate of potential human risk; the use of a compound as a potential male contraceptive, the ability to design chemicals without reproductive problems and lastly the use of specific compounds to be utilised as probes to study normal testicular function.

Figure 2.
Why is it important to understand how compounds affect the testis?

1. Potential male contraceptive.

2. To design compounds without adverse effects.

3. To utilize compounds as probes to understand normal function.

4. To improve the assessment of human
   hazard to produce a better estimate of risk.

The use of the rationale described above will be exemplified by reference to two compounds, with different testicular targets in the rat viz methoxyacetic acid, the major metabolite of the glycol ether solvent, methoxyethanol (ethylene glycol monomethyl ether) and a phthalate ester plasticizer.

Methoxyacetic Acid (MAA)

The testicular toxicity of certain members of the glycol ether class of solvents has been recognised for a number of years, in a wide variety of different species (24,28). The most potent member of the series is ethylene glycol monomethyl ether (EGME; methoxyethanol, 8). This compound is readily absorbed by a variety of routes and evenly distributed throughout body water. In the rat the major blood and urinary metabolite is methoxyacetic acid (8), moreover metabolism is essential for toxicity, since pretreatment of animals with a number of metabolic inhibitors followed by EGME dosing will protect against the compound's testicular toxicity (23). A single oral dose of MAA will result in decreases in testicular weight within 2 days, (12) with pathological evidence of damage at the light level observable within 24h and characterised by a stage-specific lesion to pachytene spermatocytes (4, 12). These effects on pachytene spermatocytes can be reproduced using a Sertoli-germ cell co-culture system (8, 12, 15) both morphologically and by the release of marker enzymes (15, 7). Structural comparisons revealed that MAA bore a close similarity to the endogenous substates for the enzyme lactate dehydrogenase-C4, the germ cell specific isoenzyme (eg lactate, pyruvate and alpha-ketovalerate) and indeed in in vitro studies the enzyme is inhibited by MAA (Fig 3). Since pachytene spermatocytes have the highest specific activity of this enzyme (22) it is possible that such an inhibition may be a contributary feature to the testicular toxicity. Chapin et al (2) has shown that in a fertility trial with EGME, the pattern of decreased fertility obtained coincided with the histological picture at different doses and supported a primary effect on pachytene spermatocytes. Holloway et al (16, this volume) have shown that this pattern of infertility can be reproduced with more sensitive functional end points.

Figure 3.

Lineweaver - Burke plot showing the inhibition of testicular LDH-C4 activity by methoxyacetic acid (MAA).

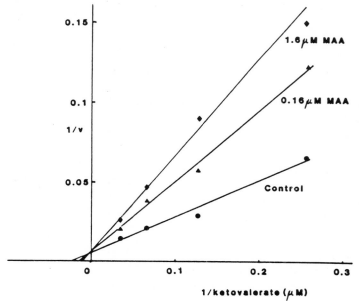

Mono-(2-ethylhexyl)pnthalate (MEHP)

Phthalate esters are a series of compounds used extensively as solvents and plasticizers in polyvinylchloride products. Although their acute toxicity is low in the rat, they can

produce detrimental effects on the testis. Testicular damage
can be elicited within 3-6 hours of a single oral dose, with
the primary effect located in the Sertoli cell (10, 6). Strict
structure - activity relationships apply with the ester
conformation being necessary in the 1,2-(ortho-) position (10)
and that it should be of a particular chain length (13, table
1). The compounds also show a predilection to affect immature
animals and to a much lesser extent their adult counterparts
(eg 27), although the adults show the same basic morphological
response (5). The phthalate esters producing testicular
toxicity are metabolised in the gut by non-specific esterases
(26) and it is the corresponding monoester metabolites which
appear responsible for toxicity. The induced testicular lesion
will also produce deficits in fertility (19, 21) and is
persistant, with incomplete recovery of spermatogenesis after 4
daily doses by 24 weeks (Fig 4). Gray and Beamand (14) were
able to show that the effects of the appropriate monoester
could be reproduced in vitro, with primary testicular cell
cultures and that these were specific, since they did not show
any effects with the parent diesters or analogues which did not
produce toxicity in vivo.

Table 1.

EFFECT OF SOME PHTHALATE MONOESTERS ON GERM CELL DETACHMENT IN RAT TESTICULAR CELL CULTURES

Phthalate monoester	Testicular toxicity	No. of germ cells detached (% of control) at (μ M)					
		1	10	100	1000	3000	10000
2-Ethylhexyl	yes	208*	213*	284*			
n-octyl	yes	130#	161#	500*			
n-hexyl	yes	132+	199*	221*			
n-pentyl	yes	111	147	206*	276*		
n-butyl	yes		113	143+	165+	228*	
tert-butyl	no				115	110	207*
n-propyl	no				100	99	259*
ethyl	no				86	81	210*
methyl	no				102	86	48*

* p< 0.001; # p<0.01; + p<0.05

[After Foster et al (1980) and Gray & Beamand (1984)]

Figure 4.

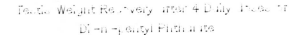

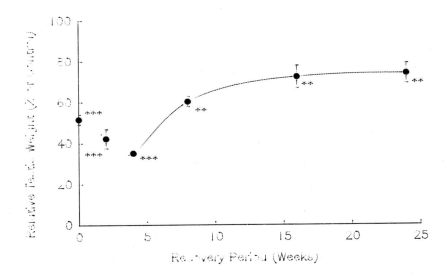

Using enriched cultures of Sertoli cells Williams and Foster (31) were able to show that one of the most potent and most used member of the series, mono-(2-ethylhexyl)phthalate (MEHP), would alter Sertoli cell function by perturbing lactate but not pyruvate production. In contrast, MEHP did not affect FSH stimulated lactate, but did significantly inhibit FSH stimulated pyruvate (32). MEHP would also interfere with FSH stimulated cAMP production (Fig 5) in contrast to another Sertoli cell toxicant (1,3-dinitrobenzene) which also affected lactate and pyruvate production (31), but not that in response to hormone. The finding that MEHP will affect the FSH responsiveness of Sertoli cells may go some way towards explaining its target cell toxicity (FSH receptors are predominantly found on Sertoli cells) and the age susceptibility in response (FSH having a greater role to play in the initiation of spermatogenesis).

Figure 5.

Effect of m-Dinitrobenzene (DNB) and mono-(2-ethylhexyl)phthalate (MEHP) treatment (24hr) on FSH-stimulated cAMP production by rat Sertoli cells.

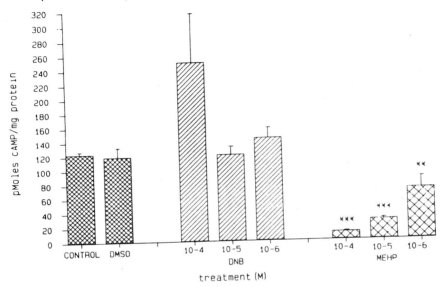

    There are, however, a number of pitfalls that can trip the unwary in the use of chemicals to probe spermatogenesis. Most of these relate to the appropriateness of the test system being used. For example, physiologists would not use a gonadotrophin that had not been adequately tested for its purity, cross-reactivity etc, by the same token they should not use a xenobiotic that has not been correctly analysed for contaminants etc, purities published on manufacturers' bottles are not always correct! The correct biological system is also of importance, is the species being tested a sensitive one to the compound, has an appropriate route of administration been chosen? If for example the compound is dosed via an intra-testicular injection, does it require metabolism? Would the testis ever see such a concentration if the compound was given parenterally? Have the pH and osmolarity of the injected solution been checked to rule out non-specific events before the compound is proposed as a potential male contraceptive?

    Many of these caveats can equally be applied to the use of testicular cell cultures, where due consideration must be given to the limitations (and advantages) of such systems. This is particularly true in the choice of compounds/metabolites, since testicular cells generally have poor xenobiotic metabolising capacity and very few show accumulation within the testis. One must exercise even greater care regarding the generation of non-specific artifacts and toxic responses through insufficient evidence being available on metabolism and tissue distribution, as well as those noted above for in vivo experiments. Unfortunately, there are a number of examples in the literature of impure substances being applied to testicular cells of a non-responsive species, at an inappropriate concentration, and from these experiments deducing the mode of action or possibilities for contraception.

These are just two of many examples of how exogenous compounds may interfere with the process of spermatogenesis. Human exposure to these materials can largely be avoided by the use of non-toxic analogues where appropriate, but they do represent examples of useful probes that physiologists may use in increasing the understanding of the normal control of spermatogenesis in mammalian species.

References

1. Blackburn, D.M., Gray, A.J., Lloyd, S.C., Sheard, C.M. and Foster, P.M.D., (1988) Toxicol Appl Pharmacol 92: 54-64.

2. Chapin, R.E., Dutton, S.L., Ross, M.D., and Lamb, J. C., (1985) Fund Appl Toxicol 14: 182-189.

3. Chapin, R.E., Morgan, K.T., and Bus, J.S., (1983) Exp Mol Pathol 38: 149-169.

4. Creasy, D.M., and Foster, P.M.D., (1984) Exp Mol Pathol 40: 169-176.

5. Creasy.D.M., Beech, L.M., Gray, T.J.B., and Butler, W.H., (1987) Exp Mol Pathol 46: 357-371.

6. Creasy D.M., Foster J.R., and Foster, P.M.D., (1983) Exp Mol Pathol 139: 309-321.

7. Foster, P.M.D., Blackburn, D.M., Moore, R.B., and Lloyd, S.C., (1986) Tox Letts 32: 72-80.

8. Foster, P.M.D., Creasy D.M., Foster, J.R and Gray, T.J.B., (1984) Environ Health Perspec 57: 207-217.

9. Foster, P.M.D., Creasy, D.M., Foster, J.R., Thomas, L.V., Cook, M.W and Gangoli, S.D., (1983) Toxicol Appl Pharmacol 69: 385-399.

10. Foster, P.M.D., Foster, J.R., Cook, M.W., Thomas L.V and Gangoli, S.D., (1982) Toxicol Appl Pharmacol 63: 120-132.

11. Foster, P.M.D., Lake, B.G., Cook, M.W., Thomas, L.V and Gangoli, S.D., (1982) Adv Exp Biol 136A: 445-452.

12. Foster, P.M.D., Lloyd, S.C and Blackburn, D., (1987) Toxicology 43: 17-30.

13. Foster, P.M.D., Thomas, L.V., Cook, M.W and Gangoli, S.D., (1980) Toxicol Appl Pharmacol 54: 392-398.

14. Gray, T.J.B and Beauman, J.A., (1984) Food Chem Toxicol 22: 123-131.

15. Gray, T.J.B., Moss, E.J., Creasy, D.M and Gangoli, S.D., (1985) Toxicol Appl Pharmacol 79: 490-501.

16. Holloway, A.J., Foster, P.M.D and Moore, H.D.M., (1986) Abstr IV European Testis Workshop p165.

17. Jackson, H., Fox, B.W and Craig, A.W., (1961) J Reprod Fert 2: 447-465.

18. Jackson, H., Partington, M and Fox, B.W., (1962) Nature (London) 194: 1184-1185.

19. Lamb, J.C., Chapin, R.E., Teague, J., Lawton, A.D and Reel, J.R., (1987) Toxicol Appl Pharmacol 88: 255-269.

20. Lei, K.Y., Abbvasi, A and Prasad, A.S., (1976) Am J Physiol 230: 1730-1732.

21. Lindsram, P., Harris, M., Ross, M., Lamb, J.C., Chapin, R., Di-n-pentyl phthalate induced infertility: correlation with serum androgen binding protein (1988) Toxicologist 8 Abst 55 p14.

22. Meistrich, M.L., Trostle, P.K., Frapart, M and Erickson, R.P., (1977) Dev Biol 60: 428-441.

23. Moss, E.J., Thaomas, L.V., Cook, M.W., Walters, D.G., Foster, P.M.D., Creasy, D.M and Gray, T.J.B., (1985) Toxicol Appl Pharmacol 79: 480-489.

24. Nagano, K., Nakayama, E,. Koyano, M., Oobayashii, H., Adachi H and Yamada, T., (1979) Japan J Ind Health 21: 29-35.

25. Romments, F.F.G., Grootenhuis, A.J., Moogerbrugger, J.W and Van Der Molen, H.J., (1985) Mol Cell Endocrinol 42: 105-111.

26. Rowland, I.R., Cottrell, R.C and Phillips, J.C., (1977) Food Chem Toxicol 15: 17-21.

27. Sjoberg, P., Lindqvist N.G and Ploen, L., (1986) Environ Health Perspec 65: 237-242.

28. Stenger, E.G., Aeppli, L., Miller, D., Peheim, E and Thomann, P., (1971) Arzneim Forsch 21: 880-885.

29. Thompson, J.N., Howell, J.M., and Pitt, G.A.J., (1964) Proc R Soc London B 159: 510-535.

30. Van Thiel, D.M., Gaveler, J.S., Cobb, C.F., Santucci, L and Graham, T.O., (1983) Pharmacol Biochem Behav 18: 317-323.

31. Williams, J and Foster, P.M.D., (1988) Toxicol Appl Pharmacol (in press).

32. Williams J and Foster P.M.D., (1988) Abstracts of 5th European Testis Workshop, Brighton. Abstract F7.

Effects of Xenobiotics on Glutathione and ATP Levels in Isolated Round Spermatids from Rats

P.J. den Boer, A. Verkerk[1] and J.A. Grootegoed

*Departments of Biochemistry II and [1]Cell Biology and Genetics,
Medical Faculty, Erasmus University Rotterdam,
P.O. Box 1738, 3000 DR Rotterdam, The Netherlands*

Introduction

Glutathione (L-gamma-glutamyl-L-cysteinylglycine; GSH) is the most abundant nonprotein thiol in mammalian cells. It is involved in many biological processes including transport of amino acids, enzyme activities and protection of cells against toxic compounds. Glutathione-supported defense mechanisms of cells include the elimination of peroxides and the detoxication of xenobiotics via conjugation (10). There is little information about the possible roles of glutathione during spermatogenesis. However, recent observations show that GSH depletion of the male reproductive tract potentiated the mutagenic effect of the alkylating agent ethyl methane sulfonate on spermatozoa (14). High concentrations of GSH have been found in rat and mouse testes (2,5). The concentration of GSH in rat testis increases approximately 3-fold between 8 and 29 days of age coinciding with the initial wave of meiosis, and is then maintained during further testis development (2).

In the present study different aspects of the role of glutathione in cellular defense mechanisms were studied using isolated round spermatids. These cells might be useful as an *in vitro* model to study the mechanism of action of toxic compounds which interfere with spermatogenesis through a direct effect on spermatids. For example, the (−) enantiomer of the male antifertility agent gossypol, which is effective *in vivo* acting on mitochondria in spermatids and spermatozoa, is also effective in decreasing the ATP content of isolated spermatids, probably as a result of an effect on the coupling between electron transport and ATP synthesis in the mitochondria (1).

Estimation of glutathione

Round spermatids from rats were isolated by sedimentation at unit gravity and further purified by density gradient centrifugation, as described previously (3). The GSH content of the isolated spermatids was determined by a flow cytometric assay described by Poot et al. (12), using monobromobimane as a thiol staining agent. After incubation for 18 h the relative fluorescence intensity (RFI) of the intact spermatids was measured. Propidium iodide (PI) was added to the cell suspension before analyzing the cells, and only spermatids which excluded PI were analyzed. The average RFI of the cell population was calculated. Furthermore, the cellular ATP content was also estimated and expressed as $nmol/10^6$ intact cells (cells excluding PI).

Peroxides

Cumene hydroperoxide (CHP) was used as a model compound to study the glutathione redox cycle (13). CHP is converted by glutathione peroxidase to the corresponding alcohol (reaction 1).

$$CumeneOOH + 2\ GSH \longrightarrow CumeneOH + GSSG + H_2O \quad (1)$$

The oxidized glutathione (GSSG) is then reduced by the enzyme glutathione reductase, at the expense of reducing equivalents from NADPH (reaction 2).

$$GSSG + NADPH + H^+ \longrightarrow 2\ GSH + NADP^+ \quad (2)$$

$NADP^+$ can be reduced to NADPH via the pentose phosphate pathway and a number of other reactions.

It was observed that spermatids, incubated for 18 h with low concentrations of CHP, maintained their GSH and ATP levels (Table 1). Concomitantly, the activity of the pentose phosphate pathway was increased (not shown). The data from the flow cytometer showed a population of cells containing approximately equal amounts of GSH (Fig.1). The result indicate that the GSH redox cycle was active in the cells, and that metabolism of low concentrations of the peroxide did not lead to glutathione depletion in intact cells. However, at higher concentrations of CHP the capacity of this defense mechanism was inadequate to prevent cell degeneration, as indicated by the loss of both GSH

TABLE 1. Effect of cumene hydroperoxide (CHP) on GSH and ATP levels in round spermatids from rats.

[CHP] (μM)	GSH (RFI)	ATP (nmol/10^6 cells)	% of cells excluding PI*
0	125.0 ± 1.0	5.95 ± 0.23	95.0 ± 1.0
5	129.7 ± 0.6	5.81 ± 0.33	92.3 ± 2.1
10	130.0 ± 1.7	5.73 ± 0.28	89.3 ± 1.5
15	130.0 ± 1.0	5.78 ± 0.77	86.3 ± 5.5
20	131.1 ± 4.5	5.62 ± 0.14	72.3 ± 4.0
40	n.d.**	0.38 ± 0.29	<5

*propidium iodide
**too low a number of intact cells to determine RFI
Round spermatids were isolated as described previously (3) and incubated for 18h at 32°C in phosphate-buffered saline (PBS) supplemented with 6 mM sodium L-lactate, 5.6 mM glucose, 0.4% BSA and antibiotics, in the presence of different concentrations of CHP. The ATP content at t=0 h was 6.72 ± 0.16 nmol/10^6 cells. The results represent the mean ± SD of triplicate incubations.

and ATP from the cells and by the decrease of the percentage of PI excluding cells. A rate-limiting factor in the defense mechanism of spermatids against peroxides could be a relatively low activity of glucose 6-phosphate dehydrogenase, the first enzyme of the pentose phosphate pathway (4).

Conjugation.

The other defense mechanism studied involves the conjugation between GSH and electrophilic xenobiotics catalyzed by glutathione S-transferases (GST) (reaction 3).

$$GSH + X \longrightarrow GSX \quad (3)$$

This type of reaction initiates the detoxication of a number of xenobiotics. The formed conjugates can be metabolized further to mercapturic acids, which are water soluble and can be released from the cells and finally excreted by the kidney (6). This defense mechanism leads to an irreversible loss of glutathione from the cells, and therefore requires cellular uptake and/or synthesis of glutathione.

GST activities were estimated in whole testis homogenates from 5 week-old rats (344.0 ± 3.0 mU/mg protein) and in isolated round spermatids (37.5 ± 0.7 mU/mg protein), using 1-chloro-2,4-dinitrobenzene as a substrate (7). The specific activity of GST in spermatids was relatively low but indicated that spermatids contain the enzymic activity to catalyze conjugation reactions between GSH and a number of toxic compounds. GST activities have been reported to be present also in spermatozoa (11).

The effect on GSH levels in spermatids was studied using the GST substrate diethyl maleate (DEM). The glutathione level in spermatids was decreased after 18 h of incubation in the presence of low concentrations of DEM, but the ATP content was not affected (Table 2).

TABLE 2. Effect of diethyl maleate (DEM) on GSH and ATP levels in round spermatids from rats.

[DEM] (μM)	GSH (RFI)	ATP (nmol/10⁶ cells)	% of cells excluding PI[*]
0	148.0 ± 1.0	5.97 ± 0.16	96.7 ± 1.2
10	95.3 ± 1.2	5.36 ± 0.24	97.0 ± 1.0
30	67.7 ± 1.2	5.44 ± 0.78	97.0 ± 1.0
100	58.0 ± 1.0	5.05 ± 0.50	96.0 ± 1.0
300	43.3 ± 2.1	2.76 ± 0.53	92.7 ± 0.6
1000	n.d.[**]	0.05 ± 0.01	<5

[*]propidium iodide
[**]to low a number of intact cells to determine RFI
Round spermatids were isolated and incubated as described in Table 1, in the presene of different concentrations of DEM. The ATP content at t=0 h was 6.20 ± 0.10 nmol/10⁶ cells. The results represent the mean ± SD of triplicate incubations.

Approximately 97% of the cells excluded propidium iodide after incubation with 100 μM of the GST substrate. The present flow cytometric analysis indicated a decrease of the GSH content in each cell rather than GSH depletion in a part of the cell population (Fig.1).

Glutathione depleted cells are dependent on uptake of exogenous glutathione or *de novo* synthesis of glutathione to replenish their GSH content. In this context, the gamma-glutamyl cycle which includes the activity of the enzyme gamma-glutamyl transpeptidase

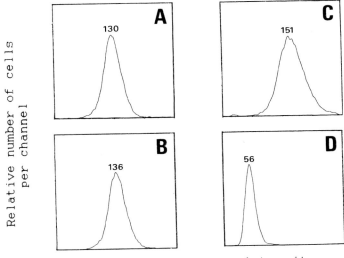

Relative number of cells per channel

Relative fluorescence intensity
(RFI; channel number)

FIG. 1. GSH contents (RFI) of isolated round spermatids from rats after 18 h of incubation in (A) the absence and (B) in the presence of 20 μM cumene hydroperoxide, and in (C) the absence and (D) presence of 100 μM diethyl maleate.

(GGT), plays an important role. GGT has been detected in Sertoli cell preparations, whereas spermatids seem to have very low activity levels of this enzyme (8,9). A low activity of the enzyme may be a rate-limiting factor in the maintenance of cellular glutathione levels in spermatids and spermatozoa if the testis and the epididymis are exposed to xenobiotics and drugs that form conjugates with glutathione by way of GST activities.

Concluding remarks

Isolated spermatids from rats are able to inactivate peroxides via the GSH redox cycle, up to a point where the rate of NADP$^+$ reduction may become rate-limiting. In contrast, irreversible cellular depletion of GSH is induced through glutathione S-transferase catalyzed conjugation of low concentrations of xenobiotics with GSH. This depletion finally may result in degeneration of the cells, and it is suggested that this is related to a limited capacity for replenishment of the intracellular GSH pool in spermatids. In the testicular tubules, it can be expected that spermatids do not succumb to low levels of aspecific toxic compounds that can be inactivated by Sertoli cells. However, epididymal sperm may be vulnerable to compounds forming conjugates with GSH. the more so because different compounds may gain access to the epididymis via passive or active transport (15).

Acknowledgement

This investigation received financial support from the World Health Organization Special Programme of Research, Development and Research Training in Human Reproduction.

References

1. Den Boer, P.J., and Grootegoed, J.A. (1988): J. Reprod. Fert., in the press.
2. Calvin, H.I., and Turner, S.I. (1982): J. Exp. Zool., 219:389-393.
3. Grootegoed, J.A., Jansen, R., and Van der Molen, H.J.(1984): Biochim. Biophys. Acta, 767:248-246.
4. Grootegoed, J.A., Oonk, R.B., Toebosch, A.M.W., and Jansen, R., (1986): In: Molecular and Cellular Endocrinology of the Testis, edited by M. Stefanini, M. Conti, R. Geremia, and E. Ziparo. pp. 215-225. Excerpta Medica, Amsterdam.
5. Grosshans, K., and Calvin, H.I. (1985): Biol. Reprod., 33:1197-1205.
6. Habig, W.H., Pabst, M.J., and Jakoby, W.B. (1974): J. Biol. Chem., 249:7130-7139.
7. Habig, W.H., and Jakoby, W.B. (1981): Meth. Enzymol.,77:398-405.
8. Hodgen, G.D., and Sherins, R.J. (1973): Endocrinology, 93:985-989.
9. Lu, C., and Steinberger, A. (1977): Biol. Reprod., 17:84-88.
10. Meister, A., and Anderson, M.E. (1983): Ann. Rev. Biochem., 52:711-760.
11. Mukhtar, H., Lee, I.P., and Bend, J.R. (1978): Biochem. Biophys. Res. Comm., 83:1093-1098.
12. Poot, M., Verkerk, A., Koster, J.F., and Jongkind, J.F.(1986): Biochim. Biophys. Acta, 883:580-584.
13. Poot, M., Verkerk, A., Koster, J.F., Esterbauer, H., and Jongkind, J.F. (1987): Eur. J. Biochem., 162:287-291.
14. Teaf, C.M., Bishop, J.B., and Harbison, R.D. (1987): Teratogenesis, Carcinogenesis, and Mutagenesis, 7:497-513.
15. Wong, P.Y.D., Lau, S.K.D., and Fu, W.O. (1987): J. Reprod. Fert. 81:259-267.

Rat *In Vitro* Fertilization Can Detect Testicular Toxicity Induced by Low Doses of Ethylene Glycol Monomethyl Ether

A.J. Holloway, H.D.M. Moore and P.M.D. Foster*

*Institute of Zoology, Zoological Society of London,
Regent's Park, London 4RY and
*Central Toxicology Laboratory, Imperial Chemical Industries plc,
Alderley Park, Macclesfield, Cheshire, SK10 4JT*

INTRODUCTION

There are many chemicals known to cause testicular damage in laboratory animals and there is a growing number of reports of reduced fertility in man after exposure to such chemicals (for reviews see 8, 10, 12, 14). Conventionally, single and multigeneration breeding trials are used to assess reproductive performance after toxic insult. These trials use large numbers of animals over relatively long periods and so are time consuming and expensive. It would be useful to have a quicker, relatively cheap assay so that potential testicular toxicants can be prescreened before launching a major investigative programme. A robust in vitro fertilization (IVF) system, sensitive enough to detect subtle changes in the fertilizing capacity of spermatozoa, could provide such an assay. In such a system, males would be exposed to appropriate levels of a toxicant and their fertility monitored at suitable intervals. Allowing the toxicant to act in vivo ensures that it reaches the target cells via normal metabolic avenues. By assessing fertility in vitro, the morphological, physiological and biochemical parameters of spermatozoa obtained for IVF can be rapidly and directly correlated with fertilizing capacity.

To be of practical use, the IVF assay must be carried out using the rat, since this is the main animal used in toxicological testing. Although IVF was first described in the rat by Toyoda and Chang in 1974 (13), it has for many years proved to be a notoriously unreliable procedure. Recently, the finding that oocyte fertilizing potential could be adversely affected by the dose of pregnant mares serum gonadotrophin used to induce superovulation (4) and the introduction of a number of other minor changes have improved the reliability of the technique.

Ethylene glycol monomethyl ether (EGME), an intermediate in the food and chemical industry, is a known testicular toxicant (9, 15). In the rat it causes cellular degeneration, particularly arrecting pachytene spermatocytes; late stage spermatids, leptotene and zygotene spermatocytes are also affected, but to a lesser extent (5, 6). In this study, single, low doses of EGME were used to induce specific lesions in the rat testis. Cauda epididymal spermatozoa were then obtained at twice weekly intervals to investigate whether changes in fertility could be detected using an IVF system.

MATERIALS AND METHODS

Animals

Animals were maintained on a light regime of 14 hours light and 10 hours darkness, with the light period starting at 06.00 hours. They were fed ad libitum with Diet M & R1 (Special Diet Services).

Treatment of males

Adult male rats (54) (AP/ALPK, Wistar derived, Central Toxicology Laboratories, Imperial Chemical Industries, plc), weighing between 475g - 625g were housed in pairs. The animals were lightly anaesthetized with sodium pentobarbitone (Sagatal, May and Baker Ltd, UK) and randomly assigned to four treatment groups. EGME (>99% pure) was diluted by 1:5 in 50% ethyl alcohol. The animals were given single, oral doses of 50, 100 or 200mg EGME/kg or 1ml/kg 50% ethyl alcohol.

The fertilizing capacity of cauda epididymal spermatozoa from between one and three males per treatment group was assessed twice a week for eight weeks after treatment. To increase the number of observations one epididymis was surgically removed from some males up to two weeks before these animals were culled for recovery of the spermatozoa from the remaining epididymis. Hemi-epididymectomy did not adversely affect the fertility of spermatozoa from the contralateral tract.

In vitro fertilization

The method used was a modification of that described by Toyoda and Chang (13). A diagram of the schedule for rat IVF using spermatozoa from males treated with EGME is given in figure 1.

Fertilization medium

The working medium was a combination of two stock solutions. All chemicals were supplied by BDH Chemicals, Ltd. (England) unless otherwise stated. Solution A was comprised of 6.636g NaCl/l, 427mg KCl/l, 302mg $CaCl_2.2H_2O/l$, 194mg KH_2PO_4/l, 172mg $MgSO_4$ /l, 2mg phenol red/l. Solution B was comprised of 12.94g $NaHCO_3/l$ and 2mg phenol red/l. The working medium comprised 83.35ml Solution A, 16.28ml Solution B, 0.37ml sodium lactate, 5.5mg sodium pyruvate, 100mg dextrose, 5mg penicillin (Sigma), 5mg streptomycin (Sigma) and 400mg bovine serum albumin (Sigma). The medium was sterilized by filtration through a 0.22μm Millipore filter. Plastic petri dishes (35mm) containing 0.4ml medium under silicone fluid (Dow Corning) were equilibrated overnight in an atmosphere of 5% carbon dioxide in air at 37°C in a humidified incubator.

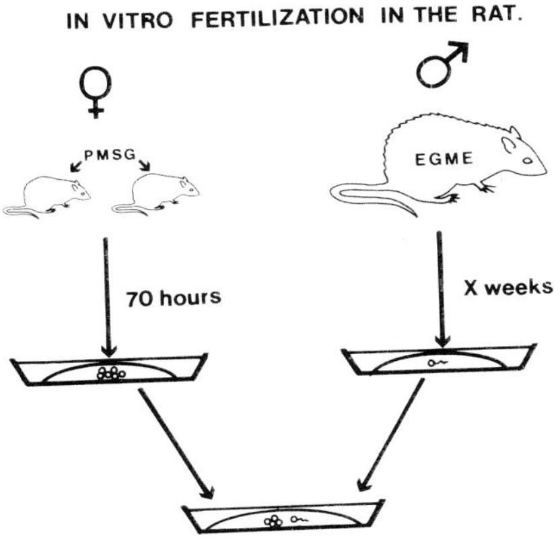

FIG. 1. Schematic representation of IVF using spermatozoa from males treated with EGME.

Oocyte collection

Immature female rats weighing between 60g and 85g were housed in groups of ten. Ovulation was induced by a subcutaneous injection of 15 IU pregnant mares serum gonadotrophin (Intervet) at 17:30 hours. The ovaries and oviducts were excised 68 to 70 hours later. They were washed in Dulbecco's phosphate buffered saline (PBS) at 37°C and blotted to remove any blood. The oviducts were placed in fresh PBS and ruptured to release the oocytes. The oocytes in their cumulus mass were transferred to dishes containing working medium.

Preparation of spermatozoa

Males were anaesthetized with sodium pentobarbitone. The right testis and epididymis were pulled up through a midline incision. The cauda epididymidis was excised after ligating the caput epididymis and blood vessels. The testis was returned to the scrotal sac and the body cavity closed by sutures. Spermatozoa were gently expressed from the distal cauda region into the equilibrated medium, allowed to disperse and were transferred to the oocyte dishes to give a final concentration between 500,000 and 1×10^6 spermatozoa/ml.

The left cauda epididymidis and testis were subsequently removed between four and fourteen days later. The male received a lethal dose of sodium pentobarbitone and spermatozoa were obtained from the cauda region as described above.

Examination of oocytes and embryos

The oocytes and embryos were examined 19 - 24 hours after collection. They were washed in clean medium to remove unattached spermatozoa and transferred to microscope slides. They were gently compressed by coverslips supported by wax spots at each corner and examined using a Nikon inverted phase contrast microscope for the presence of a decondensing sperm head or pronucleus and sperm tail in the vitellus. Degenerate oocytes were discarded.

Statistics

Fertilization rates for rats treated with EGME were compared with those of the control rats using Chi squared analysis.

RESULTS

The data for the number of oocytes examined and the number of males from the four treatment groups for each assessment are summarized in table 1.

TABLE 1. The number of oocytes and the number of males examined for each treatment group.

Weeks after treatment	No. of oocytes (no. of males) for each treatment group			
	Control	200mg/kg	100mg/kg	50mg/kg
1.0	142 (3)	127 (1)	39 (2)	20 (1)
1.5	92 (2)	74 (2)	29 (1)	30 (1)
2.0	37 (2)	41 (1)	110 (2)	9 (1)
2.5	43 (2)	75 (2)	44 (2)	–
3.0	167 (3)	44 (2)	66 (1)	41 (2)
3.5	64 (1)	89 (1)	59 (1)	34 (1)
4.0	50 (1)	70 (1)	29 (2)	47 (3)
4.5	82 (2)	77 (2)	53 (1)	43 (2)
5.0	85 (2)	58 (1)	99 (2)	32 (2)
5.5	132 (3)	107 (2)	84 (2)	63 (2)
6.0	110 (2)	84 (2)	78 (1)	–
6.5	109 (2)	40 (2)	45 (1)	73 (2)
7.0	60 (1)	84 (2)	63 (1)	9 (1)
7.5	27 (1)	60 (1)	53 (1)	–
8.0	23 (1)	32 (1)	27 (1)	44 (2)

The percentage of oocytes fertilized by the control males was consistently greater than 65% throughout the experiment, with a mean of 73.8% ± 5.2%. The mean fertilization rate for males given 50mg EGME/kg was 68.8% ± 6.8%. 56% oocytes were fertilized five

weeks after treatment with 50mg EGME/kg, this was significantly
less than the 73% oocytes fertilized by control males. The mean
fertilization rate for males given 100mg EGME/kg was 68.9% ± 14%.
Males given 100mg EGME/kg had significantly lower fertility than
controls at 3.5 weeks (49% compared with 65.5%), 4.5 weeks (60%
compared with 77%), 5 weeks (36% compared with 73%); 6 weeks (51%
compared with 69%) and 6.5 weeks after treatment (60% compared
with 77%). The mean fertilization rate for males given 200mg
EGME/kg was 55.9% ± 21%. Males given 200mg EGME/kg had
significantly lower fertility than control males at 2 weeks (34%
compared with 73%), 3 weeks (48% compared with 65%), 4.5 weeks
(28% compared with 77%), 5 weeks (26% compared with 72%), 5.5
weeks (62% compared with 69%), 6 weeks (9.5% compared with 77%)
and at 7 weeks after exposure (55% compared with 75%) (figure 2).

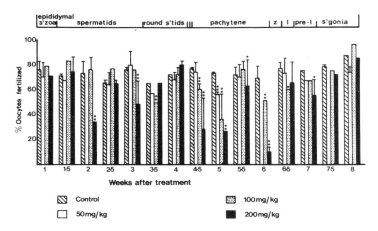

FIG. 2. The percentage oocytes fertilized after IVF with
spermatozoa from males treated with 50, 100 and 200mg EGME/kg.
* Significantly different from controls (p < 0.05)

DISCUSSION

Consistently high rates of fertilization (>65%) were obtained
for the control males using this in vitro fertilization system.
The mean rate for control males was 73% (882/1200) which was
slightly lower than the 75 - 88% fertilization rate obtained by
Toyoda and Chang (13) but considerably higher than the 53.6%
achieved by Evans and Armstrong (4).
    It was possible to demonstrate that fertility was reduced in
males treated with EGME. Poor fertility occurred at specific times
after dosing, at 2, 3 and 3.5 weeks and between 4.5 and 7 weeks
after dosing. In the Wistar rat spermatogenesis takes 53.2 days
(7) while epididymal transfer takes approximately 8.5 days (11).
Therefore, elongated spermatids exposed to EGME would be found in

the cauda epididymides at 2, 3 and 3.5 weeks after dosing. Similarly, pachytene spermatocytes exposed to EGME would be found in the distal cauda between 4.5 to 6 weeks later, and after 7 weeks the exposed leptotene and preleptotene spermatocytes would reach the cauda. There was a clear dose response to EGME, in both the extent to which fertility was reduced and in the number of cell types affected. After the lowest dose administered in this experiment (50mg EGME/kg) the pachytene spermatocytes were affected. The higher doses (100 and 200mg EGME/kg) affected the pachytenes to a greater extent and also damaged the late stage spermatids. The leptotene spermatocytes were affected in males given 200mg EGME/kg. These data are in agreement with the histological reports which showed that pachytene spermatocytes were particularly vulnerable to EGME, with leptotene and zygotene spermatocytes affected to a lesser extent (2, 3, 6, 7). Serial breeding trials have indicated that late stage spermatids and spermatogonia were damaged by EGME (1).

Previous studies have shown that pachytene spermatocytes affected by EGME become necrotic (6). However, when a single dose was given, as in this study, enough mature spermatozoa could be expressed from the distal cauda after five weeks to ensure that the concentration in the oocyte dishes was between 500,000 and 1×10^6/ml. Therefore, the loss of fertility was not due to insufficient numbers of spermatozoa, but was a result of the production of infertile spermatozoa from germ cells sublethally affected during sensitive phases of spermatogenesis.

The IVF system was more sensitive than serial breeding in detecting changes in fertility. Using serial breeding, it was not possible to detect any reduction in fertility after dosing rats with 50mg EGME/kg/day for five days (1). However, using IVF, there was a slight, but significant reduction in fertility after a single dose of 50mg EGME/kg.

In conclusion, in vitro fertilization provides a sensitive but reliable method of measuring the fertilizing capacity of rat spermatozoa. It was possible to detect dose related reductions in fertility after exposure to EGME, even using levels of the toxicant which, using conventional assays would be regarded as below the "no effect" dose. Furthermore, it was shown that the induced infertility was due to impaired sperm function rather than a reduction in sperm numbers.

REFERENCES

1. Chapin, R.E., Dutton, S.L., Ross, M.D., Lamb, J.C. (1985): Fundam. and Appl. Toxicol., 5:182–189.

2. Creasy, D.M., Flynn, J.C., Gray, T.J.B. and Butler, W.H. (1985): Exp. and Mol. Pathol., 43:321–336.

3. Doe, J.E., Samuels, D.M., Tinston, D.J. and de Silva Wickramaratne, G.A. (1983): Toxicol. and Appl. Pharmacol.,

69:43-47.

4. Evans, G. and Armstrong, D.T. (1984): J. Reprod. Fert., 70:131-135.

5. Foster, P.M.D., Creasy, D.M., Foster, J.R., Thomas, L.V., Cook, M.W. and Gangolli, S.D. (1983): Toxicol. and Appl. Pharmacol., 69:385-399.

6. Foster, P.M.D., Creasy, D.M., Foster, J.R. and Gray, T.J.B. (1984): Env. Health Perspectives, 57:207-217.

7. Huckins, C. (1965): Anat. Rec., 151:364.

8. Lee, I.P. and Dixon, R.L. (1978): Env. Health Perspectives, 24:117-127.

9. Miller, R.R., Ayres, J.A., Calhoun, L.L., Young, J.T. and McKenna, M.J. (1981): Toxicol. and Appl. Pharmacol., 61:368-377.

10. Moore, H.D.M. (1986): Food and Chem. Toxicol., 24:607-613.

11. Robb, G.W., Amann, R.P. and Killian, G.J. (1978): J. Reprod. Fert., 54:103-107.

12. Sever, L.E. and Hessel, N.A. (1985): In: Endocrine Toxicology, edited by J.A. Thomas et al, pp. 211-248, Raven Press, New York.

13. Toyoda, Y. and Chang, M.C. (1974): J. Reprod. Fert., 36:9-22.

14. Waller, D.P., Killinger, J.M. and Zaneveld, L.T.D. (1985): In: Endocrine Toxicology, edited by J.A. Thomas et al, pp. 269-333, Raven Press, New York.

15. Wiley, F.H. (1938): J. Industrial Hygiene and Toxicology, 20:4.

ACKNOWLEDGMENTS

This study was supported by a collaborative project grant from the Medical Research Council and Imperial Chemical Industries plc.

Germ Cell - Sertoli Cell Interactions in Vertebrates

B. Jégou, B. Le Magueresse, P. Sourdaine, C. Pineau,
J.F. Velez de la Calle, D.-H. Garnier, F. Guillou*
and C. Boisseau

*Laboratoire de Biologie de la Reproduction, UA CNRS 256,
Université de Rennes I, Campus de Beaulieu
35042 Rennes Cédex, France.
*Physiologie de la Reproduction, INRA
3730 Monnaie, France*

INTRODUCTION

In the last decade it has become well established that in addition to the regulation by FSH, LH and testosterone, cell to cell interactions within the testis play a crucial role in the control of spermatogenesis. Thus, interactions between Leydig cells, Sertoli cells and myoid cells as well as the existence of a major influence of Sertoli cells upon germ cells have been demonstrated (see review 39).

Germ cells represent approximately 75% of the total cell composition of the testis (45) and are the end point of the endocrine and paracrine regulations within this organ. Para- doxically, despite these facts, the role that they may play in the local regulation of the testis has, until recently, received very little attention. This is partly due to the complex organization of the mammalian seminiferous tubules which makes it very difficult to isolate and culture most of the germ cell types that they contain.

With regard to what can be considered as part of "the most complex cell interactions in the testis" (39) and to the important role that germ cells may play in the paracrine, control of testicular function, several experimental approaches have been developed for unravelling germ cell influences upon Sertoli cell function : 1) the study of Sertoli cell morphology and function in relation to the different stages of spermatogenesis in the rat (see review 32). 2) the study of germ cell effects on rat Sertoli cell cultures (8, 13, 24-27). 3) the selective removal of sub-classes of germ cells in adult rats in vivo using various experimental means and the study of the consequences on several parameters of Sertoli cell function (14-15, 18-20).

GERM CELL - SERTOLI CELL INTERACTIONS

Recently, a fourth type of approach in this field has been initiated : the use of non-mammalian models whose particular organization of the testis provides unique possibilities to explore germ cell contributions to the paracrine regulation of testicular function (3).

In this paper we will present data from our group demons- trating the usefulness of these four types of in vitro and in vivo experimental approaches to demonstrate the crucial importance of germ cells in the development and the regulation of Sertoli cell function.

MATERIALS AND METHODS

Studies In The Rat

In vitro

Sertoli cell cultures.

Sertoli cells were prepared from Sprague-Dawley rats at different ages (10, 15 and 20 days old) according to a method previously described (28). For 45-day-old rats, this method was slightly modified; incubation time in the 0.1 M glycine buffer and the two successive collagenase-dispase solutions (0.05%) were 20, 30, and 40-45 min, respectively. All Sertoli cell-enriched suspensions were plated (day 0 of culture) in 10 cm^2 Nunc dishes at the density given in the figure legends. The cells were incubated at 32°C in a humidified atmosphere of 5% CO_2 and 95% air. Ham's F-12-Dulbecco's Modified Eagle's Medium was supplemented, after the first 24 h of incubation, with insulin (10 μg/ml), transferrin (5 μg/ml) and epidermal growth factor (10 ng/ml). When specified, 1 μg of oFSH S16 or 0.5 mM of dibutyryl cAMP (dbcAMP) was added per culture dish after the first 24 h of culture. Culture media were replenished daily and FSH or dbcAMP was replaced until the end of the experiment.

On day 2 of culture, some dishes were exposed to a Tris-HCl buffer solution (20 mM; pH 7.4) to remove contaminating germ cells (9). The remaining cells were observed under phase contrast microscopy. This was routinely set at 2-2.5 min, except for Sertoli cell cultures recovered from 45-day -old rats, for which a 15 min exposure was used.

Preparation of the crude and enriched germ cell fractions.

Germ cells were prepared from adult Sprague-Dawley rat testes by trypsinization (29). The crude germ cell suspensions obtained were added to Sertoli cells (hypotonically treated or not) on day 3 of culture at a concentration of 3×10^6 cells/culture dish. Germ cell viability, assessed by the erythrosine red exclusion test, was greater than 97%. In some experiments. enriched fractions of pachytene spermatocytes, early spermatids (steps 1-8) and cytoplasts from elongated spermatids (CES). were prepared from the crude germ cell suspensions by centrifugal elutriation (29). Pachytene spermatocytes and early spermatids were added to Sertoli cells on day 2 or 3 of culture at concentrations of 2×10^6 and 8×10^6 cells/culture dish, respectively. Twenty-four hours after adding crude or enriched germ cell suspensions, culture and coculture media were collected and fresh media were then added to each of the dishes.

Assay of Sertoli cell parameters.
Culture and coculture media from days 3-4 or 5-6 of culture were collected and centrifuged (10,000 x g; 4°C; 30 min). Super-natants supplemented with 10% glycerol were kept at -20°C before measurement of ABP by equilibrium dialysis (7). Testosterone (150 ng/dish) was added as a substrate for aromatization 24 hours before the oestradiol assay. Oestradiol 17β was measured by RIA using a specific antibody, as previously described (41). Transferrin released into the culture or coculture media for 24 hours was also measured by a specific RIA. ABP, oestradiol 17β and transferrin levels were expressed as picomoles, picograms and micrograms respectively, per μg Sertoli cell DNA or per dish. In Sertoli cell cultures prepared from 45-day-old rats, micrograms of Sertoli cell DNA were estimated from measurement of the DNA content in the dish corrected for germ cell contamination estimated by a flow cytometric technique (25).

In vivo

Sprague-Dawley rats 90 days old were used. Except for short servicing periods, exposed rats were continuously whole body irradiated with ^{60}Co γ rays at a low dose rate (7cGy/day; total of 588 cGy; 1 cGy = 1 rad). During the irradiation (Days 14, 28, 41, 54, 62, 84) and post-irradiation (Days 7, 20, 35, 42, 60, 86) periods, groups of 5 experimental and 5 control rats were sacrificed by decapitation. Testes and epididymides were dissected out and weighed. Testes were then processed for histological observations. Cells were counted in 20 cross sections (5 μm) per testis at stage VII of the cycle according to Leblond and Clermont's classification (23). ABP contents in the caput epididymides were measured by SS-PAGE as previously described (37).

Studies In The Dogfish (Scyliorhinus canicula).

Dissociation and identification by transillumination of the seminiferous lobules.
As shown in Fig. 1, the structure of the dogfish testis is zonate and is made up of lobules in successive bands at different stages of spermatogenesis.

These lobules are composed of cysts, each of the cysts consisting of one Sertoli cell associated with 1-64 germ cells at an identical stage of spermatogenesis.

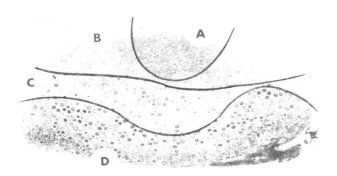

FIG. 1. Photomicrograph of a transverse section of a testis from an adult dogfish (Scyliorhinus canicula L.). A : zone of genesis (spermatogonia); B : spermatocytes; C : round and elongating spermatids; D : elongated spermatids and spermiation.

In order to dissociate the seminiferous lobules, sections from adult dogfish testes were incubated with collagenase (0.025%) and pronase (0.08%) at 4°C. The tissue was then dissociated mechanically at 17°C in a Ca^{++} and Mg^{++} free Gautron's buffer (GB; 10). The lobules were collected in GB supplemented with DNAse and BSA before being rinced with GB. Based on differences in light absorption and size as well as on comparison with the corresponding histological and ultrastructural cell composition, the seminiferous lobules were identified and classified according to Mellinger (31) after individual collection.

RESULTS

In Vitro Experiments In The Rat

Effects of a crude germ cell preparation on ABP, oestradiol-17β and transferrin secretion by Sertoli cells collected from 20-day-old-rats.

As indicated in Fig. 2, the addition of increasing numbers of germ cells induced a dose-related stimulation of ABP and transferrin secretion and a dose-related inhibition of oestradiol production.

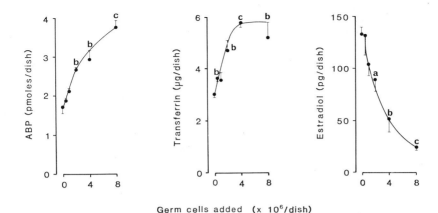

Germ cells added (x 10⁶/dish)

FIG. 2. Effects of the addition of a crude germ cell preparation on FSH-stimulated ABP, transferrin and oestradiol secretion by Sertoli cells in culture. Germ cells were added in increasing amounts to the Sertoli cell cultures on Day 2 and the assays were performed on media from Day 6-7 of culture. Values are means ± s.e.m.; n = 3; a : P < 0.05; b : P < 0.01; c : P < 0.001; when compared to production by Sertoli cells alone.

Effects of animal age and of hypotonic treatment on ABP and oestradiol production.

An age-related increase of basal and of FSH-induced ABP secretion per Sertoli cell was observed in both hypotonically and non-hypotonically treated cultures (Fig. 3 a,b). Conversely, an age dependent decrease of FSH-induced oestradiol secretion was noted under both culture conditions (Fig. 3c).

Whereas the removal of germ cells contaminating the Sertoli cell cultures by hypotonic treatment had no effect on the younger Sertoli cells (10 and 15 days), such treatment caused a significant decrease in basal and FSH-induced ABP production by Sertoli cells prepared from rats aged 20 and 45 days (Fig. 3 a,b; P < 0.05 to P < 0.001).

In the untreated cultures, FSH-stimulated ABP production of Sertoli cells prepared from 10, 15 and 20 day-old donors (+63-71%; P < 0.01) but had no effect on the older Sertoli cells (Fig. 3 b). Interestingly, our data indicate that the relative stimulation induced by FSH in hypotonically treated culture from 20-day-old rats (i.e. FSH/hypotonically treated cultures v.s hypotonically treated cultures) was significantly greater (stimulation of 141%; P < 0.001) compared to the stimulation observed in untreated cultures of the same age (stimulation of 70%, P < 0.01, Fig. 3 a,b).

Similarly, whereas FSH did not stimulate ABP production by untreated Sertoli cells prepared from rats of 45 days of age (see above), this hormone significantly stimulated this parameter after hypotonic treatment (stimulation of 36%; $P < 0.05$).

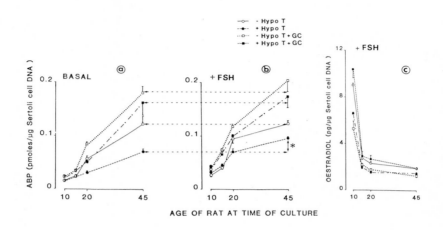

FIG. 3. <u>In vitro</u> production of ABP and oestradiol-17β by rat Sertoli cells as a function of age, FSH and the presence or absence of germ cells (contaminating or added germ cells). Sertoli cells were isolated at different ages and cultured under basal or FSH-stimulated conditions. Some of the dishes were exposed to hypotonic treatment (Hypo T) 48 h later, to remove contaminating germ cells. On day 3, 3×10^6 cells from a crude germ cell suspension (GC; from adult rat testes) were added to some dishes. Media were changed daily and culture media from days 5-6 were assayed for parameters of Sertoli cell function. Values are means $\pm$ s.e.m. of 3 to 5 dishes, each assayed in duplicate and are representative of the results obtained in 3 experiments. * : $P < 0.05$.

It must be noted that oestradiol production was not affected by the hypotonic treatment at all the ages investigated (Fig. 3 c).

<u>Effects of the addition of a crude germ cell preparation on Sertoli cell function at different ages.</u>
The addition of a crude preparation of germ cells to untreated and hypotonically treated Sertoli cells induced a significant stimulation of basal ABP production (Fig. 3 a; $P < 0.05$ to $P < 0.01$) and a significant inhibition of FSH-induced oestradiol secretion (Fig. 3 c; $P < 0.05$ to $P < 0.01$). In the presence of FSH, germ cells also increased ABP production except

after 10 days when no effect was observed (Fig. 3 b; $P < 0.05$ to $P < 0.001$). When comparing culture conditions in which an equivalent number of added germ cells adhered to the Sertoli cell monolayers (hypotonically treated cultures and basal conditions), the stimulatory effect of germ cells on ABP secretion increased with the age of the Sertoli cell donor : 24%, 26%, 66% and 135%, at 10, 15, 20 and 45 days of age respectively (Fig. 3 a). It is also noteworthy that the addition of germ cells to hypotonically treated cultures from rats of 20 and 45 days of age, induced a decrease in the relative response to FSH. In particular, whereas Sertoli cells from 45-day-old donors became responsive to FSH after removal of the contaminating germ cells (see above), they returned to a refractory state to this hormone when germ cells were added to such cultures (Fig. 3 b).

Effects of pachytene spermatocytes on Sertoli cell secretory activity.
The effects of increasing concentrations of dbcAMP on ABP, transferrin and oestradiol secretion by Sertoli cells prepared from 20-day-old rats are presented Fig. 4. Our results indicate that dbcAMP stimulates these three parameters of Sertoli cell function.

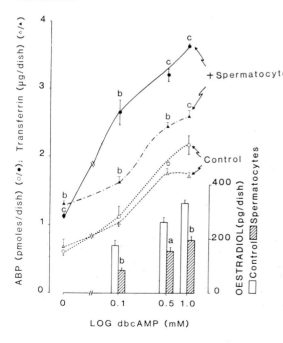

Fig. **4.** Effects of an enriched fraction containing pachytene spermatocytes (2×10^6/dish) on dbcAMP-stimulated ABP, transferrin and oestradiol secretion by Sertoli cells recovered from 20-day-old rats. Germ cells were added on day 2 of culture and Sertoli cell parameters were assayed in day 3-4 culture media. Values are means $\pm$ s.e.m. for 3 dishes, each assayed in duplicate. a : $P < 0.05$; b : $P < 0.01$; c : $P < 0.001$. (When compared to production by Sertoli cells alone).

The addition of 2×10^6 pachytene spermatocytes per culture dish caused a highly significant stimulation of both basal and dbcAMP-induced ABP and transferrin secretion (Fig. 4).

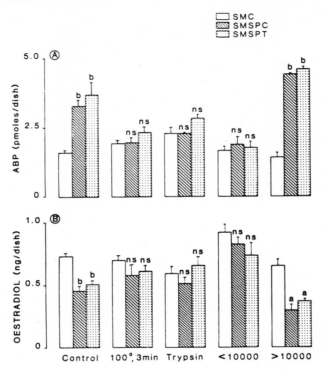

FIG. 5. Preliminary characterization of germ cell factor(s) acting upon Sertoli cell function. Enriched fractions of pachytene spermatocytes ($1 \times 10^6/400$ µl) or of early spermatids ($4 \times 10^6/400$ µl) were incubated for 20 hours at 32°C, after which spent media were harvested by centrifugation. They are referred to as SMSPC and SMSPT respectively. Culture medium incubated without cells served as control (SMC). Spent media (400 µl) were submitted to no treatment (control), to 100°C for 3 min, to a trypsin digestion or to an ultrafiltration (filtrate : Molecular weight (MW) $\leqslant$ 10,000 and retentate : MW $\geqslant$ 10,000) before being added to the Sertoli cell cultures on Day 4 of culture in the presence of 1 µg NIH-oFSH-S16 per dish (final volume of 1 ml). Half of the dishes also received 150 ng testosterone as a substrate for aromatization. ABP (A) and oestradiol (B) levels were assayed in Day 4-5 culture media. Values are means $\pm$ s.e.m. for duplicate determinations of each of the 3 dishes used. a : P $\leqslant$ 0.01; b : P $\leqslant$ 0.001; ns : not significant when compared to respective controls (open columns).

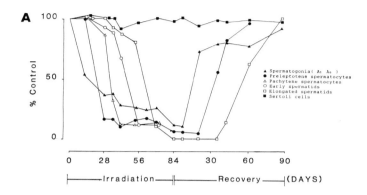

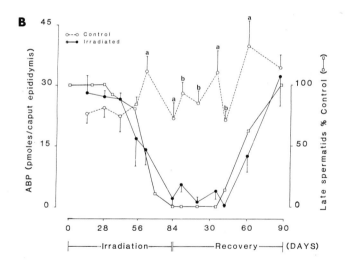

FIG. 6A. Temporal changes in the number of Sertoli cells and germ cells per testis during and after low dose-rate continuous Y irradiation (7 cGy/day)

FIG. 6B. Temporal changes in epididymal ABP content of adult rats in relation to late spermatid numbers during and after continuous Y irradiation at 7 cGy/day. Values represent means ± s.e.m. for 5 rats per group. a : P < 0.01; b : P < 0.001.

Conversely coculture of the Sertoli cells with this germ cell type induced a marked decrease of oestradiol secretion (Fig. 4).

Stimulation and inhibition of ABP, transferrin and oestradiol respectively were also observed when early spermatids were added to the Sertoli cell cultures whereas cytoplasts from elongated spermatids had little (ABP, transferrin) or no effect (oestradiol) on these parameters (data not shown).

Effects on germ cell conditioned media on Sertoli cell secretory activity.

Fig. 5 shows that media conditioned either by pachytene spermatocytes (SMSPC) or by early spermatids (SMSPT) stimulated and inhibited ABP and oestradiol levels respectively. Stimulations of smaller amplitude of transferrin production were also observed when SMSPC and SMSPT were added to Sertoli cell cultures (data not shown).

A preliminary characterization of the factor(s) responsible for these effects indicates that it is/they are heat and trypsin sensitive and present in the fraction of ultrafiltration containing the molecular weights $>$ 10,000 (Fig. 5).

In Vivo Experiment In The Rat.

In this experiment, the effects of germ cell depopulation and repopulation of the seminiferous tubules of adult rats, following continuous γ irradiation at low dose-rate, was investigated on Sertoli cell ABP production.

Our results indicate that under such conditions, irradiation of the animals led to a decrease in the weight of the testes whereas following cessation of the exposure to the γ rays the weight of this organ partially recovered (results not shown).

The target cells of irradiation were spermatogonia (Fig. 6a). Their progressive disappearance resulted in a sequential decrease in the number of the other germ cell types, following a maturation-depletion process (Fig. 6a). The number of Sertoli cells was unaffected (Fig. 6a). After cessation of the irradiation, a progressive and total recovery of the different germ cell categories from spermatogonia to late spermatids was observed (Fig. 6a).

This study confirms earlier work from our group (18, 34) showing that in the adult rat, Sertoli cells can sustain the disappearance of most germ cells from spermatogonia to early spermatids, without any significant change in ABP production. However, it is noteworthy that when the late spermatid number decreased, a sharp drop in the epididymal content of ABP was observed (Fig. 6 b). Conversely, this study reveals that ABP levels remained very low until a recovery was observed which closely paralleled the recovery in the number of late spermatids (Fig. 6 b). A highly significant positive correlation (r = 0.908; P $<$ 0.001; n = 30) was found between these two parameters.

Experiment In The Dogfish.

Following enzymatic and mechanical dissociation isolated seminiferous lobules of the dogfish were obtained. Their light absorption and size varied markedly. The transillumination pattern of these freshly isolated lobules related to the schematic representation of the different stages of spermatogenesis is shown in Fig. 7. Due to their small size lobules at stages I to III were not collected. Lobules at stage IV were recognizable by the presence on their surface of a small dark ring, corresponding to the central cavity. At stage V-VI lobules display little pale grey spheres. During the early prophase of meiosis (stage VIIa) the lobule size increases significantly and the spheres visible over their surface, corresponding to germ cells, enlarge. At stage VIIb the chromosomes of the primary spermatocytes at the diplotene-diakinesis stage cause a darkening of the lobule centre. Due to their relative rarity lobules at stage VIII-X (end of meiosis and secondary spermatocytes) were not collected.

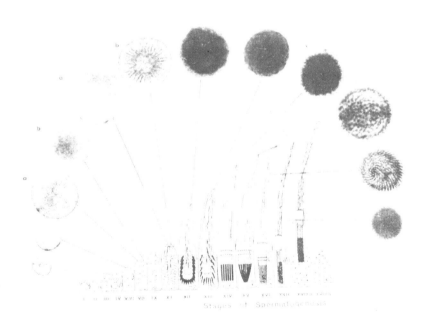

FIG. 7. Transillumination of the freshly isolated seminiferous lobules of the dogfish in relation to the schematic representation of the stages of spermatogenesis of Mellinger (3). Drawing modified from Stanley, (1966, Zeitsch. für Zell-forshung 75:453) and Collenot and Damas, (1975, Cahiers de Biologie Marine 16:39).

The transillumination pattern at stage XIa, which corresponds to the beginning of spermiogenesis, is homogeneously pale with small spots appearing over the lobule surface. At stage XIb the size of the lobules reaches its maximum (400 μm) and plateaus until stage XVI. The radial arrangement of the round spermatids at this stage causes a sunflower like appearance over the lobule surface. Thereafter (stage XII), the condensation of the spermatid nuclei induces the appearance of a dark crown. At stage XIII spermatids elongate and their nuclei condense further developing a large dark area with an irregular border. In the following stage (XIV) the centre of the lobule remains dark; the arrangement of the spermatids in loose bundles causes the appearance of faint stripes within their clear periphery. At stage XV, large grey spots, caused by compaction of the spermatid bundles, are clearly visible over the lobule surface. At stage XVI the size of the lobules begins to decrease and the bundles of spermatids with curved flagella form spiral arrays. The transillumination pattern at stage XVII shows a marked darkening of the lobules and a further decrease of their size. Lobules at the time of spermiation (XVIII) and degenerated lobules were not collected.

DISCUSSION AND CONCLUSION

During sexual maturation Sertoli cells undergo morphological and functional modifications. In fact, from approximately 15-20 days of age in the rat : 1) Sertoli cells cease dividing, they progressively acquire their mature type of morphology and tight junctions appear thus forming the blood-testis barrier (4, 11, 35, 43); 2) Secretion of important Sertoli cell parameters such as ABP, fluid production, transferrin, plasminogen activator, begins and increases rapidly (1, 16, 17, 22, 33, 42); 3) Sertoli cell aromatase activity as well as other Sertoli cell steroïdogenic enzyme activities decrease dramatically (44). 4) Sertoli cell responsiveness to FSH declines (30). All these important changes take place and develop while primary spermatocytes and early spermatids appear and strikingly increase in number (4, 5). This temporal correlation in vivo and the in vitro results herein presented showing that germ cells and media conditioned by these cells, in particular pachytene spermatocytes and early spermatids, stimulate ABP and transferrin production and inhibit oestradiol secretion and that germ cells greatly interfere with Sertoli cell responsiveness to FSH, strongly suggest that these germ cells play, in conjunction with FSH and testosterone, a key role in the maturation of Sertoli cells. Several additional experimental observations support this hypothesis : 1) oestradiol secretion by Sertoli cells isolated from adult rats (70 days) prenatally irradiated (Sertoli cell only tubules) is similar to oestradiol secretion by normal 7-10 day-old rats

(38); 2) production of ABP and of·seminiferous tubule fluid by the testis of immature rats (23-35 day-old), that were depleted of spermatocytes and of early spermatids, following various treatments (prenatal irradiation or experimental cryptorchidism at 14-17 days of age) is comparable to that of 15-20 day-old animals (20, 21, 36); 3) oestrogen synthesis in adult seminiferous tubules has only been reported in germ cell depleted testes of men and dogs containing Sertoli cell tumors (2, 12, 40).

Preliminary characterization of the spermatocyte and spermatid factor(s) detected in the culture media indicates that it is/they are proteinaceous, like the factor(s) previously detected in media conditioned with a crude germ cell preparation (24). Whether or not single or several different factors are involved in the regulation of ABP, transferrin and oestradiol production and to what extent the contacts between membranes of germ cells and Sertoli cells also contribute to the paracrine regulation await further investigation.

It is noteworthy that whereas pachytene spermatocytes and early spermatids appear to strongly influence ABP secretion in immature rats (present data, 18, 25-27), in this study, using . irradiation, no correlation was found between the numbers of these cell types and testicular and epididymal contents of the biologically active binding protein. Instead, the results herein presented and our previous experiments (15, 18, 34) demonstrate the existence of a very close relationship between the number of late spermatids and ABP levels. This may indicate that changes occur in the paracrine control of Sertoli cells by germ cells between the period of establishment of spermatogenesis and once the spermatogenic process is fully developed. This hypothesis is presently being investigated in our laboratory.

Taken together, these results reinforce the concept of a paracrine regulation of Sertoli cell function by germ cells both in immature and mature rat testes. Isolation and characterization of the germ cell factor(s), study of the possible contribution in this paracrine control of membrane mediated mechanisms and the development of new experiments in vivo and in vitro on mammals of different ages, are the prime targets for future research in this important field of intratesticular cell to cell communications.

It must however be noted that though promising, research in mammals on this aspect of the regulation of testicular function is restrained by : 1) the very complex structure of the mammalian seminiferous tubules; 2) the impossibility of preparing germ cells without destroying their anatomical relationship with Sertoli cells; 3) the impossibility of isolating, with a high rate of enrichment, other categories of germ cells other than pachytene spermatocytes and round spermatids. Consequently, the methods herein described to isolate and identify the freshly isolated seminiferous lobules of the dogfish constitute powerful means to extend the investigation of germ cell - Sertoli cell interactions to areas that are not presently accessible in mammals. Furthermore, taking into account the fact that cartilaginous fish appeared at least 350 million years ago (6), studies on this model should also provide important information on the evolution of germ cell - Sertoli cell communications within the testis of vertebrates.

ACKNOWLEDGMENTS

We acknowledge the collaboration of Dr PINON-LATAILLADE and Dr J. MASS in the γ irradiation experiment and of Miss COQUIL in the exploratory stages of the work on the dogfish. We wish to thank Mrs A.M. TOUZALIN and Mrs J. CHAUVIN for their expert technical assistance and Mrs M. MATHELIER for the preparation of the manuscript.

REFERENCES

1. Au, C.L., Robertson, D.M. and de Kretser, D.M. (1983): Endocrinology, 112:239-244.
2. Berthrong, M., Goodwin, W.E. and Scott, W.W. (1949): J. Clin. Endocrinol., 9:579-592.
3. Callard, G.V., Pudney, J.A., Mak, P. and Canick, J.A. (1985): Endocrinology, 117:1328-1335.
4. Clermont, Y. and Perey, B. (1957): Am. J. Anat., 100:241-266.
5. de Jong, F.H. and Sharpe, R.M. (1977): J. Endocr., 75:197-207.
6. Dodd, J.M. (1983): In: Fish Physiology, Vol. IX, Reproduction, Part A, Endocrine Tissues and Hormones, edited W.S. Hoar, D.J., Randall and E.M. Donalson, pp. 31-95. Academic Press. New York.
7. Fritz, I.B., Rommerts, F.F.G., Louis, B.G. and Dorrington, J.H. (1976): J. Reprod. Fertil., 46:17-24.
8. Galdieri, M., Monaco, L. and Stefanini, M. (1984): J. Androl., 5:409-415.
9. Galdieri, M., Ziparo, E., Palombi, F., Russo, M.A. and Stefanini, M. (1981): J. Androl., 5:249-254.
10. Gautron, J. (1978): Biol. Cell., 31:31-44.
11. Gilula, N.B., Fawcett, D.W. and Aoki, A. (1976): Dev. Biol., 50:142-168.
12. Huggins, C. and Moulder, P.V. (1945): Cancer Res., 5:510-514.
13. Ireland, M.E. and Welsh, M.J. (1987): Endocrinology, 120:1317-1326.
14. Jégou, B., Laws, A.O. and de Kretser, D.M. (1983): J. Reprod. Fertil., 69:137-145.
15. Jégou, B., Laws, A.O. and de Kretser, D.M. (1984): Int. J. Androl., 7:244-256.

16. Jégou, B., Le Gac, F. and de Kretser, D.M. (1982): Biol. Reprod., 27:590-595.
17. Jégou, B., Le Gac, F., Irby, D.C. and de Kretser, D.M. (1983): Int. J. Androl., 6:249-260.
18. Jégou, B., Le Magueresse, B., Pinon-Lataillade, G., Velez de la Calle, J.F., Garnier, D.H., Mass, J. and Boisseau, C. (1986): In: Molecular and Cellular Endocrinology of the testis, edited by M. Stefanini, M. Conti, R. Geremia and E. Ziparo, pp. 63-73. Excerpta Med. Int. Congr. Ser 716, Elsevier, Amsterdam.
19. Jégou, B., Peake, R.A., Irby, D.C. and de Kretser, D.M. (1984): Biol. Reprod. 30:179-187.
20. Jégou, B., Risbridger, G.P. and de Kretser, D.M. (1983): J. Androl., 4:88-94.
21. Karpe, B., Ploën, L., Hagenäs, L. and Ritzén, E.M. (1981): Int. J. Androl., 4:145-160.
22. Lacroix, M., Smith, F.E. and Fritz, I.B. (1982): Mol. Cell. Endocrinol., 75:197-207.
23. Leblond, C.P. and Clermont, Y. (1952): Am. N.Y. Acad. Sc., 55:548-573.
24. Le Magueresse, B. and Jégou, B. (1986): Biochem. Biophys. Res. Commun., 141:861-869.
25. Le Magueresse, B. and Jégou, B. (1988a): Endocrinology, 122: Nº4, (in press).
26. Le Magueresse, B. and Jégou, B. (1988b): Mol. Cell. Endocrinol, (in press).
27. Le Magueresse, B., Le Gac, F., Loir, M. and Jégou, B. (1986): J. Reprod. Fertil., 77:489-498.
28. Mather, J.P. and Philips, D.M. (1984): In: Methods for Serum-free culture of cells of the Endocrine Systems, edited by D.W. Barnes, A.D. Sirbasku and G.H. Sato, pp. 29-45. Alan R. Liss, Inc., New York.
29. Meistrich, L.M., Longtin, J., Brok, W.A., Grimes, S.R. and Myles, L.M. (1981): Biol. Reprod., 25:1065-1077.
30. Means, A.R., Fakunding, H.L., Huckins, C., Tindall, D.J. and Vitale, R. (1976): Recent Prog. Horm. Res., 32:477-522.
31. Mellinger, J. (1965): Zeitsch. Für Zellforschung, 67:653-673.
32. Parvinen, M. (1982): Endocr. Rev., 3:404-417.
33. Perez-Infante, V., Bardin, C.W., Gunsalus, G.L., Musto, N.A., Rich, K.A. and Mather, J.P. (1986): Endocrinology, 118:383-392.
34. Pinon-Lataillade, G., Vélez de la Calle, J.F., Viguier-Martinez, M.C., Garnier, D.H., Folliot, R., Maas, J. and Jégou, B. (1988): Mol. Cell. Endocrinol., (in press).
35. Ramos, A.S. Jr and Dym, M. (1979): Biol. Reprod., 21:909-922.
36. Rich, K.A. (1979): PhD thesis, Monash University, Melbourne, Australia.

37. Ritzén, E.M., French, F.S., Weddington, S.C., Nayfeh, S.N. and Hansson, V. (1974): J. Biol. Chem., 249:6597-6604.

38. Rommerts, F.F.G., de Jong, F.H., Brinkmann, A.O. and Van der Molen, H.J. (1982): J. Reprod. Fertil., 65:281-288.

39. Sharpe, R.M., Kerr, J.B., Cooper, I. and Bartlett, J.M.S. (1986): In: Molecular and Cellular Endocrinology of the Testis, edited by M. Stefanini, M. Conti, R. Geremia and E. Ziparo, pp. 15-26. Excerpta Med. Int. Congr., Ser. 716, Elsevier, Amsterdam.

40. Teilum, G.M.D. (1949): J. Clin. Endocrinol., 9:301-318.

41. Terqui, M., Dray, F. and Cotta, J. (1973): C. R. Acad. Sci. (Paris) D, 277:1795-1798.

42. Tindall, D.J. and Means, A.R. (1976): Endocrinology, 99:809-818.

43. Vitale-Calpe, R., Fawcett, D.W. and Dym, M. (1973): Anat. Rec., 176:333-344.

44. Welsh, M.J. and Wiebe, J.P. (1978): Endocrinology, 103:838-844.

45. Wing, T.Y. and Christensen, A.K. (1982): Am. J. Anat., 165:13-25.

The Role of FSH in the Maintenance of Spermatogenesis

J.M.S. Bartlett, G.F. Weinbauer and E. Nieschlag

Max Planck Clinical Research Unit for Reproductive Medicine and Institute of Reproductive Medicine, Westfälische-Wilhelms Universität Steinfurter Straße 107, D4400 Münster, Federal Republic of Germany

REQUIREMENTS FOR SPERMATOGENESIS IN RATS AND PRIMATES

Whilst the ability of testosterone to maintain spermatogenesis in the absence of gonadotrophins in adult rats and monkeys is widely accepted (1, 2, 14, 16), the role of FSH is still open to debate. A number of studies have suggested that withdrawal of FSH has no effect on spermatogenic function in the adult animal. However alternative studies argue equally strongly for a specific role of FSH in maintaining spermatogenesis (6, 9, 17, see 15 for review).

Previous studies from our laboratory suggest a role for FSH in the maintenance of spermatogenesis (20, 22, 23). In rhesus monkeys actively immunised against FSH spermatogenic function was impaired within 4 weeks of immunisation and remained significantly lower than controls for up to 4.5 years, provided booster innoculations against FSH were given to maintain the anti-FSH titre (20, 22). Immunisation resulted in reduced sperm counts per ejaculate (when compared with pretreatment values), reduced motility and a reduction in the numbers of normally formed spermatozoa (20, 22). However, following long-term observations it was found that whilst sperm counts remained impaired in immunised animals, morphology and motility recovered to within the normal range within a period of 4.5 years (21). Passive immunisation also resulted in reduced spermatogenesis (23). These data would suggest that FSH has a major role to play in spermatogenesis in the adult rhesus monkey.

This finding contradicts that previously described for the adult rat, where immunisation against FSH produced no significant effect on spermatogenic function (6) apart from a transient decrease in numbers of preleptotene spermatocytes, although no booster injections were given in this instance. In experiments with hypophysectomised rats, Russell and Clermont (18) showed that whilst FSH alone had apparently no effect on the numbers of degenerating cells present post hypophysectomy, treatment with LH alone was not sufficient to restore numbers of degenerating cells to control levels; and only treatment with both FSH and LH reduced numbers of degenerating cells to control levels. They concluded that complete maintainance of spermatogenesis requires both FSH and LH/androgens in the adult.

Recently attempts have been made to clarify whether androgens alone can maintain fully quantitative spermatogenesis. However, even if such studies should prove successful, via the use of supraphysiological testosterone injections, the question remains –does FSH play a physiological role in the maintenance of spermatogenesis in the adult rat?. Recent studies have suggested that by using testosterone injections (10, 19) producing high intratesticular testosterone concentrations, fully quantitative spermatogenesis can be maintained. However, work by Maddocks et al (12, 13) suggests that the intratesticular concentrations of testosterone measured post mortem may not reflect the in vivo situation, and that such high levels of androgen may not be available in vivo. If this is so, then the question remains can FSH, in conjunction with low levels of intratesticular testosterone, maintain spermatogenesis in the adult rat or monkey?

Although the majority of such studies have been performed in the rat, a recent study in GnRH antagonist treated primates suggests that even with intratesticular testosterone levels maintained at around 30-50% of normal values spermatogenesis was almost completely inhibited (21), arguing strongly for a role of FSH in these animals. It is clear, therefore, that differences exist in the relative importance of FSH in primates and rodents, and we have therefore studied the role of FSH in adult hypophysectomised rats treated with low doses of testosterone, or FSH alone.

EFFECT OF PURIFIED hFSH ALONE AND IN COMBINATION WITH TESTOSTERONE ON MAINTENANCE OF SPERMATOGENESIS IN ADULT HYPOPHYSECTOMISED RATS

Recently a highly purified, LH-free FSH preparation has become available (8), and we have used this preparation to investigate the role of FSH and testosterone in maintenance of spermatogenesis in the adult rat. Groups of adult rats were hypophysectomised and treated with either: a subcutaneous testosterone implant, designed to maintain serum testosterone in the normal range; twice daily injections of an LH-free FSH preparation; or a combination of these treatments. One group of hypophysectomised and one group of normal animals were included as controls.

In animals treated with FSH no stimulation of testicular steroidogenesis and no increase in epididymal weights when compared with untreated hypophysectomised animals could be demonstrated, indicating that the FSH preparation used was free of LH. Therefore it was concluded that the effects on testicular function induced by FSH treatment alone were due to direct FSH action. Treatment with FSH maintained testicular weights and numbers of preleptotene spermatocytes, pachytene spermatocytes and round spermatids at levels significantly higher than those seen in untreated hypophysectomised animals. The failure of FSH to stimulate the development of elongated spermatids in our study is consistent with the early observation that this event is androgen-dependent (4, 5).

The administration of testosterone implants maintained spermatogenesis, in a purely qualitative fashion, as reported previously by other groups (1-4). The combination of testosterone and FSH treatments maintained spermatogenesis and testicular weights at almost normal levels, with levels of round spermatids, pachytene spermatocytes and testis weights all approximately 80% of control values. This effect of FSH in the presence of testosterone was not due to increased conversion of testosterone to dihydrotestosterone, since no change in DHT:T ratios was observed throughout the study. The effect of FSH treatment also was apparently not related to an increase in intratesticular testosterone or seminiferous tubular testosterone content. It is possible that testosterone synergises with FSH in the priming of Sertoli cell enzymes which synthesise factors aiding the process of spermatogenesis, for example, **production** of lactate, which is an energy substrate for spermatocytes and round spermatids (7, 11).

In conclusion, there is evidence supporting a central role for FSH in the maintenance of spermatogenesis in adult rats and primates, although FSH might be of greater importance for spermatogenesis in primates than in rodents.

ACKNOWLEDGEMENTS

The authors gratefully acknowledge the technical assistance of K. Brunswicker, M. Heuermann, M, Möller & R. Sandhowe, and the secretarial assistance of S. Baha and B. Dinkhoff. The work was carried out whilst J. Bartlett was in reciept of a Max-Planck Research Fellowship.

REFERENCES

1. Ahmad, N., Haltmeyer, G.C., and Eik-Nes, K.B. (1973): Biol. Reprod., 8:411-419.

2. Ahmad, N., Haltmeyer, G.C., and Eik-Nes, K.B. (1975): J. Reprod. & Fertil., 44:103-107.

3. Buhl, A.E., Cornette, J.C., Kirton, K.T., and   Yuan, Y.D. (1982): Biol. Reprod., 27:183-188.

4. Cunningham, G.R., and Huckins, C. (1979): Endocrinology, 105:177-186.

5. Clausen, O.P., Purvis, K., and Hansson, V. (1979): Arch. Androl., 2:59-66.

6. Dym, M., Raj, H.G.M., Lin, Y.C., Chemes, H.E., Kotite, N.J., Nayfeh, S.N., and French, F.S. (1979): J. Reprod. & Fertil. Suppl., 26:175-181.

7. Grootegoed, J.A., Jansen, R., and van der Molen. H.J. (1984): Ann. NY Acad. Sci., 438:557-560.

8. Harlin, J., Khan, S.A., and Diczfalusy, E. (1986): Fertil. Steril., 46:1055-1061.

9. Hodgson, Y., Robertson, D.M., and de Kretser, D.M. (1983): In: International Review of Physiology, Vol. 27 Edited by R.O. Greep, pp 275-237. American Physiological Society, New York.

10. Huang, H.F.S., Marshall, G.R., Rosenberg, R., and Nieschlag, E. (1987): Acta Endocrinol. 116:433-444.

11. Jutte, N.P.H.M., Jansen, R., Grootegoed, J.A., Rommerts, F.F.G., Clausen, O.P.F., and van der Molen, H.J. (1983): J. Reprod. & Fertil. 65:431-438.

12. Maddocks, S., and Setchell, B.P. (1987): J. Physiol. 392:69P.

13. Maddocks, S., and Setchell, B.P. (1988): Oxford Reviews of Reproductive Biology 10: in press.

14. Marshall, G.R., Jöckenhovel, F., Lüdecke, D., and Nieschlag, E. (1986): Acta Endocrinol. 113:424-431.

15. Marshall, G.R., and Nieschlag, E. (1987): In: "Inhibins: Isolation, estimation and physiology": Vol I. Edited by A.R. Sheth pp 3-15. CRC Press, Boca Raton, Florida.

16. Marshall, G.R., Wickings, E.J., Lüdecke, D.K., and Nieschlag, E. (1983): J. Clin. Endocrinol. Metab. 57:152-159.

17. Matsumoto, A.M., and Bremner, W.J. (1987): Bailliere's Clinical Endocrinology and Metabolism 1:71-87.

18. Russell, L.D., and Clermont, Y. (1977): Anat. Rec. 187:347-366.

19. Sharpe, R.M., Donachie, K. and Cooper, I.: (1988) J. Endo. 117:19-26.

20. Srinath, B.V., Wickings, E.J., Witting, C., and Nieschlag, E. (1983): Fertil. Steril. 40:110-117.

21. Weinbauer, G.F., Gökeler, E., & Nieschlag, E. (1988): J. Clin. Endocrinol. Metab. In press.

22. Wickings, E.J., and Nieschlag, E. (1980): Fertil. Steril. 34:269-274.

23. Wickings, E.J., Usadel, K.H., Dathe, G. and Nieschlag, E. (1980): Acta Endocrinol. 95:117-128.

Expression of a Testis-Specific hsp 70 Gene-Related RNA in Defined Stages of the Rat Seminiferous Epithelium

Z. Krawczyk*, P. Mali and M. Parvinen

*Institute of Biomedicine, Department of Anatomy, University of Turku, Kiinamyllynkatu 10, SF-20520 Turku, Finland, and *Department of Tumor Biology, Institute of Oncology, 44-100 Gliwice, Poland*

INTRODUCTION

Heat shock proteins are a set of specific proteins synthesized in cells exposed to elevated temperature and a number of other stressing factors. The most prominent and most thoroughly investigated is the heat shock protein of molecular weight of about 70000 (hsp70). Besides the genes which are strictly heat inducible, the hsp70 family may contain genes that are heat inducible but also become expressed at certain levels in the absence of stress (2,3). The function of these genes is poorly understood although recent observations suggest that they may be involved in stabilization and assembly of nascent proteins in various cellular compartments, as well as in the recovery of cellular structures from injuries (13). In addition, some hsp70 related proteins may have a function in cellular growth and differentiation (5,6,11).

Recently Krawczyk et al. (8) and Zakeri and Wolgemuth (16) reported that testes of the adult rat and mouse contain abundant levels of the transcript related to the hsp70 gene. This transcript, called hst70 RNA, differs in size from other hsp70-related heat shock transcripts and its level is not affected by hyperthermia (8,16, Krawczyk and Wisniewski, in preparation). Its expression is developmentally regulated: it is absent in newborn animals but appears in testes that have initiated spermiogenesis (7,16). In testes depleted of germinal cells after experimental cryptorchidism (7), busulphan treatment, increased age (Krawczyk and Szymik, unpublished observation), or certain mutations affecting the reproductive tract (16), the hst70 RNA is not detectable. In testicular cells separated by gravity sedimentation, the highest level of the transcript was detected in fractions enriched in round and elongated spermatids as well as in residual bodies, but a very low amount was detected in pachytene spermatocytes (16). Therefore, the main localization of this transcript has been proposed to be during the haploid phase of spermatogenesis.

To gain a more accurate localization of the cellular expression of the hst70 mRNA in the seminiferous epithelium, we have utilized the possibilities provided by the slot-blot hybridization technique in microdissected seminiferous tubules in which the exact stage of the epithelial cycle was identified by transillumination and phase contrast microscopy, and the results were compared with in situ hybridization of testis sections.

MATERIALS AND METHODS

Slot-blotting of RNA

Pools of seminiferous tubule segments from Sprague-Dawley rats at different stages of the cycle were isolated by transillumination- assisted microdissection (12). For a more accurate analysis, 2 mm segments of seminiferous tubules were cut sequentially under a stereomicroscope and the exact stage was determined by intermediate squash preparations (15). RNA was isolated by the heparin-DNase method as described by Krawczyk and Wu (9) and filtered through nitrocellulose using a Bio-dot apparatus (Bio-Rad) with 48 slots. To detect the testis-specific hsp70 gene related transcript we used the SmaI-BamHI (1.6 kb) fragment of the plasmid pM1.8. The plasmid contains a 5'-end fragment of the mouse hsp70 gene cloned into the pBR322 vector (R. Morimoto, unpublished work; for partial restriction map see 8). The SmaI-BamHI restriction fragment was labelled by random priming with ^{32}P-dCTP (Amersham, U.K.). After hybridization, the autoradiograms were scanned by a densitometer and the relative intensities of hst70 hybridizations were compared with those of 28S ribosomal RNA (plasmid pI-19) in the same filter.

In situ hybridization

The testes were fixed in 10 % buffered formalin, embedded in paraffin and 5 μm sections were cut on microscope slides. The in situ hybridization procedure was performed as described by Sandberg and Vuorio (14) using the SmaI-BamHI restriction fragment labelled by random priming with ^{35}S-dATP (Amersham, U.K.). The slides were dipped in a Kodak NTB-2 emulsion and exposed for 7-14 days. The stages were identified from adjacent sections using the criteria of Leblond and Clermont (10) and the grain densities determined above defined cell types.

RESULTS

The slot-blot hybridizations of total RNA isolated from ten pools of seminiferous tubule segments showed a lower level of hst70 RNA in stages VIII and IX-XI than in other stages. The hybridization of successive 2 mm segments showed a similar pattern of hst70 RNA distribution: The level was highest in stages I-VI, decreased at stages VII and VIII reaching a minimum at stages IX-XI. Then the level of the hst70 RNA increased again and reached a high value at stage XII-XIV which was only slightly lower than that observed at stages I-VI. When the same filter was rehybridized with mouse ribosomal 28 S RNA, maxima were found in the region of stages VII and VIII of the cycle.

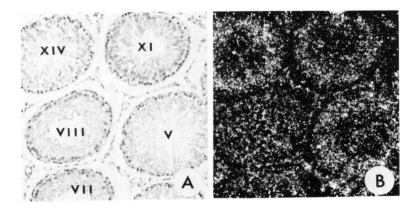

Fig. 1. Low power (100 x) photomicrographs of rat testis sections hybridized in situ with ^{35}S-labelled hst70 cDNA probe. The stages of the seminiferous epithelial cycle are indicated in (A), and the same field was rephotographed in dark field illumination to visualize the autoradiographic silver grains (B). A lower hybridization level is found above stages VII and VIII of the cycle than above stages XIV and V. Stage XI shows an intermediate grain density.

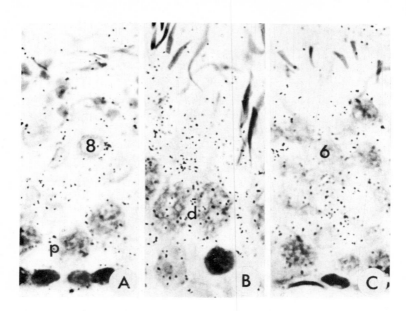

Fig. 2. High power (1000 x) photomicrographs of stages VIII (A), XIII (B) and VI (C) of rat seminiferous epithelium to show the cellular localization of hst70 RNA. Low grain densities are found above pachytene spermatocytes (p) and step 8 spermatids (8) at stage VIII, whereas diakinetic primary spermatocytes at stage XIII (d) and round spermatids at stage VI (6) contain higher levels of hst70 RNA.

The in situ hybridization was in agreement with the slot blot analyses. Stages I, XII, XIII and VI displayed higher grain densities over the seminiferous epithelium than stages VIIc, VIId and IX (Fig. 1). A detailed analysis (Fig. 2) revealed that late pachytene primary spermatocytes at stage XII, diakinetic and dividing spermatocytes at stages XIII and XIV and early round-nucleated spermatids at stages I - VI of the cycle were significantly more densely labelled than other cell types. Control hybridization with lambda-phage vector cDNA showed evenly distributed low grain densities over all stages of the cycle.

DISCUSSION

It is important to determine at what step of spermatogenesis a given gene is activated and transcribed. The most common approach has been the fractionation of cells by sedimentation velocity at unit gravity. Although this technique is useful in analyses of haploid gene expression (4), the accurate timing and developmental stage of the onset of transcription of certain genes is not always possible. This cell fractionation applied to the determination of the hsp70 gene related transcript resulted in the conclusion that it is primarily expressed postmeiotically (16).

We present evidence that the gene coding for the hst70 RNA is activated and transcribed before formation of round spermatids. The results solve at least partially the controversy that could arise about the origin of the heat shock-related testis-specific RNA. The former results on the transcript level during the maturation of rat testes indicated an expression in late spermatocytes or early spermatids since it first appeared at detectable levels in testes of 3 weeks old rats (7). However, reappearance of the transcript during restoration of spermatogenesis after busulphan treatment was correlated with the appearance of the spermatids in certain seminiferous tubules (Krawczyk and Szymik, submitted for publication). These data excluded the possibility of the transcription of the hst70 RNA in the leptotene and zygotene spermatocytes and strongly suggested its postmeiotic origin. However they also suggested a possibility of the late meiotic activation of this gene.

The function of the possible translational product of the hst70 mRNA remains obscure. Recently, Allen and Eddy (1) have described a testis-specific hsp70 related protein which is present in spermatocytes as well as in early spermatids. It is not known whether this protein is translated from hst70 mRNA but if this is the case one could speculate about its involvement in the differentiation of spermatocytes into spermatids.

ACKNOWLEDGEMENTS

We thank Mr. Henrik Wikgren and Miss Maija Parvinen for excellent technical assistance. This work was supported by grants from The Academy of Finland (Project no. 200 at the MRC) and by the Finnish Ministry of Education. The plasmids pM1.8 and pI-19 were generous gifts from Drs. R. Morimoto and Norman

B. Hecht, respectively.

REFERENCES

1. Allen, R.L. and Eddy, E.M. (1986): J. Cell Biol. 103: 81a.
2. Carper, S.W., Duffy, J.J. and Gerner, E.W. (1987): Cancer Res. 47:5249-5255.
3. Craig, E.A. (1985): CRC Crit. Rev. Biochem. 18:239-280.
4. Hecht, N.B. (1986): Development, Growth and Differentiation, 28 (Suppl.): 33-34.
5. Kaczmarek, L., Calabretta, B., Kao, H., Heintz, N., Nevins, J. and Baserga, R. (1987): J. Cell Biol. 14:183-187.
6. Kao, H.T., Capusso, O, Heintz, N. and Nevins, J.R. (1985): Mol. Cell Biol. 5:628-633.
7. Krawczyk, Z., Szymik, N. and Wisniewski, J. (1987): Mol. Biol. Rep. 12:35-41.
8. Krawczyk, Z., Wisniewski, J. and Biesiada, E. (1987): Mol. Biol. Rep. 12:27-34.
9. Krawczyk, Z. and Wu, C. (1987): Anal. Biochem. 165:20-27.
10. Leblond, C.P., and Clermont, Y. (1952): Ann. N.Y. Acad. Sci. 55:548-573.
11. Milarski, K.L., and Morimoto, R.I. (1986): Proc. Natl. Acad. Sci. USA. 83:9517-9521.
12. Parvinen, M. and Ruokonen, A. (1982): J. Androl. 3:211-220.
13. Pelham, H.R.B. (1986): Cell 46:959-961.
14. Sandberg, M., and Vuorio, E. (1987): J. Cell Biol. 104:1077-1084.
15. Toppari, J., Eerola, E. and Parvinen, M. (1985): J. Androl. 6:334-343.
16. Zakeri, Z.F. and Wolgemuth, D.J. (1987): Mol. Cell. Biol. 7:1791-1796.

Differentiation of Ovarian and Testicular Cells: Intragonadal Regulation by Growth Factors

B.C.J.M. Fauser, B. Galway and A.J.W. Hsueh

Department of Reproductive Medicine, M-025 School of Medicine,
University of California, San Diego
La Jolla, California 92093, USA

INTRODUCTION

Endocrine signals from the anterior pituitary, including follicle-stimulating hormone (FSH) and luteinizing hormone (LH), are the primary regulators of gonadal differentiation. Both male and female gonads are structurally compartmentalized. The functional unit of the ovary is the follicle, consisting of an outer layer of theca cells and an inner layer of granulosa cells, separated from each other by the basement membrane. The granulosa cells, in turn, surround the innermost oocyte. In the testis, the functional unit is the seminiferous tubule where spermatogenesis takes place. The Sertoli cells that support spermatogenesis are situated inside the tubules, whereas the androgen-producing Leydig cells are situated in the interstitial area. Recent studies in the male and female have focused on the potential role of local paracrine or autocrine signalling systems in the modulation of gonadal cell differentiation induced by pituitary gonadotropins. It seems likely that the selection of the dominant follicle and atresia of the remaining follicles is largely controlled by intra-ovarian hormones. Likewise, the local differences in spermatogenesis in individual seminiferous tubules may also be regulated by local hormones.

The advancement of new techniques to purify and characterize new protein hormones, the widespread use of primary <u>in vitro</u> cell cultures, and the development of specific bioassays and radioimmunoassays to dectect various growth factors, has greatly contributed to a better understanding of the significance of growth factors in intragonadal regulatory mechanisms. Initially, attention was mainly focussed on the mitogenic activity of growth factors. More recent studies, however, also emphasize the effects of these presumptive local hormones in the regulation of gonadal cell differentiation. In particular, primary culture systems of gonadal cells have proven to be very useful in studying these effects. In the ovary, gonadal peptides (such as growth factors, and inhibin) are locally produced and are capable of modifying LH receptor induction as well as FSH-stimulated steroid biosynthesis. In the testis, growth factors produced by Sertoli cells are capable of modulating androgen biosynthesis by Leydig cells, raising the possibility of intratesticular cell to cell communications.

Intragonadal roles of ovarian steroids (such as estrogens, progesterone, and androgens), as well as several peptide hormones such as gonadotropin releasing hormone, vasoactive intestinal peptide and arginine vasopressin has been reviewed recently (15, 42, 43, 48). The present review will focus on the function and chemistry of various growth factors and recent work from this and other laboratories on the local production and action of various growth factors in the ovary and testis.

FUNCTION AND CHEMISTRY OF GROWTH FACTORS

EGF / TGF-α

Growth factors that have been shown to modulate gonadal differentiation can be categorized into several major groups (Table 1). Epidermal growth factor (EGF) was originally identified by Cohen in 1960, while testing extracts from mouse submaxillary glands for nerve growth factor (NGF) activity, and subsequently named for its capacity to induce proliferation of the basal layer of the skin (52). Another <u>in vivo</u> action of EGF is the inhibition of gastric acid secretion, and this growth factor was found to be identical to urogastrone purified from human urine. Many types of cultured cells, such as fibroblasts, cornea, glia, conjunctiva, and tumor cells respond to EGF, and several lines of evidence suggest a potential role of EGF in carcinogenesis.

EGF is a single chain peptide with 53 amino acids

Table 1. chemistry of various growth factors

	MOL WEIGHT	STRUCTURE	NOTES
EGF	6,100	single chain	share same
TGF-α	5,600	homology with EGF (17, 51, 52, 68)[*]	receptor
IGF-I (Sm-C)	7,600	2 chains (A and B)	
IGF-II (rat MSA)	7,200	single chain	
insulin	5,700	2 chains (A and B) (2, 63)[*]	
inhibin	32,000	αβ-heterodimer	α-βA, α-βB
activin	28,000	ββ-homodimer	βA-βB, βA-βA
TGF-β	25,000	homodimer (14, 55, 67)[*]	homology with inhibin-β
FGF (basic)	15,000	single chain	acidic, basic
Interleukin-1	17,500	single chain (8, 33, 50, 60)[*]	homology with FGF

EGF = epidermal growth factor, TGF = transforming growth factor, IGF = insulin-like growth factor, FGF = fibroblast growth factor.
[*] = literature reference

(only 48 amino acids are essential to exert its biological activity), and a molecular weight of 6,100 (17). Observations that sarcoma virus-induced cell transformation resulted in a specific decrease of EGF-binding capacity led to the identification of transforming growth factor-α (TGF-α) (68). TGF-α is also composed of a single, 50 amino acid chain (51) and exhibit great sequence homology with EGF. Both peptides are secreted as large, inactive precursors, that need to be cleaved by proteolytic enzymes before becoming biologically active. Although EGF and TGF-α are products of unlinked genes that are independently regulated, TGF-α binds to the same receptor as EGF and has similar biological activity. Sequence data show that a large part of the EGF receptor is highly homologous to the chicken v-erb B oncogene product and that this conserved region contains sequences shared by almost all tyrosine kinases. The oncogenic properties of v-erb B demonstrate that an altered EGF-receptor can contribute directly to tumorigenesis.

IGFs / insulin

The second group of growth factors consists of the insulin-like growth factors (IGFs) and insulin. The IGFs, identified in 1976 from human serum comprising insulin-like activity that could not be neutralized by antibodies against insulin, exhibit a great structural and functional similarity to insulin (63). Initial studies suggested that the biological effects of the IGFs were mediated through the insulin receptor. However, in addition to their weak insulin-like metabolic effects, the IGFs have potent mitogenic activities which can only be mimicked by insulin at much higher concentrations. Insulin is composed of a single chain, consisting of 2 subunits (A and B) joined by disulfide bonds, with a connecting C-peptide that is cleaved from the mature hormone upon its release. More than 45% of the amino acids of the A and B chains of the IGFs are located in the same position as in the insulin molecule. The C and D chains of the IGFs, however, are unique. Three dimensional models demonstrate that insulin and the IGFs have different antigenic domains.

The IGFs can be divided into at least two distinct groups; basic IGF, or IGF-I (identical to somatomedin-C), and neutral IGF or IGF-II (also designated as rat multiplication stimulating activity [rat MSA]). The somatomedins constitute a group of serum-derived peptides, produced by the liver which mediate growth hormone action. The molecular weights of IGF-I (a single chain, consisting of 70 amino acids), IGF-II (a single-chain with 67 amino acids), and insulin are 7,600, 7,200, and 5,700, respectively. Both the IGFs and insulin are secreted as large, inactive precursors. Specific receptors have been identified for both IGFs and insulin. The IGF-I receptor is composed of two α and two β subunits and binds IGF-I, IGF-II, and insulin with decreasing affinity. The β subunit of the receptor contains IGF-I-dependent tyrosine kinase activity, whereas the α subunit contains the binding sites. In contrast, the IGF-II receptor is a single chain peptide which binds IGF-II with greater affinity than IGF-I, and is incapable of binding insulin.

inhibin / activin / TGF-β

The controversy about the existence of a gonadal protein which specifically inhibits the secretion of pituitary FSH was recently resolved with the purification of inhibin from bovine and porcine follicular fluid. Inhibin is secreted by granulosa cells in the ovary (12), and Sertoli cells in the testis (13) as a 30,000 molecular weight protein composed of 2 dissimilar subunits. A smaller β- and a larger α-subunit are joined by cysteine disulfide bonds. In addition, two forms of the β-subunit have been identified (named βA and βB), based on minor amino acid sequence differences, allowing the formation of inhibin $\alpha-\beta A$ and $\alpha-\beta B$ dimers (for review see Bicsak & Hsueh [14]). Homodimers of two inhibin β-chains ($\beta A-\beta A$ [also known as FSH-releasing protein; FRP], or $\beta A-\beta B$ [known as activin] have a molecular weight of 28,000. Although the $\alpha\beta$-heterodimer of inhibin suppresses FSH release, the $\beta\beta$-homodimers stimulate FSH secretion.

TGF-β, which has been isolated from both tumor and normal cells, is characterized by its ability to induce a phenotypical transformation of normal cells. It has both stimulatory and inhibitory effects on proliferation and differentiation of cells in the immune system, connective tissue, and epithelium. It appears that the effect of TGF-β on mesenchymal cells is not entirely a function of the peptide itself, but depends on the action of other growth factors on a cell at a given time. Furthermore, TGF-β is also capable of regulating the mitogenic activity of other growth factors.

TGF-β is a 25,000 molecular weight homodimeric molecule that on reduction yields two identical polypeptide chains containing 112 amino acids (55). Only the dimer is biologically active. TGF-β shares sequence homology with the β-chain of inhibin, and the Mullerian duct inhibiting substance (MIF); these molecules are believed to be products of the same gene family (67). Other peptides, such as a growth inhibitor isolated from monkey kidney cells, and a cartilage-inducing substance isolated from bovine bone have also been shown to have sequence homology with TGF-β. The TGF-β receptor has been found on many cells and is a large molecule composed of two subunits. Unlike receptors for most other growth factors, the TGF-β receptor appears to have no tyrosine kinase activity.

FGF / interleukin

Fibroblast growth factors (FGFs) are single chain peptides which were originally identified in pituitary and brain extracts, based on their ability to stimulate proliferation of fibroblasts. FGFs have both mitogenic and non-mitogenic activities in a wide variety of cells throughout the body. In addition, FGF has recently been implicated in ovarian angiogenesis (the generation of new capillary blood vessels) (32). Two different forms of FGF, basic and acidic, have been identified based on their difference in isoelectric point (8, 33). Basic FGF is composed of 146 amino acids (molecular weight 15,000) and has greater biopotency. The two forms of FGF have 55% amino acid sequence homology and share the same receptor.

There is increasing evidence that a bidirectional communication exist between the endocrine and the immune systems. Interleukin-1 is an important mediator of activated macrophage function resulting in both T and B lymphocyte proliferation and differentiation. This cytokine also regulates the function of a wide range of non-immune tissues including those of liver, bone, muscles, and endocrine organs. Interleukin-1 is also a single chain peptide which consists of 116 amino acids (molecular weight 17,500). Two distinct forms have been identified based on differences in isoelectric point; interleukin-1α and interleukin-1β (50, 60). The interleukin-1β form is present in much larger quantities and a weak (approximately 25%) homology exists between interleukin-1β and FGF (31).

GROWTH FACTORS AND INTRAGONADAL REGULATION

EGF / TGF-α

Although EGF dose-dependently inhibits the FSH stimulated aromatase activity (estrogen production) in granulosa cells in culture (41) (Table 2), progesterone production is slightly enhanced by co-treatment of cells with EGF (46). EGF also inhibits the FSH induction of LH receptors on granulosa cells (57), and, surprisingly, induces oocyte maturation in isolated follicles (23). Like EGF, treatment of granulosa cells with TGF-α also causes a dose-dependent decrease of FSH-stimulated aromatase activity (4), supporting the concept of a shared receptor.

Binding sites for EGF have been identified in granulosa cells (46), and the EGF receptor number is regulated by gonadotropins (28). Theca/interstitial cell preparations produce EGF-like factors as determined by radioreceptor and biological assays (65), low levels of EGF mRNA have been shown to be present in the ovary (62), and EGF has recently been detected in follicular fluid by radioimmunoassay (40).

Table 2. Growth factors as intragonadal regulators in the ovary

	ACTION	RECEPTOR	ORIGIN
EGF	LH R↓,E$_2$↓ Prog↔, A↓	GC, EGF R	TC (EGF-like)
TGF-α	E$_2$↓ (4, 41, 46, 57)*	same (28, 46)*	same (40, 49, 62, 65)*
IGF-I	LH R↑, E$_2$↑	GC	GC
IGF-II	P↑,A↑	?	?
insulin	same (2, 20, 25, 37, 61, 71)*	GC (5, 28, 40, 46)*	? (21, 35, 39, 58)*
inhibin	E$_2$↓,A↑	?	GC
activin	E$_2$↑,Prog↓,A↓	?	?
TGF-β	LH R↑,E$_2$↑,Prog↑ (3, 19, 24, 44, 45, 74)*	?	TC (mRNA) (12, 36, 64, 73)*
FGF	E$_2$↓,Prog↑	?	GC, LC
interleukin-1	LH R↓,E$_2$↓,Prog↓ (6, 9, 29, 30, 34)*	?	? (59)*

GC = granulosa cells, TC = theca cells, LC = luteal cells
* = literature reference

Moreover, RNA for TGF-α was found in rat ovaries, and immunoreactive TGF-α was detected in the interstitial and theca cells (49). These observations show that EGF and TGF-α are locally produced in the ovary and may be involved in a paracrine communication between theca and granulosa cells to modulate differentiated ovarian functions.

EGF also inhibits human chorionic gonadotropin (hCG)-induced testosterone production by rat testis cells in culture (Table 3), and the presence of EGF binding sites in these cells has been described (72). An EGF-like substance is produced by Sertoli cells (38), suggesting paracrine intratesticular roles of this growth factor. Furthermore, EGF may regulate male reproductive functions by stimulating directly the meiotic progression of spermatogenesis (69).

IGFs / insulin

Studies from this and other laboratories demonstrate that immunoreactive and bioactive ovarian IGF-I is present in the granulosa cells (Table 2) (35). Its production is controlled by growth hormone (21), gonadotropins and estrogens (39). Furthermore, IGF-I gene expression has been observed in the ovary by

Table 3.Growth factors as intragonadal regulators in the testis

	ACTION	RECEPTOR	ORIGIN
EGF TGF-α	LH R↓ , T↓ ? (72)[*]	+ (72)[*]	SC (EGF-like) (38)[*]
IGF-I IGF-II insulin	T↑ ? T↑ (1, 53)[*]	+ ? + (16, 48a)[*]	SC ? ? (10, 18, 66)[*]
inhibin activin TGF-β	T↑ I↓ T↓ (7, 26, 44, 54)[*]	? ? ?	SC (13) ? SC (TGF-β- like) (11, 13)[*]
FGF interleukin-1	T↓ T↓ (27)[*]	+ ? (27)[*]	testis extracts (70)[*] testis extracts (47)[*]

SC = Sertoli cells   [*] = literature reference

determination of specific mRNA levels (58). IGF-I receptors has been identified in granulosa cells (5, 40), and IGF-I exerts a stimulatory effect on FSH-induced steroidogenesis and FSH-induced receptor induction by granulosa cells (2, 20) as well as androgen biosynthesis by theca cells (25, 37). Although IGF-II and insulin receptors are present in the ovary, the observed similar, but less potent, actions of insulin and IGF-II in gonadal cells (71) are probably mediated through binding to IGF-I receptors (2, 22, 61). These in vitro observations indicate that granulosa cells are the site of IGF-I production, reception, and action (Table 2), suggesting an autocrine function for this peptide in the ovary.

Although binding sites for the IGFs have also been identified in both the Sertoli cells (16) and the Leydig cells (48a) of the testis, it is generally believed that insulin and IGF-II act through the IGF-I receptors (16). Insulin and IGF-I augment testosterone production by cultured testicular cells (Table 3) (1, 48a, 53). Moreover, a peptide that binds to the IGF-I receptor is found in conditioned medium of cultured Sertoli cells by immunoblotting and radioreceptor assays (10, 18, 66). In conclusion, IGF-I represents a potential intratesticular regulator, based on its release by Sertoli cells, together with its facilitatory action on Leydig cell steroidogenesis.

inhibin / activin / TGF-β

FSH secretion by cultured pituitary cells is differentially regulated by inhibin, activin and TGF-β. Recently, the potential regulation of aromatase activity in granulosa cells by these peptides was also investigated. It was shown that basal estrogen secretion by granulosa cells is unaffected by treatment with TGF-β or inhibin alone, whereas FSH-stimulated accumulation of estrogen and progesterone is dose-dependently augmented by TGF-β (Table 2) (3, 19) and suppressed by inhibin (74). In contrast, inhibin enhances, but activin suppresses, androgen production in cultured ovarian theca-interstitial cells and explants of follicle walls (44). Moreover, the FSH induction of LH receptors in granulosa cells is also enhanced by TGF-β (24).

Theca cells in culture produce TGF-β as determined by both radioreceptor and radioimmunoassays (64), and the TGF-β gene is expressed in the rodent ovary (36). Inhibin is synthesized by granulosa cells, and its production is stimulated primarily by FSH, whereas growth factors including IGF-I and EGF, may also have direct effects on the production of inhibin (12). The demonstration of inhibin mRNA in cultured granulosa cells (73) also confirms that these cells are the site of inhibin synthesis. Activin, on the other hand, augments FSH induced aromatase activity and arrests progesterone (45) and androgen (44) secretion. These data suggest that inhibin may act as an autocrine, and TGF-β as a paracrine regulator of granulosa cell steroid production.

In contrast to the stimulatory effect of TGF-β in the ovary, TGF-β inhibits testicular testosterone production *in vitro* (Table 3) (7, 26, 54). Preliminary data suggest that TGF-β-like activity is present in Sertoli cell conditioned medium (11). Like TGF-β, activin diminishes testosterone production, whereas inhibin enhances LH-stimulated androgen formation (44). Inhibin is synthetized by Sertoli cells in the testis, and the production is primarily regulated by FSH (13). These data indicate that inhibin and TGF-β, which are released by Sertoli cells, may serve as intragonadal paracrine signals in the modulation of LH-stimulated androgen biosynthesis.

FGF / interleukin-1

FGF has major mitogenic activities and may play a role in the support of growth and development of granulosa and theca cells. Moreover, cultured bovine granulosa cells produce bioactive FGF (59) and express the gene encoding basic FGF (59). Because FGF has been identified as an angiogenic factor in the ovary (32), the possible effect of FGF on granulosa cell differentiation was investigated. Treatment of cultured granulosa cells with FGF inhibits FSH stimulation of estrogen production (IC_{50} = 10^{-12} M), but enhances progesterone secretion at low doses (Table 2) (9). Subsequent studies suggest that the inhibitory effect takes place distal, rather than proximal to cAMP formation (6).

Recently, a form of basic FGF has been purified and characterized from the bovine testis (70), suggesting that FGF may have an intratesticular regulatory role as well. FGF causes a dose-dependent inhibition of LH-induced testosterone production (IC_{50} = 1.1×10^{-9} M) by cultured neonatal rat testis cells and further studies indicate that Leydig cell 17α-hydroxylase activity may be inhibited by FGF (27). The concept of a direct testicular action of FGF is further supported by the demonstration of high-affinity, low capacity FGF receptors in these cultured testis cells (Table 3).

Recent studies support the role of interleukin-1, presumably a macrophage-derived factor, in the regulation of endocrine functions. This includes the modulation of the production of insulin, corticotropin-releasing factor (CRF), cortisol, and thyroglobulin. Interleukin-1β inhibits FSH-induced LH receptor formation and progesterone production in granulosa cells (Table 2) (29, 34). In addition, studies from our laboratory show a dose-dependent inhibition of FSH-stimulated estrogen production in primary cultures of rat granulosa cells, with IC_{50} values of 9.7×10^{-12} M (30).

Macrophages are present in large quantities in the testis and are closely associated with Leydig cells (56). Moreover, large amounts of an interleukin-1-like factor are detected in testes homogenates, based on its stimulation of lymphocyte proliferation (47), suggesting that this cytokine may also be capable of regulating testicular steroid production. Studies performed in our laboratory showed that interleukin-1 dose-dependently inhibits hCG-induced androgen production in rat testicular cells in culture with

IC_{50} values of 6×10^{-12} M (unpublished data), suggesting interaction between the immune factors and the reproductive system in the ovary as well as the testis.

CONCLUSION

Various growth factors have been shown to be secreted by ovarian theca or granulosa cells, or testicular Sertoli cells. Specific mRNA of most growth factors has been detected in the gonads, allowing studies to determine how its synthesis is regulated. Moreover, numerous studies have demonstrated that many of these growth factors are capable of modulating proliferation and differentiation of ovarian and testis functions in vitro, and their binding sites have been characterized. The major challenge for the near future is to establish the possible roles of growth factors in vivo in gonadal regulations.

ACKNOWLEDGEMENTS

Studies in this laboratory have been supported by grants from the National Institute of Health (HD-14084) and the Andrew W. Mellon Foundation. B. Fauser - permanent address; Department of Obstetrics and Gynecology, Dijkzigt University Hospital, Rotterdam, the Netherlands - is supported by grants from the Fulbright Program, the Dutch Foundation for the Advancement of Pure Research (ZWO), and by the Erasmus University of Rotterdam.

REFERENCES

1. Adashi, E.Y., Fabics, C., and Hsueh, A.J.W. (1982): Biol. Reprod., 26:270-280.
2. Adashi, E.Y., Resnick, C.E., D'Ercole, A.J., Svoboda, M.E., and van Wijk, J. J. (1985): Endocr. Rev., 6:400-420.
3. Adashi, E.Y., and Resnick, C.E. (1986): Endocrinology, 119:1879-1881.
4. Adashi, E.Y., Resnick, C.E., and Twardzik, D.R. (1987): J. Cell. Biochem., 33:1-13.
5. Adashi, E.Y., Resnick, C.E., Hernandez, E.R., Svoboda, M.E., and van Wijk, J.J. (1988): Endocrinology, 122:194-201.
6. Adashi, E.Y., Resnick, C.E., Croft, S.C., May, J.V., and Gospodarowicz D. (1988): Mol. Cell. Endocrinol., 55:7-14.
7. Avallet, O., Vigier, M., Perrard-Sapori, M.H., and Saez, J.M. (1987): Biochem. Biophys. Res. Commun., 146:575-581.

8. Baird, A., Esch, F., Mormede, P., Ueno, N., Ling, N.,
    Bohlen, P., Ying, S.-Y., Wehrenberg, W.B., and
    Guillemin, R. (1986): Rec. Progr. Horm. Res., 42:143-
    201.
9. Baird, A., and Hsueh A.J.W. (1980): Reg. Pept., 16:243-250.
10. Benahmed, M., Morera, A.M., Chauvin, M.C., and de Peretti,
    E. (1987): Mol. Cell. Endocrinol., 50:69-77.
11. Benahmed, M., Morera, A.M., Chauvin, M.A., and Cochet, C.
    (1987): 69th Annual Meeting of the Endocrine Society, p.
    22 (Ab 6).
12. Bicsak, T.A., Tucker E.M., Cappel, S., Vaughan, J., Rivier
    J., Vale W., and Hsueh, A.J.W. (1986): Endocrinology,
    119:2711-2719.
13. Bicsak, T.A., vale W., Vaughan, J., Tucker, E.M., Cappel,
    S., and Hsueh, A.J.W. (1987): Mol. Cell. Endocrinol.,
    49:211-217.
14. Bicsak, T.A., and Hsueh, A.J.W. (1988): In: The Primate
    Ovary, edited by R.M. Brenner, Plenum Press, New York,
    In Press.
15. Bicsak, T.A., and Hsueh, A.J.W. (1988): In; Cell to Cell
    Communication in Endocrinology, edited by F. Piva, and
    G. Forti, Raven Pres, New york, In Press.
16. Borland, K., Mita, M., Oppenheimer, C.L., Blinderman, L.A.,
    Massague, J., Hall, P.F., and Czech, M.P. (1984):
    Endocrinology, 114:240-246.
17. Carpenter, G., and Zendegui, J.G. (1986): Exp. Cell. Res.,
    164:1-10.
18. Chatelain, P.G., Naville, D., and Saez, J.M. (1987):
    Biochem. Biophys. Res. Commun., 146:1009-1017.
19. Dahl, K.D., Czekala, N.M., Lim, P., and Hsueh, A.J.W.
    (1987): J. Clin. Endocrinol. Metab., 64:486-493.
20. Davoren, J.B., Hsueh, A.J.W., and Li, C.H. (1985): Am. J.
    Physiol., 249:E26-E33.
21. Davoren, J.B., and Hsueh, A.J.W. (1986): Endocrinology,
    118:888-890.
22. Davoren, J.B., Kasson, B.G., Li, C.H., and Hsueh, A.J.W.
    (1986): Endocrinology, 119:2155-2162.
23. Dekel, N., and Sherizly, I. (1985): Endocrinology, 116:406-
    409.
24. Dodson, W.C., and Schomberg, D.W. (1987): Endocrinology,
    120:512-516.
25. Erickson, G.F, Magoffin, D.A., Dyer, C.A., and Hofeditz, C.
    (1985): Endocr. Rev., 6:371-399.
26. Fauser, B.C.J.M., and Hsueh, A.J.W. (1988): 35th Annual
    Meeting of the Society for Gynecologic Investigation, p.
    277 (Ab 436).
27. Fauser, B.C.J.M., Baird, A., and Hsueh, A.J.W. (1988):
    Endocrinology, In Press.
28. Feng, P., Knecht, M., and Catt, K. (1987): Endocrinology
    120:1121-1126.

29. Fukuoka, M., Mori, T., Taii, S., and Yasuda, K. (1988): Endocrinology, 122:367-369.
30. Galway, A.B., Zhou, M.-H., and Hsueh, A.J.W. (1988): 35th Annual Meeting of the Society for Gynecologic Investigation, p. 171 (Ab 223).
31. Gimenez-Gallego, G., Rodkey, J., Bennet, C., Rios Candelore, M., DiSalvo, J., and Thomas, K. (1985): Science, 230:1385-1388.
32. Gospodarowicz, D., Cheng, J., Lui, G.M., Baird, A., Esch, F., and Bohlen, P. (1985): Endocrinology, 117:2283-2391.
33. Gospodarowicz, D., Ferrara, N., Schweigerer, L., and Neufeld, G. (1987): Endocrinology, 8:95-114.
34. Gottschall, P.E., Uehara, A., Hoffmann, S.T., and Arimura, A. (1987): Biochem. Biophys. Res. Commun., 149:502-509.
35. Hammond, J.M., Baranao, L.S., Skaleris, D., Knight, A.B., Romanus, J.A., and Rechler, M.M. (1985): Endocrinology, 117:2553-2555.
36. Hernandez, E.R., Twardzik, D.R., and Adashi, E.Y. (1987): 20th Annual Meeting of the Society for the Study of Reproduction, p. 58 (Ab 35).
37. Hernandez, E.R., Resnick, C.E., Svoboda, E.M., van Wijk, J.J., Payne, D.W., and Adashi, E.Y. (1988): Endocrinology 122:1603-1612.
38. Holmes, S.D., Spotts, G., and Smith, R.G. (1986): J. Biol. Chem., 261:4076-4080.
39. Hsu, C.-J., and Hammond, J.M. (1987): Endocrinology, 120:198-207.
40. Hsu, C.-J., Holmes, S.D., and James, J.M. (1987): Biochem. Biophys. Res. Commun., 147:242-247.
41. Hsueh, A.J.W., Welsh, T.H., and Jones, P.B.C. (1981): Endocrinology, 108:2002-2004.
42. Hsueh, A.J.W. (1983): J. Reprod. Fert., 69:325-342.
43. Hsueh, A.J.W. (1986): Clinics Endocrinol. Metab., 15:117-134.
44. Hsueh, A.J.W., Dahl, K.D., Vaughan. J., Tucker, E., Rivier, J., Bardin, C.W., and Vale, W. (1987): Proc. Natl. Acad. Sci. USA, 84:5082-5086.
45. Hutchison, L.A., Findlay, J.K., de Vos, F.L., and Robertson, D.M. (1987): Biochem. Biophys. Res. Commun., 146:1405-1412.
46. Jones, P.B.C., Welsh, T.H., and Hsueh, A.J.W. (1982): J. Biol. Chem., 257:11268-11273.
47. Kahn, S.A., Soder, O., Syed, V., Gustafsson, K., Lindh, M., and Ritzen, E.M. (1987): Int. J. Androl., 10:495-503
48. Kasson, B.G., Adashi, E.Y., and Hsueh, A.J.W. (1986): Endocr. Rev., 7:156-168.
48a. Kasson, B.G., and Hsueh, A.J.W. (1987): Mol. Cell. Endocrinol., 52:27-34.

49. Kudlow, J.E., Kobrin, M.S., Purchio, A.F., Twardzik, D.R., Heranadez, E.R., Asa, S.L., and Adashi, E.Y. (1988): Endocrinology, 121:1577-1579.
50. Lachman, L.B. (1983): In: Beneficial effects of endotoxins, edited by A. Nowtny, pp. 283-305. Plenum Press, New York.
51. Lee, D.C., Rose, T.M., Webb, N.R., and Todaro, G.J. (1985): Nature, 85 313:489-491.
52. Levi-Montalcini, R., and Cohen, S. (1960): Ann. Natl. Acad. Sci. USA, 85:324-329.
53. Lin, T, Haskell, J., Vinson, N., and Terracio, L. (1986): Biochem. Biophys. Res. Commun., 137:950-956.
54. Lin, T., Blaisdell, J., Haskell, J.F. (1987): Biochem. Biophys. Res. Commun., 146:387-394.
55. Massague, J. (1985): J. Cell. Biol., 100:1508-1514.
56. Miller, S.C., Bowman, B.M., and Rowland, H.G. (1983): Am. J. Anat., 168:1-13.
57. Mondschein, J.S., and Schomberg, D.W. (1981): Science, 211:1179-1180.
58. Murphy, L.J,. Bell, G.I., and Friesen, H.G. (1987): Endocrinology, 120:1279-1282.
59. Neufeld, G., Ferrara, N., Schweigerere, L., Mitchell, R., and Gospodarowicz, D. (1987): Endocrinology, 121:597-603.
60. Oppenheim, J.J., Kovacs, E.J., Matsushima, K., and Durum, S.K. (1986): Immunol. Today, 7:45-56.
61. Poretsky, L., and Kalin, M.F. (1987): Endocr. Rev., 8:132-141
62. Rall, L.B., Scott. J., and Bell, G.I. (1985): Nature, 313:228-231.
63. Rinderknecht, E., and Humbel, R.E. (1976): Proc. Natl. Acad. Sci. USA., 73:2365-2369.
64. Skinner, M.K., Keski-Oja, J., Osteen, K.G., and Moses, H.L. (1987): Endocrinology, 121:786-792.
65. Skinner, M.K., Lobb, D., and Dorrington, J.H. (1987): Endocrinology, 121:1892-1899.
66. Smith, E.P., Svoboda, M.E., van Wijk, J.J., Kierszenbaum, A.M., and Tress, L.L. (1987): Endocrinology, 120:186-193.
67. Sporn, M.B., Roberts, A.B., Wakefield, L.M., and Associan, R.K. (1986): Science, 233:532-534.
68. Todaro, G.J., de larco, J.E., and Cohen, S. (1976): Nature, 264:26-31.
69. Tsutsumi, O., Kurachi, H., and Oka, T. (1986): Science, 233:975-977.
70. Ueno, N., Baird, A., Esch, N., Ling, N., and Guillemin, R. (1987): Mol. Cell. Endocrinol., 49:189-194.
71. Veldhuis, J.D., Kolp, L.A., Toaff, M.E., Strauss III, J.F., and Demers, L.M. (1983): J. Clin. Invest., 72:1046-1057.
72. Welsh, T.H., and Hsueh, A.J.W. (1982): Endocrinology, 110:1498-1506.

73. Woodruff, T.V., Meunier, H., Jones, P.B.C., Hsueh, A.J.W., and Mayo, K. E. (1987): Mol. Endocrinol., 1:561–568.

74. Ying, S.-Y., Becker, A., Ling. N., Ueno, N., and Guillemin, R. (1986): Biochem. Biophys. Res. Commun., 136:969–975.

The Androgen Responsiveness of Sertoli Cells Depends on a Complex Interplay between Androgens, FSH and Peritubular Cell Factors

G. Verhoeven and J. Cailleau

*Laboratory for Experimental Medicine and Endocrinology,
Gasthuisberg, Onderwijs en Navorsing, Herestraat 49, B-3000
Leuven, Belgium*

Androgens are the major factors involved in the maintenance of spermatogenesis. Nonetheless, the mechanisms by which these hormones affect germ cell development are poorly understood and attempts to study specific effects of androgens on testicular cells in vitro have yielded only mildly encouraging results. In the present report we show that prolonged exposure to androgens may be required to observe some effects of androgens on cultured testicular cells. This phenomenon might be related to the ability of androgens to stimulate the androgen receptor apparatus in their target cells. Moreover, we demonstrate that stimulatory as well as inhibitory effects of androgens on Sertoli cells may be amplified by androgen-regulated paracrine factors produced by peritubular cells.

MATERIALS AND METHODS

Sertoli cells (S) were prepared and cultured as described previously (3). These preparations contain no Leydig cells and less than 3% peritubular cells. In some experiments hypotonic treatment was used to accelerate the disappearance of germ cells. Peritubular cells (PT) were prepared essentially as described by Tung et al. (2). These cells were cultured for 6 days in medium containing 10% fetal calf serum. Thereafter they were maintained in serum-free medium. PT cells were shown to be free of contaminating Leydig cells and S cells by the absence of a cAMP, steroid, aromatase or androgen binding protein (ABP) response to LH and FSH. Fibroblasts were prepared from rat footsoles and were cultured in the same way as PT cells.

Androgen receptor concentration was measured in cultured cells using a monolayer binding assay described previously. Routinely [³H]mibolerone was used as a ligand to avoid interference of ABP in the measurements. When the cells were pretreated with androgens or FSH measurements were performed 18 h after removal of these agonists (4).

ABP was measured in the culture media using a filter disc assay (4). Routinely measurements were performed in the combined spent media from day 4, 5 and 6 of culture. Inducible aromatase activity was measured on day 7 by incubating the cells for 24 h in the presence of 0.5 μM testosterone (T), 0.1 mM MIX and FSH 100 ng/ml. The production of 17β-estradiol was measured by RIA.

In a series of experiments the influence of PT cell or fibroblast spent media on S cell function was evaluated. Spent media were derived from cells cultured in the absence of serum and were extensively dialyzed before use. S cells were cultured for 6 days in the presence of the spent media. The media were replaced on day 3 and ABP was measured in the media from the last 3 days of culture. Aromatase activity was measured on day 7 as described but in the presence of spent medium.

RESULTS

The androgen receptor concentration in testicular cells is controlled by FSH and by androgens.

In a first series of experiments (4) we demonstrated that daily pretreatment of S cells with FSH or with testosterone (T) for 6 days results in a marked increase in the concentration of the androgen receptor. The combination of these hormones had additive effects (Table 1). The increase could be shown using a monolayer binding assay on intact cells and using sucrose density gradient centrifugation of S cell cytosol. The effects of FSH could be mimicked by dbcAMP and the effects of androgens were blocked by the antiandrogen cyproterone acetate. Androgens also increased the androgen receptor concentration in PT cells. In these cells FSH was ineffective. LH had no effect in S or in PT cells. Detailed studies on the affinity, ligand specificity and sedimentation characteristics of the [³H]mibolerone binding protein in S cells and PT cells confirmed that this protein had the same characteristics as the androgen receptor in other target tissues.

Prolonged exposure of S cells to androgens results in a time and dose dependent decrease of inducible aromatase activity

Daily pretreatment of S cells for 7 days with androgens resulted in a dose-dependent decrease in FSH-inducible aromatase activity (Table 2). Half maximal inhibition was observed at 10^{-7}M testosterone (5). The inhibition was reversible and could also be observed when other inducers of the aromatase were tested (dbcAMP, L-isoproterenol, cholera toxin). The inhibition increased in a nearly linear fashion as a

function of the duration of pretreatment.   Five days were
required   to   observe   half-maximal   inhibition   with 10^{-6}M
testosterone.   The effect was observed with aromatizable and
non-aromatizable androgens   while   other   classes   of   steroid
hormones were ineffective.   The inhibition of aromatase activity
was   paralleled   by   an   increase   in   ABP   production   and   was
blocked by cyproterone acetate (5).

TABLE 1 :   Influence of testosterone (T) and FSH on androgen
              receptor   concentrations   in   Sertoli   cells   and
              peritubular cells[a].

Pretreatment	Androgen receptor concentration (fmol/mg protein)	
	Sertoli cells	Peritubular cells
Control	27.3 ± 3.2	18.3 ± 0.7
T	43.7 ± 4.7*	42.7 ± 1.3*
FSH	57.3 ± 4.4*	17.9 ± 1.7
LH	25.5 ± 2.7	18.7 ± 0.8
T + FSH	71.3 ± 6.3*	43.1 ± 2.4*
T + LH	45.8 ± 1.8*	41.3 ± 1.4*

a Cells were pretreated for 6 days with T (0.1 µM), oFSH (10
ng/ml) or oLH (10 ng/ml). Androgen receptor concentration was
measured as explained in the Experimental section. Values are
means ± SD of triplicates. Values followed by an asterisk are
significantly different (P < 0.05) from the control.

*Effects of PT cells and PT cell conditioned media on androgen
responses in S cells*

Coculture of S cells with PT cells markedly enhanced the
androgen dependent inhibition of inducible aromatase activity
and the stimulation of ABP production (Table 3).   Extensively
predialysed spent media derived from PT cells exposed for 7
days   to   testosterone   had   comparable   effects   on   aromatase
activity and ABP production.   Such effects were not observed
with   spent   media   from   identically   treated   fibroblasts.
Preliminary data suggest that the effects of PT cells are
mediated by one or more paracrine factors and that there is
some analogy between the factor responsible for ABP induction
(PMod-S) and the aromatase inhibiting factor (AIF).   Both
active principles are destroyed by heating and by trypsin and
their weight is in the 50-100 kD range.   The androgen
dependent   production   of   both   factors   is   inhibited   by
cyproterone acetate (not shown).

TABLE 2 :   Influence of prolonged exposure to steroids on Sertoli cell aromatase activity[a]

Pretreatment	17β–estradiol (ng/mg protein)	
	$10^{-7}M$	$10^{-6}M$
Control	3.98 ± 0.37	3.98 ± 0.37
Testosterone	2.11 ± 0.17[x]	1.06 ± 0.13[x]
Progesterone	3.75 ± 0.11	3.66 ± 0.23
Corticosterone	3.40 ± 0.13	3.31 ± 0.17
17α–Ethinylestradiol	3.81 ± 0.17	3.71 ± 0.33

[a] Sertoli cells were pretreated for 7 days with the indicated concentrations of steroids. FSH-inducible aromatase activity was measured on day 8. Values are means ± SD of 6 incubations.

TABLE 3 :   Influence of S cell–PT cell coculture and influence of PT cell conditioned media on aromatase activity and ABP production

Treatment	n	17β–estradiol	ABP
		pg/ml	fmol/ml
S only[1]	6	490 ± 21	271 ± 27
S : PT coculture	6	251 ± 37	721 ± 31
		ng/mg prot.	pmol/mg prot.
S + fibroblast spent medium[2]	3	3.23 ± 0.1	0.83 ± 0.11
S + PT spent medium	3	1.61 ± 0.2	3.23 ± 0.21

[1] S cells were cultured alone or in the presence of 20% PT cells. $10^{-7}M$ testosterone was added daily to the culture medium. ABP was measured in the combined media from day 5-7 of culture. FSH inducible aromatase activity was measured on day 8.

[2] S cells were maintained for 7 days in spent media from fibroblast or PT cells exposed to $10^{-7}M$ testosterone. The media were extensively dialyzed before use. ABP was measured in the combined media from day 4-6 of culture. FSH inducible aromatase activity was measured on day 7.

DISCUSSION

Three major conclusions may be derived from these data (Fig. 1) :

Firstly, both PT cells and S cells can figure as direct targets for androgen action in the testis. Both cell types contain an androgen receptor (R) with characteristics comparable to those of the receptor in other androgen target tissues. An interesting feature of this receptor is that its concentration is low in the absence of androgens but can be increased up to 3-fold in the presence of these hormones. In S cells the androgen receptor concentration is also increased by FSH. It is tempting to speculate that regulation of androgen receptor concentration may be an important mechanism controlling androgen-responses in a tissue where the receptor may be fully occupied by the high endogenous concentration of androgens (4).

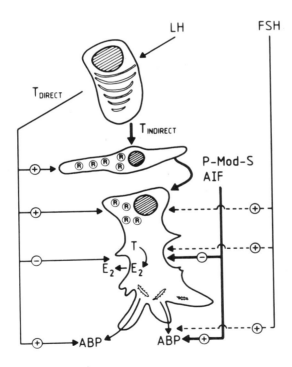

Fig. 1.   Direct and indirect effects of androgens on PT cells and S cells

Secondly, inhibition of FSH-inducible aromatase activity in S cells can be used as a novel parameter of androgen action in these cells. This inhibitory effect of androgens may explain the disappearance of aromatase activity in the tubular compartment during pubertal development and the spontaneous increase in aromatase activity observed when S cells are cultured in the absence of androgens (4). It should be noted that this effect as well as the mentioned effects of androgens on their own receptor are only observed after prolonged exposure to androgens.

Finally, our data show that androgens may also indirectly influence S cell function via one or more paracrine mediators produced under their influence by PT cells. These mediators not only mimick the direct stimulatory effects of androgens on ABP and transferrin production (P Mod-S activity) but also their inhibitory effects on inducible aromatase activity (AIF). The finding that androgens, paracrine mediators produced by S cells and paracrine factors derived from germ cells (1) – agonists with very divergent modes of action – ultimately have comparable stimulatory and inhibitory effects on S cells raises fundamental questions on the nature of androgen action in S cells.

REFERENCES

1. Le Magueresse, B., and Jégou, B. (1986): *Biochem. Biophys. Res. Commun.*, 141:861–869.
2. Tung, P.S., Skinner, M.K., and Fritz, I.B. (1984): *Biol. Reprod.*, 30:199–211.
3. Verhoeven, G. (1980): *J. Steroid Biochem.*, 12:315–322.
4. Verhoeven, G., and Cailleau, J. (1988): *Endocrinology*, 122:in press.
5. Verhoeven, G., and Cailleau, J. (1988): *Mol. Cell. Endocrinol.*, in press.

ACKNOWLEDGEMENTS

The text presents research results of the Belgian National incentive program on fundamental research in Life Sciences initiated by the Belgian State Prime Minister's Office Science Policy Programming. The scientific responsibility is assumed by its authors. This work was also supported by a Grant from the "Nationaal Fonds voor Wetenschappelijk Onderzoek" and the "Nationale Loterij".

Expression of the Pro-Opiomelanocortin (POMC) Gene in Rat Testicular Germ Cells and the Response of Sertoli Cells to POMC-Derived Peptides

C. Boitani[1], C.L.C. Chen[2], R. Canipari[1] and C.W. Bardin[2]

[1]Institute of Histology and general Embryology,
University La Sapienza of Rome, Via Scarpa 14, 00161 Rome,
and [2] The Population Council, 1230 York Avenue, New York, N.Y. 10021

INTRODUCTION

In the last few years, a large body of evidence has accumulated to indicate that in mammals the testis contains pro-opiomelanocortin (POMC), the precursor molecule for a variety of peptides such as melanocyte-stimulating hormones (α, β and τ), ACTH and β-endorphin (2). Following localization of the POMC-derived peptides and POMC messenger RNA in Leydig cells (8, 18), several studies have been reported on the secretion, regulation and possible function of these peptides in the male gonad (5, 6, 9-11, 17, 19-20).

In this study we have extended the analysis of testicular cell types which may express the POMC gene and we have further analysed the effect of POMC-derived peptides on two parameters of Sertoli cell function that are known to be regulated by cyclic AMP, namely aromatase and plasminogen activator.

METHODS

Cell preparation

Germ cells.
Seminiferous tubules from 35-day old Sprague Dawley rats were freed from interstitial tissue by collagenase treatment and dispersed into single cells as previously described (3). The total germ cell suspension was collected after sedimentation of the tubules and fractionated into several cell classes by velocity sedimentation at unit gravity on an albumin gradient. The cellular fractions composed of middle-late pachytene

spermatocytes and round spermatids (steps 1-8 of spermiogenesis) were collected and washed in MEM.

Sertoli   cells.

   Sertoli cell monolayers were obtained from 10- and 35-day old rats according to the method of Mather and Phillips (15).   At day three of culture, cells were treated with hypotonic solution to remove contaminating germ cells.   At day four of culture, cells were washed twice with fresh medium and incubated for 24 hours in the presence of various hormones.

Northern Blot Analysis

   Total RNA was isolated from whole testes, germ cells and Sertoli cells by the urea/lithium chloride precipitation method and fractionated on an agarose gel as previously described (9). POMC-like mRNAs were identified by hybridization with a radioactive POMC cDNA probe and exposed to X-ray film.   The rat POMC cDNA (pl13) contains the nucleotide sequences coding from the mid portion of the NH2-terminal glycopeptide of POMC to the poly-A   tail   (7).

Assay of aromatase and urokinase plasminogen activator (uPA) activities

   Estradiol produced by Sertoli cell cultures was measured in the media by RIA as previously described (4). uPA activity in the media was determined by incubating the sample with antiserum specific for tissue type plasminogen activator, followed by incubation with plasminogen and a chromogenic substrate (21, 2). Proteins were measured using the method of Lowry (14) with BSA as standard.

RESULTS

   Sertoli cells and spermatogenic cells were isolated to determine if other testicular cell types, in addition to Leydig cells, were responsible for expression of the POMC gene in the testis. Fig.1 shows that POMC mRNA was clearly detected in total RNA from whole mature testis as well as from germ cell preparations (lane 1 and 3).   Sertoli cells did not express any POMC transcripts (lane 2).   Purified populations of pachytene spermatocytes and round spermatids were isolated and total RNA was hybridized with the POMC cDNA probe.   Both germ cells contained POMC transcripts, the size of those in meiotic cells being smaller than that in haploid cells (data not shown).

   The finding that germ cells may also be a source of the POMC peptides in the testis, is of further interest in that Sertoli cells are capable of responding to these peptides.   We have reported a stimulatory effect of α-MSH on cAMP and estradiol production by Sertoli cell cultures (5, 6). We asked the question whether another functional parameter of Sertoli cells known to

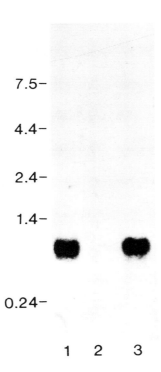

FIG. 1. Northern blot analysis of POMC mRNA in whole testis (lane 1), Sertoli cells (lane 2), and germ cells (lane 3). The same amount (25 µg) of total RNA from each preparation was loaded in each lane. Molecular size markers (Kb) are indicated on the left.

---

be regulated by cAMP such as PA activity was affected by melanocyte-stimulating hormone. When Sertoli cells from 10-day old rats were incubated for 24 h with α-MSH in the presence of methylisobutylxanthine (MIX), the uPA activity released into the media was markedly decreased. In the absence of MIX, α-MSH had no effect on PA activity (Table 1). As shown in fig.2, the effect of α-MSH on uPA activity was dose-dependent with an ED50 of approximately 0.2 nM. This observation indicates that in the presence of MIX the uPA response (10 fold decrease) was much more sensitive to α-MSH than when cAMP accumulation or aromatase activity (3 fold increase) were used as end points (table 1).

TABLE 1.   Effect of α-MSH on estradiol (E2) and uPA secretion

TREATMENT	E2 (ng/mg protein ± SEM)	uPA (PU/mg protein ± SEM)
NONE	0.25 ± 0.01(a)	0.26 ± 0.01
α-MSH (1 μM)	0.43 ± 0.02(b)	0.25 ± 0.01
MIX (0.3 mM)	0.95 ± 0.06(c)	0.32 ± 0.03(e)
α-MSH + MIX	2.88 ± 0.20(d)	0.04 ± 0.002(f)

a vs b, c vs d, e vs f: P < 0.01

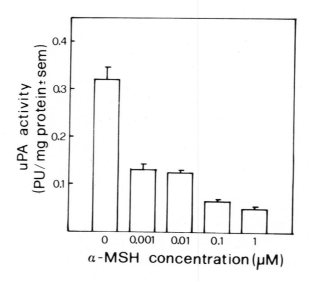

FIG. 2. Dose-response curve of α-MSH on uPA activity released into the medium by Sertoli cells. Cells were incubated with different concentrations of α-MSH plus MIX (0.3 mM). The uPA was measured in the presence of anti tPA. Each point is the mean of three plates, each assayed in duplicate.

When the response of Sertoli cells to FSH in terms of uPA activity was studied, we observed the same magnitude of change as α-MSH (Fig.3). In contrast, the two hormones displayed a differential effect, FSH being more potent than α-MSH, when cAMP production and aromatase activity were used as end points of response to the hormones.

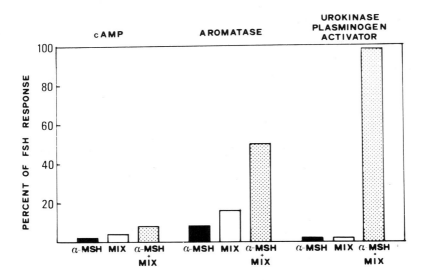

FIG. 3. Comparison of the Sertoli cell response to FSH and α-MSH in terms of cAMP production, aromatase activity and uPA activity. The response to α-MSH is expressed as percent of FSH response.

DISCUSSION

The data reported here show that rat germ cells, but not Sertoli cells are a site of testicular POMC gene expression. Among the cell types in the testis, Leydig cells have also been shown to express this molecule (8, 18). It is not clear at this time to what extent germ cells and Leydig cells account for the presence of POMC mRNA in the male gonad. Purified populations of these cell types would allow a quantitative comparison. Mouse germ cells have also been shown recently to be a source of POMC as well as proenkephalin mRNA (12, 13). Taken together, these observations are in keeping with the hypothesis that POMC peptides produced by either germ cells or Leydig cells may play a role in interaction with the Sertoli cells. However the actual secretion of POMC-derived peptides by germ cells remains to be demonstrated.

Of particular interest is the finding that α-MSH, one of the POMC-derived peptides has divergent effects on two cAMP-dependent parameters of Sertoli cell function. It stimulates an increase in aromatase activity and a decrease in urokinase plasminogen activator activity. The reason for this differential response of Sertoli cells to the same peptide is not known. Another notable observation of the present study was that α-MSH in the presence of MIX was as effective as FSH in terms of the uPA response, but was less potent in stimulating aromatase activity. Since an increase in cAMP occurs with either α-MSH (5) or FSH (16), this observation indicates that the peptide and the gonadotropin have differential effects on various parameters that cannot be explained by cAMP accumulation per se.

From these data we conclude that MSH peptides do influence Sertoli cell function. The finding that germ cells also express the POMC gene suggests an even greater role for these peptides as regulators of testicular function than was previously thought.

ACKNOWLEDGMENTS

We wish to thank Miss Tiziana Menna for her skilled technical assistance in preparing purified populations of germ cells.

REFERENCES

1. Andrade-Gordon, P. and Strickland, S. (1986): Biochemistry, 25:4033-4040.
2. Bardin, C.W., Chen, C.L.C., Morris, P.L., Gerendai, I., Boitani, C., Liotta, A.S., Margioris, A. and Krieger, D.T. (1987): Recent Prog. Horm. Res., 43:1-28.
3. Boitani, C., Geremia, R., Rossi, R., and Monesi, V. (1980): Cell Differentiation, 9:41-49.
4. Boitani, C., Ritzen, E.M. and Parvinen, M. (1981): Molec. Cell. Endocr., 23:11-22.
5. Boitani, C., Mather, J.P. and Bardin, C.W. (1986): Endocrinology, 118:1513-1518.
6. Boitani, C., Farini, D., Bardin, C.W. and Stefanini, M. (1986): In: Molecular and cellular endocrinology of the testis, edited by M. Stefanini, M. Conti, R. Geremia and E. Ziparo, pp.37-42. Elsevier, Amsterdam.
7. Chen, C.L.C., Dionne, F.T., and Roberts, J.L. (1983): Proc. Natl Acad. Sci. U.S.A., 80:2211-2215.
8. Chen, C.L.C., Mather, J.P., Morris, P.L. and Bardin, C.W. (1984): Proc. Natl Acad. Sci. U.S.A., 81:5672-5675.
9. Chen, C.L.C. and Madigan, M.B. (1987): Endocrinology, 121: 590-596.
10. Fabbri, A., Knox, G., Buczko, E., and Dufau, M.L. (1988): Endocrinology, 122:749-756.
11. Gerendai, I., Shaha, C., Gunsalus, G.L. and Bardin, C.W. (1986): Endocrinology, 118:2039-2044.
12. Gizang-Ginsberg, E. and Wolgemuth, D.J. (1987): Proc. Natl Acad. Sci. U.S.A., 84:1600-1604.
13. Kilpatrick, D.L., Borland, K. and Jin, D.F. (1987): Proc. Natl Acad. Sci. U.S.A., 84:5695-5699.
14. Lowry, O.H., Rosebrough, N.J., Farr, A.L. and Randall, R.J. (1951): J. Biol. Chem., 193:265-275.
15. Mather, J.P. and Phillips, D.M. (1984): In: Methods for serum-free culture of cells of the endocrine system. Edited

by D.W. Barnes, D.A. Sirbasku and G.H. Sato, pp.29-46. Allan Liss, New York.

16. Means, A.R., Dedman, J.R., Tash, J.S., Tindall, D.J., Sickle, M. van and Welsh, M.J. (1980): Ann. Rev. Physiol., 42:59-70.

17. Morris, P.L., Vale, W.W. and Bardin, C.W. (1988): Biochem. Biophys. Res. Comm., 148:1513-1519.

18. Pintar, J.R., Schachter, B., Herman, A.B., Durgerian, S. and Krieger, D.T. (1984): Science, 225:632-634.

19. Shaha, C., Margioris, A., Liotta, A.S., Krieger, D.T. and Bardin, C.W. (1984): Endocrinology, 115:378-384.

20. Valenca, M.A. and Negro-Vilar, A. (1986): Endocrinology, 118:32-37.

21. Verheijen, J.H., Mullaart, E., Chang, G.T.G., Kluft, C. and Wijngaards, G. (1982): Tromb. Haemostas. 48:266-269.

Characterization of Peritubular Myoid Cells in Highly Enriched In Vitro Cultures

F. Palombi, D. Farini, P. De Cesaris and M. Stefanini

Istituto di Istologia ed Embriologia Generale
Via A. Scarpa 14, 00161 Roma, Italy

In recent years increasing interest has been dedicated to peritubular cells as both agents and targets of paracrine interactions in the testis (for a review see 2). Yet, in the absence of specific markers, cultures of peritubular cells, composed of myoid and non-myoid cells in highly heterogeneous combinations, are waiting to be characterized. Very recently two markers have become available for myoid cell recognition: a) desmin, shown to be a component of intermediate filaments in these cells (6) and b) alkaline phosphatase, a cell surface enzyme cytochemically detected in desmin-containing peritubular cells (4).

When primary cultures of peritubular cells from three week old Wistar rats were screened for the presence of myoid cells by either marker, we found that the latter cells only represented 30%- 35% of the entire population, the majority of which is therefore presumably composed of fibroblasts, lymphatic endothelial cells and perhaps other interstitial elements. With the aim of characterizing myoid cells and obtaining more precise information on the functions of the various cell types present in the peritubulum we have tried to fractionate the tissue through Percoll density gradients. The data we report here refer to the purification and preliminary characterization of a cell fraction highly enriched in myoid cells and the isolation of a different cell population, possibly still heterogeneous, but highly enriched in non-myoid peritubular elements.

ACKNOWLEDGMENT: Work supported by CNR grant 870046356

MATERIAL AND METHODS

Cell preparation

Peritubular tissue was·obtained from testes of three-week old Wistar rats. After removing the interstitium by trypsin treatment, the seminiferous tubules were subject to collagenase digestion to detach the peritubulum from the seminiferous epithelium which was discarded by sedimentation. The supernatant was sequentially centrifuged at 40g to yield small fragments of peritubular tissue (preparation A) and at 200g to collect single peritubular cells (preparation B) (5). Cells were cultured at 32°C or 37°C in MEM in the presence or absence of 10% Fetal Calf Serum (FCS).

Cytochemical identification of myoid cells

Cells were fixed for 10 mins in 1:1 cold acetone-ethanol. Desmin-containing intermediate filaments were localized using indirect immunofluorescence by means of a primary monoclonal antibody raised against porcine stomach (Amersham, 1:5 dilution), and a FITC-conjugated anti-mouse antibody (Zymed). Alkaline phosphatase activity was detected by the cytochemical method of Ackerman (1) after incubating the cells for 30 mins in the dark in 0.5 mg/ml Fast Blue RR and 40 μl/ml Naphthol AS-MX phosphate 0.25% ′pH 8.6) (Sigma).

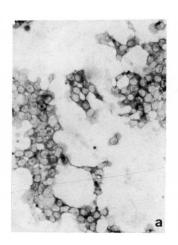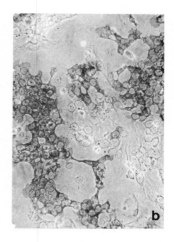

FIG.1. Primary culture of tubular wall fragments (preparation A) after 5 days in serum free medium at 32°C. a) alkaline phosphatase positive myoid cells; b) alkaline phosphatase negative Sertoli cells are apparent in phase contrast (480x)

Percoll density gradient

10 to 30 x 10[6] cells from preparation B or from preparation A (in the latter case dissociated through further trypsin digestion) were layered onto a discontinuous Percoll density gradient (3). The gradient was prepared by diluting 87% Percoll in MEM to obtain 12 solutions of 17% to 70% (density 1.04 to 1.1 g/ml) which were stratified in a 12 ml plastic tube. After centrifugation at 800g for 20 mins at 18°C, cell fractions were collected and numbered consecutively from bottom to top, thoroughly washed and cultured in MEM at 32°C or 37°C in the presence or absence of 10% FCS.

[3]H-thymidine incorporation

Cells were labelled for 18 hr on culture day 3 with 1 µCi/ml ^{3}H-thymidine (89 Ci/mmol Amersham). After a 1 hr chase, cells were solubilized and the radioactivity incorporated into acid-precipitable material was measured in a scintillation counter.

RESULTS AND DISCUSSION

Composition of the crude cell preparation subject to fractionation

When preparations of small-size cell clusters from collagenase treated seminiferous tubules (preparation A, see Material and Methods) were explanted in vitro and screened for the presence of myoid cells, they appeared to be composed of 50% desmin-containing, alkaline phosphatase positive cells, most of the remaining population being Sertoli cells. In these explants myoid cells can be cultured for days in the total absence of serum, displaying an arrangement in patches and a stable polygonal morphology (Fig 1) which becomes fibroblast-like on addition of serum (not shown). This preparation is therefore particularly enriched in myoid cells and a promising starting material for their purification. As for peritubular cell suspension (preparation B, see Material and Methods) it is composed of single cells, of which about 70% are non-myoid; it is virtually devoid of Sertoli cells, and requires serum for cell attachment and survival. In the latter cultures myoid cells display a polygonal shape only during the first day of culture, becoming subsequently elongated and indistinguishable from the other, fibroblast-like components (4). The analysis of myoid cell behaviour in the different conditions described above shows that these cells in culture can be distinguished from other peritubular elements by their specific morphology, which is stable

in the absence of serum. Moreover, myoid cell attachment and survival in serum-free cultures of tubular
wall explants, as opposed to the serum dependence of
the peritubular cell population, suggest that myoid
and non-myoid components of the peritubulum may differ
in serum requirement. Alternatively, the different
behaviour observed in the two culture systems could
reflect a specific influence of Sertoli cell products
or a response of myoid cells to dispersion into single
elements.

<u>Analysis of the cell fractions obtained through
Percoll gradient centrifugation</u>
    When centrifuged on a discontinuous Percoll density
gradient, both crude cell preparations were resolved
into 11 cell fractions, apparent as bands of different
thickness (Fig 2). Of these, appreciable numbers of
cells were present in fractions 4 to 10. Screening of
the fractions for the presence of myoid cells by
desmin and alkaline phosphatase cytochemistry showed
that these cells migrated into bands 4, 5 and 6,
whereas bands 7 and 8 appeared highly impoverished in
positive cells . In particular, fraction 5 was highly
homogeneous containing 75% and 90% myoid cells respectively from starting preparations B and A (Figs 3-4).
Crude preparation A (small clusters of tubular wall)
had usually been discarded during peritubular cell
isolation (5), because it is highly contaminated by
seminiferous epithelium. On the other hand with the
aim of yielding pure myoid cells it appears a very
favourable starting material, since Sertoli cells
differ in density and migrate to fractions 7 and 8,
while germ cells migrate to fraction 10.

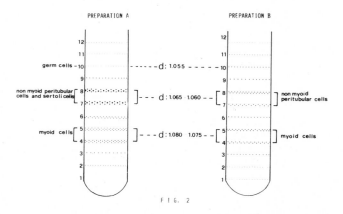

FIG. 2

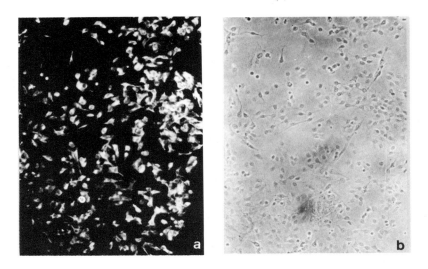

FIG.3. Fraction 5 from gradient A after culturing for 48 hr at 37°C in MEM-FCS. a) desmin positive myoid cells; b) phase contrast. Only a minority of the cells are negative for the marker (400x)

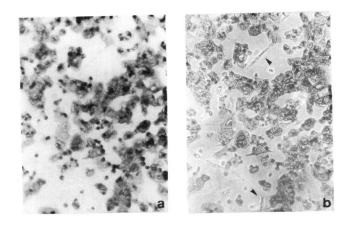

FIG.4. Positive staining for alkaline phosphatase in myoid cells from fraction 5 (gradient A). After 20 hr culture at 37°C in the presence of serum myoid cells appear polygonal while non-myoid contaminants apparent in b), phase contrast, (arrowheads) appear elongated (330x)

A second interesting cell population, though possibly heterogeneous, is represented by fractions 7 and 8 from the peritubular cell suspension (crude preparation B), a starting material virtually devoid of Sertoli cells. The two fractions, extremely poor in myoid cells (Fig 5), constitute a promising source of non-myoid peritubular elements.

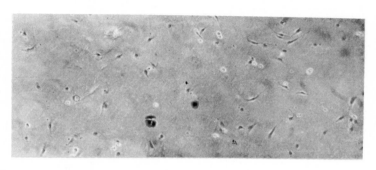

FIG.5. Fraction 8 from gradient B. Only very few alkaline phosphatase positive cells are present. The cells were cultured for 24 hr at 37°C in MEM-FCS. Phase contrast (170x)

Preliminary characterization of purified myoid cells
    When isolated in vitro, myoid cells can be cultured in the absence of serum. Under these conditions they display a stable polygonal shape (Fig 6a) and do not proliferate (Fig 7). On the other hand in medium containing 10% FCS the cells become fibroblast-like (Fig 6b) and proliferate, slowly reaching confluence (Fig 7). These data, in line with our observations on mixed cultures, show a behaviour distinctive of myoid cells and strongly suggest that the well known serum dependence of peritubular cells in vitro reflects requirements of non-myoid elements, which are numerically preponderant. Moreover the decribed highly enriched cultures offer an opportunity to study the factors regulating myoid cell proliferation and the maintenance of the contractile differentiated state.
    In conclusion we hope that 1) the dissection of the peritubulum into different cellular components, 2) the availability of myoid cells in homogeneous preparations, and 3) the possibility of maintaining isolated myoid cells in culture, will allow further characterization of peritubular tissue and its role in intragonadal interactions.

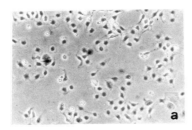
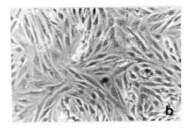

FIG.6. Fraction 5 from gradient A. Phase contrast morpholgy of myoid cells after 3 days in culture at 37°C a) in absence of serum; b) in presence of 10% FCS (110x)

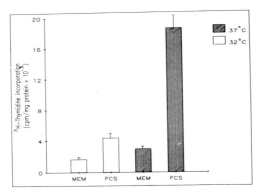

FIG.7. ^{3}H-thymidine incorporation into isolated myoid cells from fraction 5 (gradient A) under different cultural conditions

REFERENCES

1. Ackerman, G.A. (1962): Lab. Invest., 11:563-566.
2. Fritz, I.B. and Tung, P.S. (1986): in "Gametogenesis and the Early Embryo", edited by J.G. Gall, pp. 151-173. Alan Liss Inc.
3. Lefevre,A., Saez,J.M. and Finaz,C. (1983): Hormone Res., 17:114-120
4. Palombi,F. and Di Carlo, C., Biol. Reprod.,in press
5. Tung,P.S. and Fritz,I.B. (1977): in "Techniques of Human Andrology", edited by E.S.E. Hafez, pp. 125-143, Elsevier/North Holland Biomedical Press
6. Virtanen,I., Kallajoki,M., Narvanen,O., Paranko,J., Thornell,L.E., Miettinen,M., Lehto,V.P., (1986): Anat. Rec., 215:10-20

Comparison of the Effects of Transforming Growth Factor-ß and Porcine Sertoli Cell Conditioned Medium on Porcine Leydig Cell Function

O. Avallet, M.H. Perrar-Sapori, M. Vigier, M. Skalli and
J.M. Saez

INSERM U 307, Hôpital Debrousse, 69322 Lyon, France

The paracrine regulation of Leydig cell function by Sertoli cells is well established (16, 17), and probably most of these regulatory effects are exerted by Sertoli cell secreted proteins. Recent studies have shown that Sertoli cell conditioned medium (SCCM) has at least two effects on Leydig cells : an acute steroidogenic action (14, 23) and a long-term trophic effect (hCG receptor number and hCG responsiveness), the nature of which depends upon the conditions in which Sertoli cells are cultured. SCCM from Sertoli cells cultured in the presence of FSH and insulin is stimulatory, whereas SCCM from Sertoli cells cultured without hormones is inhibitory (14). Since transforming growth factor-β (TGF-β) has an inhibitory effect on both porcine (3) and rat (11) Leydig cell functions, in the present study we have compared the effect of pure TGF-β and SCCM from porcine Sertoli cells on porcine Leydig cell function. In addition the presence of TGF-β mRNA in porcine Sertoli cells was investigated.

MATERIALS AND METHODS

Human chorionic gonadotropin (hCG) was a gift of Dr. R.E. Canfield (New York) and was radioiodinated (21) and purified as described previously (4). TGF-β purified from human platelets (2) was a generous gift from Dr. A.B. Roberts (National Cancer Institute, Bethesda, MD). Heparin-Sepharose was obtained from Pharmacia, Sweden. Human TGF–β cDNA probe was provided from R. Derynck (Genetech, South San Francisco) (6).

Cell preparation and culture

Sertoli and Leydig cells were isolated from immature pig testes, and purified as previously described (5). Sertoli cells were plated in 75 cm^2 culture flasks, and Leydig cells in 24-well tissue culture dishes, containing Ham's F12/Dulbecco's modified Eagle's (DME) medium supplemented with 20 mM Hepes pH 7.4, 10 µg/ml transferrin, 5 µg/ml insulin, ascorbic acid 10^{-4}M, 10 µg/ml vitamin E and antibiotics. Testicular cells were cultured at 33°C.

Porcine Sertoli cell conditioned medium (SCCM)

On day 3 after seeding, the medium was removed and replaced by fresh medium. Spent medium was collected at day 5 and at day 7. Medium was centrifuged for 10 min (4°C) at 2500 g to remove cells. Then the medium was immediately concentrated using an Amicon membrane (YM_2, cut off : 2000 Da), dialyzed (Spectra/Por 6, cut off 2000 Da) against Tris buffer 10 mM pH 7.4 and lyophilized.

Proteins were resuspended in Tris buffer 10 mM pH 7.4 ; one half was acidified to pH 2.0 at 4°C with glacial CH_3COOH and after 1 h was neutralized with 2N NaOH (10) ; the other half was loaded onto a heparin-Sepharose column. The column was eluted with a discontinuous gradient of NaCl (0.1-0.6-1.1-2.0 M).

Leydig cell treatment with TGF-β or SCCM

On day 4 of culture, Leydig cell medium was removed and replaced by fresh medium containing different amounts of TGF-β or of proteins derived from SCCM or one of its fractions. After 40 h, the medium was removed and the binding of hCG and the acute response to this hormone (cAMP and testosterone production) were measured.

Analysis of total RNA from Sertoli cells

Sertoli cells were collected with a rubber policeman in PBS 1 mM EDTA without Ca^{2+} and Mg^{2+}. Total RNA was prepared by the guanidium thiocyanate method and purified by sedimentation through 5.7 M CsCl (12). Total RNA was then analysed by electrophoresis and blotted onto nitrocellulose (20) and hybridized with labeled TGF—β cDNA (6).

RESULTS AND DISCUSSION

The long-term effects of TGF-β and several fractions derived from SCCM on Leydig cell function are shown in Fig. 1. As reported before (3) pretreatment with TGF-β reduced the hCG receptor number and the hCG-induced testosterone response. Total SCCM had a small inhibitory effect on both parameters, confirming previous results (14), but these inhibitory actions were more pronounced following acidification. Neither the 0.1M nor the 1.1M NaCl eluates from the heparin-Sepharose column had any effect on Leydig cell function. In contrast, the 0.6M NaCl fraction had a strong inhibitory effect, which was enhanced after acidification. The 2M NaCl fraction had an inhibitory effect, which disappeared after acidification.

Since TGF-β is secreted by virtually all cell types in a biologically inactive form (10, 13, 19, 24) which can be transformed to an active form by acid treatment, the enhanced inhibitory effects of the 0.6M NaCl fraction after acidification might suggest that this fraction contains TGF-β. On the other hand, the inhibitory effect of the 2M NaCl fraction could be related to the presence of a fibroblast growth factor (FGF)-like peptide, since FGF has been identified in the testis (22), FGF had some inhibitory long-term effects on pig Leydig cells (15) and the activity of FGF is destroyed by acid treatment (8).

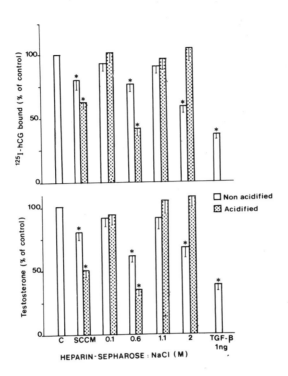

Fig. 1. Effects of SCCM and TGF- β on Leydig cell function. Leydig cells were treated for 40 h with total SCCM or with fractions eluted from a heparin-Sepharose column with 0.1, 0.6, 1.1 and 2M NaCl. Each fraction was tested before and after acid treatment.
* p < 0.05 compared to non pretreated cells (C).

The inhibitory effects of increasing concentrations of SCCM and 0.6M NaCl fraction after acid treatment and TGF-β on Leydig cell hCG binding sites are shown in Fig. 2. Treatment of Leydig cells for 40 h with the three fractions reduced the hCG binding to Leydig cells in a concentration-dependent manner with a 50% decrease at 0.2 ng/ml, 25 µg/ml and 400 µg/ml for TGF-β, 0.6M NaCl fraction and SCCM respectively. Similarly the cAMP (Fig. 3A) and the testosterone (Fig. 3B) acute response to hCG of pretreated cells was reduced. Half-maximal and maximal inhibition were observed at about 0.1 ng/ml and 1 ng/ml for TGF-β and at 5 µg/ml and 25 µg/ml protein for the acidified 0.6M NaCl fraction.

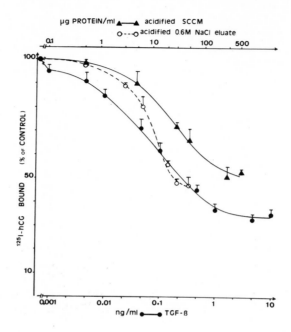

Fig. 2. Effects of TGF-β , acidified SCCM and the acidified 0.6M NaCl fraction on ^{125}I-hCG binding to Leydig cells. Cells were pretreated for 40 h.

Since at maximal concentrations the inhibitory effects of TGF-β and acidified SCCM were not additive (data not shown), the above results suggest that SCCM and the 0.6M NaCl fraction might contain TGF-β . In favour of the secretion of this peptide by porcine Sertoli cells is the presence of TGF-β mRNA in porcine Sertoli cells demonstrated by using a human TGF-β cDNA (Fig. 4). The presence of some inhibitory action of SCCM and 0.6M NaCl fraction before acid treatment might be due to the presence of some active TGF-β in these fractions and/or to partial activation of the latter form during the 40 h incubation with Leydig cells.

In conclusion the present study shows that 1) TGF-β has a strong inhibitory effect on Leydig cell function ; 2) Porcine Sertoli cells contain TGF-β mRNA ; 3) SCCM contains TGF-β-like activity. Taken together, the present results suggest that Sertoli cells secrete TGF-β which may play a role in the endocrine/paracrine/autocrine regulation of testicular function and this is also probably true for other stroidogenic tissues in which it has been shown that TGF-β is able to have a regulatory effect (1, 7, 9, 18).

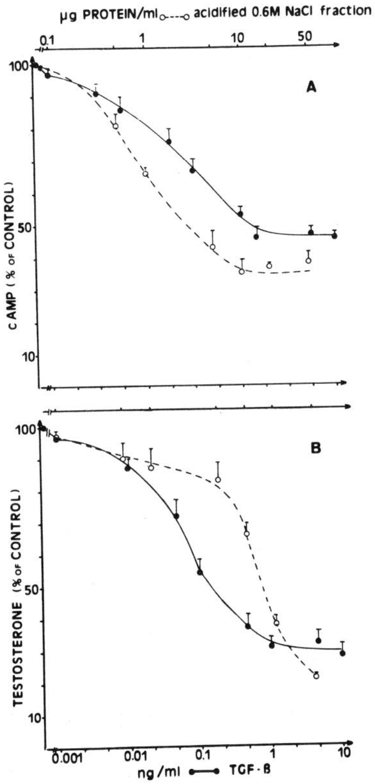

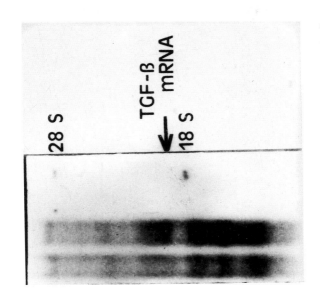

Fig. 4. Northern blot analysis of RNA from pig Sertoli cells.

Fig. 3. Effects of TGF-β and the acidified 0.6M NaCl fraction on the acute response to hCG (A : cAMP, B : Testosterone).

We thank Drs. A. Roberts and R. Derynck for generous gifts of TGF-β and TGF-β cDNA, Dr. M.G. Forest for supplying testosterone antibodies and J. Bois for her expert secretarial assistance. This work was supported by grants from la Ligue Nationale contre le Cancer and GEFLUC.

REFERENCES

1. Adashi, E.Y. and Resnick, C.E. (1986): Endocrinology, 119:1879-1881.
2. Assoian, R.K., Komoriya, C.A., Meyers, C.A., and Sporn, M.B. (1983): J. Biol. Chem., 258:7155-7160.
3. Avallet, O., Vigier, M., Perrard-Sapori, M.H., and Saez, J.M. (1987): Biochem. Biophys. Res. Commun., 146:575-581.
4. Bernier, M., Clerget, M., Mombrial, C.F., and Saez, J.M. (1986): Eur. J. Biochem., 155:323-330.
5. Bernier, M., Laferrere, B., Jaillard, C., Clerget, M., and Saez, J.M. (1986): Endocrinology, 118:2254-2261.
6. Derynck, R., Jarret, J.A., Chen, E.Y., Eaton, D.H., Bell, J.R., Assoian, R.K., Roberts, A.B., Sporn, M.B., and Goeddel, D.V. (1985): Nature, 316:701-705.
7. Feige, J.J., Cochet, C., Rainey, W.E., Mabani, C., and Chambaz, E.M. (1987): J. Biol. Chem., 262:13491-13495.
8. Gospodarowicz, D., Ferrera, N., Schweigerer, L., and Neufeld, G. (1987): Endocrine Rev., 8:95-114.
9. Hotta, M. and Baird, A. (1986): Proc. Natl. Acad. Sci. USA, 83:7795-7799.
10. Lawrence, D.A., Pincher, R., Krycève-Martinerie, C., and Jullien, P. (1984): J. Cell. Physiol., 121:184-188.
11. Lin, T., Blaisdell, J., and Haskell, J.F. (1987): Biochem. Biophys. Res. Commun., 146:387-394.
12. Maniatis, T., Fritsch, E.F., and Sambrook, J. (1982): Molecular Cloning (A Laboratory Manual). Cold Spring Harbor Laboratory, Cold Spring Harbor, NY.
13. O'Connor-McCourt, M.D. and Wakefield, L.M. (1987): J. Biol. Chem., 262:14090-14094.
14. Perrard-Sapori, M.H., Chatelain, P.G., Rogemond, N., and Saez, J.M. (1987): Mol. Cell. Endocrinol., 50:193-201.
15. Raeside, J.I., Berthelon, M.C., Sanchez, P., and Saez, J.M. (1988): Biochem. Biophys. Res. Commun., 151:163-169.
16. Saez, J.M., Perrard-Sapori, M.H., Chatelain, P.G., Tabone, E., and Rivarola, M.A. (1987): J. Steroid Biochem., 27:317-324.
17. Sharpe, R.M. (1983): Q. J. Exp. Physiol., 68:265-287.
18. Skinner, M.K., Keski-Oja, J., Osteen, K.G., and Moses, H.L. (1987): Endocrinology, 121:786-792.
19. Sporn, M.B., Roberts, A.B., Wakefield, L.M., and de Combrugghe, B. (1987): J. Cell Biol., 105:1039-1045.
20. Thomas, P.S. (1980): Proc. Natl. Acad. Sci. USA, 77:5201-5205.
21. Tuszynski, G.P., Knight, L.C., Kornecki, E., and Srivastava, S. (1983): Anal. Biochem., 130:166-170.
22. Ueno, N., Baird, A., Esch, F., Ling, N., and Guillemin, R. (1987): Mol. Cell. Endocrinol., 49:189-194.
23. Verhoeven, G. and Cailleau, J. (1985): Mol.Cell.Endocrinol., 40:57-68.
24. Wakefield, L.M., Smith, D.M., Masui, T., Harris, C.C., and Sporn, M.B. (1987): J. Cell Biol., 105:965-974.

Testicular Interleukin-1-Like Factor

O. Söder, V. Syed[1], P. Pöllänen[2], K. Gustafsson,
K. Granholm, S. Khan[1], S. Arver[3], M. Holst[4], M. von Euler
and E.M. Ritzén

[1]Max Planck Society Clinical Research Institute for Reproductive Medicine,
44 Münster, FRG;
[2]Department of Anatomy, University of Turku, SF-207 20 Turku 70, Finland;
Pediatric Endocrinology Unit and [3]Department of Endocrinology, Karolinska
Hospital;
[4]Department of Medical Cell Biology, Karolinska Institute,
S-104 01 Stockholm, Sweden

The testicular microenvironment stimulates germ cell precursors in the seminiferous tubules to initiate growth and differentiation, resulting in a cell proliferation which is among the most rapid known for mammalian tissues. How this intense cell proliferation in the testis is initiated and maintained remains to be clarified. The observation that relapses of childhood lymphoblastic leukemia often start in the testis (20) indicates that the testis provides a favorable milieu for growth not only of germ cells but also of other cell types. One possible explanation for these observations might be the presence in the testis of locally produced growth factors. Indeed, many defined peptide growth factors have been isolated from the testis during the last couple of years (6,12,22). Recently, we have reported on the isolation of an interleukin-1 (IL-1)-like factor from the rat testis and suggested it to play a role in germ cell growth and maturation (13). We here summarize our studies on the testicular IL-1-like factor and discuss its possible role in the testis. In our own work cited, IL-1 activities were determined by utilizing a murine thymocyte proliferation assay (9,23).

Interleukin-1

IL-1 is a family of hormone-like polypeptides originally isolated from macrophage culture supernatants (7,9). Production of IL-1 by macrophages is believed to be a consequence of macrophage activation by a variety of stimuli. IL-1 has multiple functions involved in cellular activation and inflammatory processes including, e.g., chemotactic action on leukocytes, stimulation of prostaglandin synthesis as well as mitogenic effects on lymphocytes and a wide variety of other target cells (7,8). In man as well as in other species, IL-1 is the product of two genes encoding two different IL-1 proteins termed IL-1α and IL-1ß (18). Human IL-1α and IL-1ß both have a relative molecular mass (M_r) of 17,000 (17K) but they differ in charge, with an isoelectric point (pI) of 5 for IL-1α and 7 for IL-1ß (11,18). Although the amino acid sequences of human IL-1α and IL-1ß show only 25% homology they share biological effects in most systems (11,18). Macrophages produce mainly IL-1ß which constitutes more than 80% of the secreted macrophage IL-1 (18). The above observations have formed the basis for the generally accepted view of macrophage IL-1 as an important host-defence factor to infection and injury (7,11).

Constitutive Production of IL-1-Like Factors by Normal Tissues

It has recently become apparent that several cell types in addition to macrophages are capable of producing IL-1-like factors in vitro and in vivo. In contrast to macrophage-derived IL-1, these IL-1-like factors are produced under non-inflammatory conditions and consist mainly of IL-1α-like factors. Thus, e.g., the epidermis, thymus, nasal pharyngeal carcinoma cells and EBV-transformed B lymphocytes have been reported to produce IL-1-α-like factors (4,14,16,27). We have investigated different organs and tissues in the rat for constitutive production of factors with IL-1-like activity. Our results demonstrate that macrophage-rich organs such as the liver, spleen, and lung produce IL-1-like factors to a low and variable degree, probably representing a low degree of macrophage activation in vivo. By contrast, extracts of normal rat skin and testis contained much higher amounts of IL-1 activity whereas most other tissues contained no IL-1 activity (FIG. 1 and ref. 13).

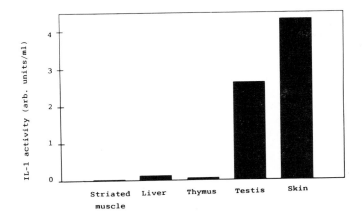

FIG. 1. IL-1 activity of rat tissue extracts. Pooled specimens of the indicated tissues from ten adult rats were homogenized in culture medium (3 ml/g tissue) and centrifuged. After 0.2 μm filtration, the supernatants were analyzed for IL-1 activity in murine thymocyte cultures. The IL-1 concentration is expressed as arbitrary units per ml as calculated from the obtained dose response curves. For methodological details, see references 13 and 23.

IL-1 Activity in the Male Genital Tract

Aqueous extracts of normal adult rat and human testes contain large amounts of IL-1 activity, demonstrating a constitutive production in vivo. IL-1 activity has also been detected in human and rat spermatozoa (13,25). On the other hand, no IL-1 activity was detected in extracts of rat and human prostate, rat seminal vesicles together with the coagulating glands, human vas deferens and epididymis or in rat and human seminal plasma (13,25).

Cellular Origin and Secretory Pathways of the Testicular IL-1-Like Factor

Extracts of isolated seminiferous tubules and conditioned media produced by 24-h cultures of seminiferous tubules, but not extracts of interstitial cells or conditioned media produced by crude interstitial cells or peritubular cells, contained IL-

1 activity (13,25). Compared to intact rat testes, higher concentrations of IL-1 activity were detected in experimentally cryptorchid and prenatally irradiated testes (devoid of germ cells) (25). Rete testis fluid collected from efferent ducts, and interstitial fluid collected by in vivo perfusion of the interstitial compartment also contained IL-1 activity (10). Removal of peritubular cells did not influence the production of IL-1-like activity by the seminiferous tubules (25). From these observations we have concluded that most of the testicular IL-1-like factor is produced by the seminiferous tubules, most probably by Sertoli cells, and, similarly to other Sertoli cell products, is secreted bidirectionally into the seminiferous tubular lumen and into the testis interstitial tissue.

Ontogeny of the Testicular IL-1-Like Factor

The demonstration of an IL-1-like factor in the adult rat testis has prompted us to investigate whether it is developmentally expressed during rat testis ontogeny. Seminiferous tubules were isolated from testes of rats of different age groups and their 24-h conditioned media analyzed for IL-1 activity in murine thymocyte cultures. No, or very low, IL-1 activity was produced by seminiferous tubules isolated from testes of 10- and 20-day-old rats. Increasing amounts were detected from day 30, reaching plateau levels at 60 days of age (25). Cultures of Sertoli cells isolated from 10-day-old rats did not contain any IL-1 activity (13). These results indicate that the testicular IL-1-like factor is produced by Sertoli cells of adult but not immature rat testes, and that it appears in the testis for the first time in parallel with the most rapid increase in germ cell proliferation.

Regulation of the Testicular IL-1-Like Factor

The developmental regulation of the production of the testicular IL-1-like factor indicated that it might be under hormonal control. This possibility has been studied by examining the IL-1 activity in testes from intact and hypophysectomized rats, with and without hormonal substitution. The results demonstrate that hypophysectomy lowers the tesicular IL-1 activity by more than 50%. LH, but not FSH or testosterone, could partially restore the activity (26). These findings may indicate that the testicular IL-1 activity is regulated by LH via a testosterone-independent mechanism. This assumption is supported by our finding that treatment of intact rats with HCG increases the IL-1 activity in testicular interstitial fluid (unpublished data).

IL-1 possesses potent inflammatory effects which might be potentially harmful to testicular tissue. Therefore, there is a need for intratesticular control mechanisms regulating the activity of the testicular IL-1-like factor. Several IL-1 inhibitors have recently been demonstrated in different tissues. Of such factors, α-melanocyte-stimulating hormone is particularly interesting as it has also been detected in the testis (2,5). Leydig cells have been reported to exert immunosuppressive effects (3). It is therefore possible that Leydig cells are involved in the regulation of the testicular IL-1-like activity as we have shown that they can inhibit testicular as well as recombinant IL-1 activity in murine thymocyte cultures (to be published). Seminal plasma also inhibits IL-1 activity but the origin of the inhibitory factor in seminal plasma in the genital tract is unknown (unpublished observations). Recently, an immunosuppressive protein has been isolated from rat testis interstitial fluid (19), but whether this factor is involved in the regulation of IL-1 activity remains to be studied.

Biochemistry of the Testicular IL-1-Like Factor and Comparison to IL-1 Isolated from Other Sources

Chromatofocusing of human testicular extracts on a Polybuffer Exchanger column revealed a single peak of IL-1 activity, eluting at an apparent pI of 5.2 (24). Rat testicular extract and rat interstitial fluid showed IL-1 activity in one peak eluting at a pI of 5.7-6.3 (10,13). There was no evidence of more basically charged IL-1 species in human or rat testicular extracts.

Ultrogel AcA 54 gel chromatography demonstrated similar molecular size profiles of the IL-1 activity in the human and rat testicular extracts. Thus, in both cases a low molecular weight peak of IL-1 activity was found, eluting at an apparent M_r of 16-20K. In addition, there was also a high molecular weight peak with an apparent M_r of 60-80K (13,24). This latter peak probably consisted of aggregated material as it was not detected when rat testicular extract was subjected to HPLC gel permeation chromatography or when a human testicular extract was run on polyacrylamide gels under reducing and denaturing conditions and visualized by immuno-detection with antibodies against human monocyte IL-1 (24). HPLC gel chromatography of rat testis interstitial fluid revealed, in addition to the major 15-18K peak, a low molecular weight peak with an apparent M_r of 5-7K (10). This low M_r material might represent a bioactive degradation product of the major peak as has been described for macrophage IL-1 (1). The reported molecular properties of the human testicular IL-1-like factor are identical to those described for human monocyte-derived IL-1α (11,18). The size and charge profile of the corresponding rat testicular factor are very close to those reported for an IL-1-like factor isolated from rat skin (21). Table 1 compares the molecular properties of the testicular IL-1-like factors with IL-1 isolated from other sources.

TABLE 1. Biochemical comparison of rat and human inter-leukin-1-like factors from different sources

Species	Source	M_r x 10^{-3}	pI
Rat	Testis	15-18	5.7-6.3
	[a]Skin	17; 30	5.7
	[b]Macrophages	14-20	4.7; 5,5; 7.3
Human	Testis	17-20	5.2
	[c]Skin	17	5.2; 7.0
	[d]Macrophages	17	5.2; 7.0

References a: 21; b: 17; c: 15; d: 18

Functional Aspects of the Testicular IL-1-Like Factor

The function of the testicular IL-1-like factor is unknown. The IL-1α-like factors isolated from skin, tumor cells and other sources discussed above have been proposed to act as autocrine or paracrine growth factors with a potential role in tumorigenesis and in the regulation of normal growth (4,14,16,27,17). Our finding that the testicular IL-1-like factor is constitutively produced in bioactive amounts and that its appearance in the testis is parallel with the increase in germ cell proliferation makes it tempting to speculate that it might act as a growth factor during spermatogenesis. Ongoing studies examining the effect of IL-1 on the proliferation of testis cells in vitro and in vivo will hopefully resolve this question. IL-1 is a potent growth factor for normal and leukemic lymphocytes. Our finding that the IL-1-like factor is secreted into the testicular interstitium might give a clue to the mechanisms behind the tendency to testicular relapse of childhood acute lymphoblastic leukemia.

ACKNOWLEDGMENTS

This work was supported by grants from the Swedish Medical Research Council (proj. no. 8282 & 3168), the King Gustaf V Jubilee Foundation, the Swedish Society of Medicine, and Magn. Bergvall Foundation.

REFERENCES

1. Bird, J., Shen, Y.J., Florentin, I., and Giroud, J.P. (1985): Br. J. exp. Path., 66:271-277.
2. Boitani, C., Farini, D., Bardin, C.W., and Stefanini, M. (1986): In Molecular and cellular endocrinology of the testis, edited by M. Stefanini, M. Conti, R. Geremia, and E. Ziparo, pp. 37-42, Elsevier Scientific Publications, Exerpta Medica, Amsterdam.
3. Born, W, and Wekerle, H. (1982): Am. J. Reprod. Immunol., 2: 291-295.
4. Busson, P., Braham, K., Ganem, G., Thomas, F., Grausz, D., Lipinski, M., Wakasugi, H., and Tursz, T. (1987): Proc. Natl. Acad. Sci. USA, 84:6262-6266.
5. Cannon, J.G., Tatro, J.B., Reichlin, S., and Dinarello, C.A. (1986): J. Immunol., 137:2232-2236.
6. Chatelain, P.G., Naville, D., and Saez, J.M. (1987): Biochem. Biophys. Res. Commun., 146:1009-1017.
7. Dinarello, C.A. (1984): Rev. Infect. Dis., 6:51-95.
8. Dinarello, C.A., Cannon, J.G., Mier, J.W., Bernheim, H.A., LoPreste, G., Lynn, D.L., Love, R.N., Webb, A.C., Auron, P.E., Reuben, R.C., Rich, A., Wolff, S.M., and Putney, S.D. (1986): J. Clin. Invest., 77:1734-1739.

9. Gery, I., Gershon, R.K., and Waksman, B.H. (1972):
    J. exp. Med., 136:128-142.
10. Gustafsson, K., Söder, O., Pöllänen, P., and
    Ritzén, E.M. (1988): In manuscript.
11. Hopp, T.P., Dower, S.K., and March, C.J. (1986):
    Immunol. Res., 5:271-280.
12. Holmes, S.D., Spotts, G., and Smith, R.G. (1986):
    J. Biol. Chem., 261:4076-4080.
13. Khan, S., Söder, O., Syed, V., Gustafsson, K,
    Lindh, M., and Ritzén, E.M. (1987): Int. J.
    Androl., 10:494-503.
14. Kupper, T., Guber, U., Ballard, D., Chua, A.O.,
    Langdon, R., Flood, T., Horowitz, M., and
    McGuire, J. (1986): Clin. Res., 34:640A.
15. Kupper, T., Ballard, D., Chua, A.O., McGuire, J.,
    Flood, P., Horowitz, M., Langdon, R., Lightfoot,
    L., and Gubler, U. (1986): J. exp. Med.,
    164:2095-2100.
16. Le, P., Tuck, D., Dinarello, C., Haynes, B., and
    Singer, K. (1987): J. Immunol., 138:2520-2526.
17. Lovett, D.H., Szamel, M., Ryan, J.L., Stertzel,
    R.B., Gemsa, D., and Resch, K. (1986): J.
    Immunol., 136: 3700-3705.
18. March, C.J., Mosley,. B., Larsen, A., Pat Ceretti,
    D., Braedt, G., Price, V., Gillis, S., Henney,
    C.S., Kronheim, S.R., Grabstein, K., Conlon,
    P.J., Hopp, P.T., and Cosman, D. (1985): Nature,
    315:641-47.
19. Pöllänen, P., Söder, O., and Uksila, J. (1988):
    Submitted for publication.
20. Saiontz, H.I., Gilchrist, G.S., Smithson, W.A.,
    Burgert, E.O., and Cupps, R.E. (1978): Mayo
    Clin. Proc., 53:212-216.
21. Schmitt, A., Hauser, C., Jaunin, F., Dayer, J.M.,
    and Saurat, J.H. (1986): Lymphkine Res., 5:105-
    118.
22. Smith, E.M., Svoboda, M.E., van Wyk, J.J.,
    Kierszenbaum, A.L., and. Tres, L.L. (1987):
    Endocrinology, 120:186-193.
23. Söder, O., and Madsen, K. (1988): Br. J.
    Rheumathol., 27:21-26.
24. Söder, O., Arver, S., Holst, M., Gustafsson, K.,
    and Ritzén, E.M. (1988): In manuscript.
25. Syed, V., Söder, O., Arver, S., Lindh, M., Khan,
    S., and Ritzén, E.M. (1988): Int. J. Androl., in
    press.
26. Syed, V., Söder, O., Khan, S., and Ritzén, M.
    (1988): In manuscript.
27. Wakasugi, H., Rimsky, L., Mahe, Y., Kamel, A.M.,
    Fradelizi, D., Tursz, T., and Bertoglio, J.
    (1987): Proc. Natl. Acad. Sci. USA, 84:804-808.

Subject Index